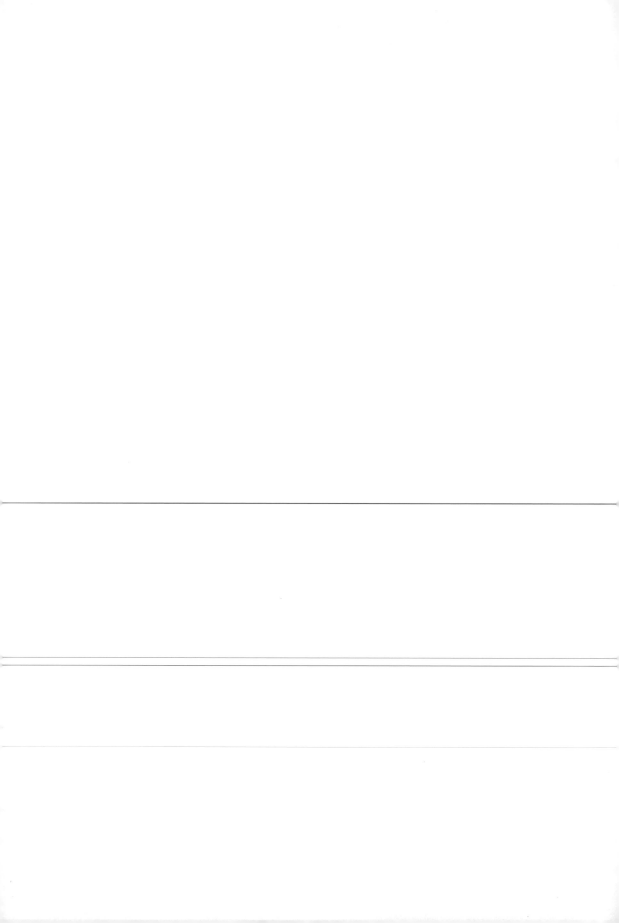

The motoneurone and
its muscle fibres

Monographs of the Physiological Society

The motoneurone and its muscle fibres

Daniel Kernell
University of Groningen

OXFORD
UNIVERSITY PRESS

OXFORD
UNIVERSITY PRESS

Great Clarendon Street, Oxford OX2 6DP

Oxford University Press is a department of the University of Oxford.
It furthers the University's objective of excellence in research, scholarship,
and education by publishing worldwide in

Oxford New York

Auckland Cape Town Dar es Salaam Hong Kong Karachi
Kuala Lumpur Madrid Melbourne Mexico City Nairobi
New Delhi Shanghai Taipei Toronto

With offices in

Argentina Austria Brazil Chile Czech Republic France Greece
Guatemala Hungary Italy Japan Poland Portugal Singapore
South Korea Switzerland Thailand Turkey Ukraine Vietnam

Oxford is a registered trade mark of Oxford University Press
in the UK and in certain other countries

Published in the United States
by Oxford University Press Inc., New York

British Library Cataloguing in Publication Data

Data available

Library of Congress Cataloging in Publication Data
Kernell, Daniel
The motoneurone and its muscle fibres/Daniel Kernell.
   p. ; cm
   Includes bibliographical references and index.
   1. Motor neurons. 2. Myoneural junction. 3. Striated muscle. I. Title.
[DNLM: 1. Motor neurons—physiology. 2. Neuromuscular Junction—physiology.
WL 102.7 K39m 2006]
   QP369.5.K47 2006 612.7—dc22 2006015483

Typeset by Newgen Imaging Systems (P) Ltd., Chennai, India
Printed in Great Britain
on acid-free paper by
Biddles Ltd., King's Lynn

ISBN 0–19–852655–5 (Hbk.:alk.paper) 978–0–19–852655–1 (Hbk.)

10 9 8 7 6 5 4 3 2 1

Preface

After about 40 years of research in the field of neuromuscular physiology, I wanted to summarize essential features of this landscape in which I have lived for so long. I believe that it is a landscape worth the effort because of its unique features which have given it a central position in classical neurobiological research and should continue to do so in the future (see Chapter 1 for further comments on this issue). Therefore I was very glad when I was offered the opportunity of writing a book on this subject for the series *Monographs of the Physiological Society*.

My ambition when writing this book has been to give a critical, balanced, and reasonably complete survey of the most essential facts about motoneurone and muscle unit physiology, including both new and older observations, provided that they are all still valid. Consequently, the illustrations cover research performed over a long period of time. A few very limited historical comments have been inserted in places in order to help the reader to use information from the older literature which is still valid and to understand the present-day impact of some of the older insights. However, it should be stressed that my account is not at all meant to be concerned with the history of science. My main aim is to summarize the present state of affairs in a generally understandable manner and thus, I hope, help (new) researchers, neuroscience students, and others to become familiar with this system and, perhaps, inspire them to find out more about it in further investigations.

The quantity of available information concerning the subject matter of this book can be indicated by searching, for instance, for items concerning 'motoneuron*' or 'motor neuron*' in the invaluable PubMed database. Such an action delivers a list of about 19 700 references from roughly the last 55 years, and this increases to about 22 900 with the addition of the search-term 'motor unit*'. This huge collection of references is still very incomplete with regard to the muscle side of the story, as well as with respect to various special features requiring other keywords. In a book of present type, a selection obviously has to be made with regard to the information sources utilized, and this process is necessarily personal and influenced by chance as well as by the author's own past experiences. If I have missed important results and failed to cite essential articles from the vast sea of neuromuscular research, I ask the respective colleagues/authors to forgive me (and to amend my mistake by displaying the omitted findings in reviews of their own).

While writing this book I was generously supported by the Department of Medical Physiology and the Faculty of Medical Sciences at the University of Groningen. I am grateful for the many interesting discussions I have had during the course of the writing process with various colleagues within the department, including Rob Bakels, Erik Boddeke, Sjef Copray, and Inge Zijdewind who all made valuable contributions by reading and commenting upon various chapters of the manuscript. Finally, the book could never have been written without the strong and continuous support of my wife, Hilda Kernell, to whom I dedicate the results of my efforts.

Groningen

November 2005

Contents

Abbreviations

This list covers those abbreviations that occur many times in the text. Other abbreviations are used in only one or a few consecutive paragraphs, and such 'local' abbreviations are defined where they appear. Certain common abbreviations have acquired the status of independent words and are used as such in this text (e.g. various compounds in molecular biology and synaptic physiology, such as AMPA, DNA, GABA, NMDA, RNA, TRH). Furthermore, standard chemical notation for ions is used throughout, such as Ba^{2+} (barium), Ca^{2+} (calcium), Cl^- (chloride), Cs^+ (caesium), H^+ (hydrogen), K^+ (potassium), Mg^{2+} (magnesium), Mn^{2+} (manganese), and Na^+ (sodium).

5HT	5-hydroxytryptamine or serotonin: a neurotransmitter
ACh	acetylcholine: the transmitter at the vertebrate neuromuscular junction (and at various other central and peripheral synapses)
AChE	ACh esterase: an enzyme that hydrolyses ACh
AChR	ACh receptor: a ionotropic ligand-gated membrane channel
AHP	after-hyperpolarization: a hyperpolarizing after-potential following single spikes in the soma of a motoneurone (analogous to 'medium-duration' AHP (mAHP))
ALS	amyotrophic lateral sclerosis
ATP	adenosine triphosphate: an energy-rich compound
BDNF	brain-derived neurotrophic factor
CGRP	calcitonin gene related peptide
C_m	capacitance of membrane per unit area (F/cm^2)
CNS	central nervous system, i.e. brain and spinal cord
EM	electron microscopy
EMG	electromyogram: extracellular recording of action potentials generated in an active muscle
EPP	endplate potential: the EPSP of the neuromuscular junction
EPSP	excitatory postsynaptic potential: a depolarizing potential evoked in the postsynaptic cell by activity of excitatory synapses
F	fast-twitch muscle unit
FF	fast-twitch fatigue-sensitive muscle unit
Fint	fast-twitch muscle unit with fatigue resistance intermediate between FF and FR
FR	fast-twitch fatigue-resistant muscle unit
f–I relation	frequency–current relation: the relation between spike frequency and the intensity of a stimulating current (e.g. in a motoneurone)
f–I slope	slope of the f–I relation (Hz/nA): a measure of the 'gain' of the neuronal input– output relation
F_{min}	minimum rate (Hz) of maintained regular repetitive firing in a motoneurone
G_{in}	input conductance (S): reciprocal value of R_{in}
G_m	specific membrane conductance ($S\ cm^{-2}$): reciprocal value of R_m
HRP	horseradish peroxidase: a plant enzyme (protein) used for retrograde and intracellular labelling of (moto)neurones
I_{rh}	rheobase (nA): minimum current intensity needed to generate a single action potential
I_{rep}	threshold current intensity (nA) for generating maintained repetitive spike-firing
IPSP	inhibitory postsynaptic potential: a hyperpolarizing potential (at least at membrane potentials close to threshold) evoked by activity of inhibitory synapses
IS–SD spike	initial segment–soma-dendrite spike: the full-sized action potential recorded from the cell body of a motoneurone; the small IS spike is presumably generated in membrane

	regions close to the origin of the axon; the SD spike is elicited by the IS spike and is generated by more proximal membrane regions; only the SD spike is succeeded by an AHP
mATPase	myofibrillar ATPase: enzyme for hydrolysis of ATP, part of myosin molecule
mEPP	miniature endplate potential: a small version of the EPP, evoked by spontaneously released single quanta of ACh
MHC	myosin heavy chain: part of the myosin molecule
MLC	myosin light chain: part of the myosin molecule
MN	motoneurone: a cell with its cell body and dendrites inside the CNS and its axon connected to peripheral targets outside the CNS; unless otherwise specified, the term refers (in this monograph) to a mammalian alpha motoneurone, innervating skeletal muscle fibres
mRNA	messenger RNA (ribonucleic acid): transcribed from DNA and containing the code for a protein
MVC	maximum voluntary contraction
M wave	muscle compound action potential: evoked by electrical stimulation and recorded using EMG techniques
NMJ	neuromuscular junction
NT-3, NT-4/5	neurotrophin-3, neurotrophin-4, or neurotrophin-5 (last two equivalent)
P_0	maximal isometric tetanic force of a muscle, muscle unit, or muscle fibre (i.e. force at zero velocity)
PIC	persistent inward membrane current (excitatory)
PSP	postsynaptic potential (EPSP or IPSP)

R_{in}	input resistance of a cell, i.e. electrical resistance measured between an electrode inside the cell and the extracellular fluid
R_m	membrane resistivity (specific membrane resistance): resistance of membrane unit area ($\Omega\, cm^2$)
S	slow-twitch muscle unit (fatigue-resistant)
SDH	succinate dehydrogenase: mitochondrial enzyme used in oxidative metabolism
SR	sarcoplasmic reticulum in muscle fibres: membrane-enclosed space around the myofibrils containing stores of Ca^{2+} used in excitation–contraction coupling
T–f relation	tension–frequency relation: for a muscle (or muscle unit or muscle fibre), the relation between activation rate and the resulting contractile tension
TTX	tetrodotoxin: blocks generation of action potentials in many types of membrane, acts by blocking voltage-gated Na^+ channels of the fast and rapidly inactivating type
TwCT	twitch contraction time: time from onset to peak of a twitch
type I	histochemical class of muscle fibres (mATPase classification): slow and fatigue resistant
type II	histochemical class of muscle fibres (mATPase classification): fast and with variable fatigue sensitivity (for subtypes see Table 2.2)
V_0 or V_{max}	maximum unloaded shortening velocity of a muscle or muscle fibre
V_{th}	voltage threshold: membrane potential at threshold for generating an action potential

Chapter 1

Why bother about motoneurones?

1.1. General layout and functions of the vertebrate neuromuscular system

The vertebrate **neuromuscular system** is schematically depicted in Figure 1.1A. It includes the following.

1 The **skeletal muscles**, i.e. the 'ordinary' muscles which are generally attached to the skeletal system of bones and joints, and which produce the forces needed for movements and the maintenance of body posture.

2 The **skeletal motoneurones (MNs)**, whose long and slender tube-like processes, the peripheral **axons**, innervate and command the muscles and whose 'receptive' portions (**cell body, dendrites**) are located within the central nervous system (CNS), the spinal cord, or the brainstem. The MNs receive their commands from numerous other kinds of neurones, most of which are completely situated within the CNS.

This monograph concerns the functional properties of skeletal MNs and associated aspects of the muscular system.

One of the major differences between animals and plants is the capacity for movements. With some notable exceptions (e.g. *Mimosa pudica*), plants typically move only slowly over hours and days, whereas animals are capable, at least during some of their developmental stages, of moving around much more quickly (seconds to minutes). With the exception of sponges, all multicellular animals can be said to show a motor behaviour, which is generated and controlled by a nervous system (not needed in the slower life of plants or sponges) and mediated by contractions of muscle(-like) cells which are commanded via specialized nerve cells, the MNs. All motor behaviours have to be expressed via the activation of these neurones, the 'final common path' of the CNS (Sherrington 1906). This, in itself, makes it essential to know and understand the properties of MNs, even though they constitute only <0.0005 per cent of all the neurones of the human CNS (Fig. 1.1B). However, there is a second reason why MNs are interesting; probably no other type of mammalian nerve cell is so well known and understood.

Spinal MNs are unusually accessible for physiological experiments. The central cell bodies are comparatively large and easy to record from with microelectrodes. During such recordings, individual MNs may unambiguously be identified by electrical stimulation of their peripheral axon. Of major importance is the fact that the main target cells of MNs, the skeletal muscle fibres, are readily identifiable and their properties have been thoroughly explored. Thus MNs are one of the very few types of central neurones whose functional tasks are clearly understood, even at the level of individual cells. Furthermore,

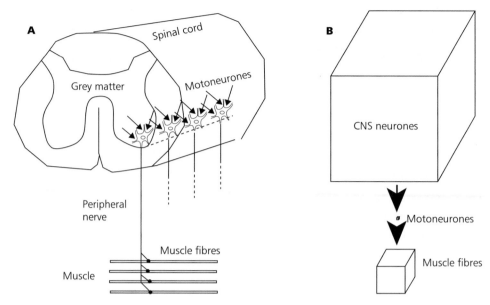

Figure 1.1 Schematic representation of the neuromuscular system. (**A**) In vertebrates, the MN cell bodies and dendrites and all the synapses controlling them lie within the CNS. For muscles below the head, MNs lie in the ventral grey matter (ventral horn) of the spinal cord, and their axons leave the CNS via the ventral roots and travel to skeletal muscles. In this book, the term 'neuromuscular system' is used to denote the (alpha) MNs and their skeletal muscle fibres which together constitute the output elements of the CNS, the **motor units**. (**B**) Each MN controls many muscle fibres; thus the MNs are in a numerical minority within the neuromuscular system. Their minority position is even more extreme in relation to all the other cells within the CNS; in humans, <0.0005 per cent of all neurones are MNs. However, their contribution is probably more important than that of any other neuronal category; all CNS control of muscles, and thus of behaviour, must be executed via the MNs.

MNs are unique with regard to the possibilities for monitoring their single-unit activity during ongoing behaviour, as can be done in animals and humans using simple electrical recordings from skeletal muscles (electromyography (EMG)).

The tasks and working conditions of MNs cannot be understood without a thorough knowledge of the properties of their target cells. Therefore this book also reviews many aspects of the organization and physiology of skeletal muscle. However, the MNs remain the main characters of the story and the treatment of muscle is limited to aspects that are relevant for understanding MN–muscle interactions. Readers interested in more information about, for instance, the basic biophysical and biochemical mechanisms of muscle contraction will have to look elsewhere (e.g. McComas 1996; Gordon *et al.* 2000; Lieber 2002; Jones *et al.* 2004).

Textbooks typically deal primarily with 'acute' neuronal and muscular functions, i.e. processes seen on the timescale of ongoing motor behaviour (milliseconds–seconds– minutes). However, equally important functions exist that take place more slowly; on time scales varying from minutes to months the MN and muscle properties may change, thereby keeping them adapted to altering functional needs. Such slow processes are often indicated by terms like 'plasticity'. The earliest, and also most dramatic, expressions of plasticity are, of course, the changes taking place during pre- and postnatal development. In such contexts of 'long-term physiology' modern molecular biology is providing increasingly important tools for the analysis of underlying mechanisms.

1.2. **Motoneurones as 'model neurones'**

Because of their accessibility for experimental research, MNs have long had an important role as 'model neurones', providing a useful starting point for analysing and understanding general issues of neuronal function. Many of the basic concepts of neurophysiology (e.g. synapse, inhibition and excitation, reflex loops, recruitment gradation, etc.) were originally defined by Sherrington and his colleagues in the course of experimental work on the MN output, as monitored by the recording of muscle contractions (Sherrington 1906; Creed et al. 1932; Bennett and Hacker 2002). The first (indirect) observations of the discharge activity of single mammalian neurones were EMG recordings in animals and man (Adrian and Bronk 1929; Denny-Brown 1929). The first types of central mammalian neurones to be extensively studied using intracellular recording techniques were lumbar MNs of the cat (Brock et al. 1952), and during the 1950s general descriptions of how nerve cells work were centred around MN physiology, often analysing other cells with regard to their similarities or differences compared with the increasingly solid database for spinal MNs (e.g. Eccles 1957).

The introduction of successful techniques for recording from brain slices *in vitro* (e.g. from the hippocampus or neocortex (Andersen and Langmoen 1980)) was very important for the further analysis of general neuronal functions and membrane properties. Unfortunately, such techniques are difficult to apply to spinal MNs of adult mammals and, partly for this reason, MNs became less popular as standards for comparison in neuronal physiology. Neurones encountered in unanaesthetized cortical slices seemed to possess more complex response properties than those familiar to classical MN investigators. However, since the 1980s an accumulating amount of experimental evidence has shown that, when investigated under appropriate conditions, MNs also have highly complex and modifiable response properties (Schwindt and Crill 1980b; Hounsgaard et al. 1986; Russo and Hounsgaard 1999; Rekling et al. 2000; Powers and Binder 2001; Heckman et al. 2003; Hultborn et al. 2004). Furthermore, a careful choice of preparations has also made it possible to study MNs under *in vitro* conditions, for example spinal cord in neonatal or young mammals (Takahashi 1990; Thurbon et al. 1998), brainstem MNs of neonatal or young postnatal mammals (Viana et al. 1994), spinal MNs of cold-blooded vertebrate species, such as turtles (Hounsgaard et al. 1988b), and mammalian MNs maintained in tissue culture (Larkum et al. 1996).

Despite all the impressive slice work from various brain portions, MNs still belong to the best and most broadly known types of neurones in the mammalian CNS. For no other central nerve cell category are functional populations and neuronal tasks so well defined (although also here intriguing questions remain). Thus MNs continue to offer unique possibilities for unravelling important principles of short- and long-term neuronal function, as seen in relation to neuronal control and command tasks.

1.3. **What will readers find where?**

This book was written with the idea that it might be of use for several different categories of readers. Some potential readers might already have a solid general knowledge of neuromuscular physiology; these readers might include graduate students in neuroscience and researchers specialized on particular subjects within this broad field. Others may have another background (e.g. experimental psychology, molecular genetics) but still want to know more about MNs in relation to questions within their own field. Furthermore, undergraduate students might be interested in selected aspects of MN function in the context of course work in neuroscience. In order to make the book easier to use for these various latter categories of readers, a chapter at general textbook level, providing some basic background information about the neuromuscular system, is included at the onset (Chapter 2).

With regard to all the chapters it should be noted that this book is meant to summarize and critically discuss lines of thought concerning MN and muscle function, as supported by experimental evidence. It was not the intention to list references to all the work ever published on MNs; such a reference list would fill more than the space allotted to the whole book.

The book concentrates on what is known about MNs and skeletal muscles (particularly limb muscles with twitch muscle fibres) in a few well-investigated mammalian species (humans, cats, and rats) together with some supplementary information from other animals such as subhuman primates, rabbits, mice, and turtles. Although the neuromuscular system works along similar principles for all vertebrate species, there are also important (mainly quantitative) differences between them. These differences will be mentioned when directly appropriate. With regard to comparative points of view, it should be remembered that some classes of invertebrates have highly effective neuromuscular machineries that are organized according to other principles than those of vertebrates (reviewed by Hoyle 1983). For instance, compared with vertebrates, arthropods (e.g. flies and crayfish) have very few MNs, different MNs are used for evoking different effects in the same muscle fibres (including inhibition), and glutamate is used instead of acetylcholine as the excitatory neuromuscular transmitter substance. The mammalian neuromuscular system clearly represents only one out of several solutions to the problem of how to interface the CNS to muscles. However, it is a solution of great importance for ourselves, as functioning mammalian organisms and as investigators of mammalian physiology.

Chapter 2

Basic neuromuscular properties

2.1. Introduction

This tutorial chapter is mainly intended as an initial support for readers who are not already familiar with the neuromuscular system. Some of the items discussed are needed as background knowledge for later chapters. These include, for instance, various basic aspects of muscle physiology (for further information see McComas 1996; Gordon *et al.* 2000; Lieber 2002; Jones *et al.* 2004), axonal spike conduction and transport mechanisms (Hille 2001; Almenar-Queralt and Goldstein 2001), and, very briefly, some general points concerning the CNS organization of motor functions (Kandel *et al.* 2000). Other items are introduced in this chapter but will receive more detailed treatment elsewhere. In such cases, illustrations and more extensive literature references may be found in one or several of the later chapters (cross-references are added in the text when appropriate).

2.2. Skeletal muscles and peripheral nerves

2.2.1. Numbers and dimensions of muscles

As a whole, the skeletal muscles of a lean person are collectively responsible for about 40 per cent of the body weight. About 85 per cent of the wet weight of each muscle represents the thin and elongated contractile cells, the **muscle fibres**, and the rest includes tendon, other connective tissue, and blood vessels (Gollnick *et al.* 1981). Anatomy textbooks list about 300 muscles per side for the human trunk and extremities (the count includes all separately named or numbered heads and muscle portions). Many of these muscles consist of several more or less distinct portions with separate pulling directions, and the same names are sometimes used for whole series of repeated muscles (e.g. valid for several back and intercostal muscles). Individual sizes may vary widely, from the tiny muscles of the larynx and the middle ear to the massive muscle groups of the hip and knee.

2.2.2. Muscle contractions

Skeletal muscles **contract** when activated by their MNs. A contracting muscle produces a force in a shortening direction; muscles can only be used for pulling on things, not for pushing. Most skeletal muscles are fixed to bones at both ends, and extend across one or (often) several joints. Muscles located on different sides will move a joint in opposite directions. Such muscles are said to be **antagonists** of each other (e.g. the elbow flexor **biceps brachii** versus the elbow extensor **triceps brachii** of the upper arm). Muscles located such that they tend to move joints in about the same direction are called **synergists** (e.g. the three elbow flexors **biceps brachii, brachialis**, and **brachioradialis** of the upper arm).

Whether a muscle will actually change its external length when it contracts depends on the forces resisting its contractile shortening force. If the opposing forces are smaller than the contractile force, the muscle will indeed shorten (shortening or **concentric** contraction). Alternatively, the external resistance to shortening may be such that the contracting muscle cannot change its external length at all (e.g. pulling on a wall, **isometric** contraction), or the opposing forces may be pulling on the contracting muscles strongly enough to make them lengthen (e.g. for knee extensors when walking down a hill, lengthening or **eccentric** contractions). All these three major types of contraction are frequently used in normal motor behaviour. In well-controlled precision movements, antagonists on both sides of joints are typically used together, whereby one set of muscles cause the movement (**prime movers**) and the other co-contracting set simultaneously brakes it. Thus, so-called 'antagonist' muscles very often work together as a team.

It should be remembered that the cellular force generators of muscles, the muscle fibres, are connected to bones via **elastic** tendinous links. Thus, even under isometric conditions, which allow no shortening between the muscular endpoints, the muscle fibres themselves will shorten to stretch the tendons, thereby transmitting their contractile force to the skeleton. This internal shortening takes time and, together with other important factors, has an influence on the time course of isometric force development.

Movements of selected joints can only be well controlled against the background of a stable **posture** in the rest of the body (e.g. stable back and legs when throwing a ball with hand and arm). This often means that weight-carrying or force-resisting joints that are not being moved should be stabilized using (near-)isometric co-contractions of muscles on one or both sides of these joints (**postural** contractions). Such postural contractions will often need dynamic adjustments (e.g. for keeping the rest of the body stable while moving an arm or a leg). Stabilizing contractions may sometimes have to be continuously active for very long periods (e.g. neck muscles keeping the head upright for hours at a time).

2.2.3. **Muscle fibres**

The force-generating cells of skeletal muscles, the **muscle fibres**, are about as thin as a hair (often 50–100 μm in diameter) and of varying lengths. In human extremities, muscle fibres are often between 30 and 80 mm long and some are substantially longer (Wickiewicz *et al.* 1983; Friederich and Brand 1990; Heron and Richmond 1993); an extreme example of long fibres (up to 600 mm) is found in human sartorius muscle (Harris *et al.* 2005). Each muscle fibre has a large number of cell nuclei distributed along its length (e.g. several tens of nuclei per millimetre in rat muscles (Schmalbruch and Hellhammer 1977; Tseng *et al.* 1994; Bruusgaard *et al.* 2003)), and it is attached to a specialized elastic connective tissue (**tendon**) at each end. The **elastin** and **collagen** fibres of the tendons also proceed inside muscles, and each muscle fibre is enclosed by a thin network of protective connective tissue. In most muscles, the muscle fibres are markedly shorter than the total length of the muscle as a whole. Such muscles have a **pennate** construction with muscle fibres lined up obliquely inside (Fig. 2.1A).

When seen under a microscope with appropriately polarized light, skeletal muscle fibres have a 'cross-striated' appearance, showing a transverse pattern of stripes: light non-polarizing 'I bands' (isotropic) and dark 'A bands' (anisotropic) recurring with a periodicity of about 2–3 µm at rest. If a muscle shortens during a contraction, the

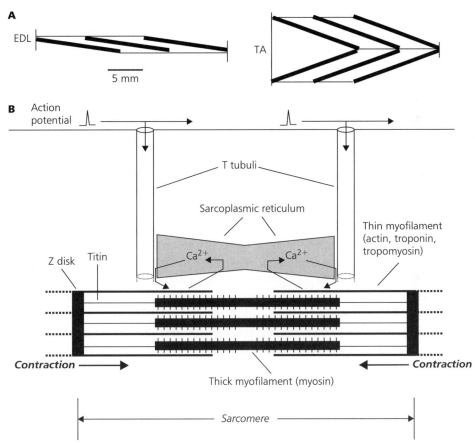

Figure 2.1 Internal structure of muscles and muscle fibres. (**A**) Examples of muscle architecture: extensor digitorum longus (EDL) and tibialis anterior (TA) of rat hindlimb. In these schematic drawings, thick lines indicate the average length and direction (pennation angle) of muscle fibres in relation to the muscle as a whole (proximal to the left). In EDL the muscle fibres go from a proximal latero-posterior tendon sheet to a distal medio-anterior one, and in TA from medial, anterior, and lateral proximal sheets to a central distal one. (Reproduced with permission, from Wang and Kernell 2000.) (**B**) Diagram of muscle fibre structures involved in excitation–contraction coupling and contraction.

I bands become thinner and the width of the A bands remains constant. The A and I bands reflect the orderly intracellular arrangement of protein structures which are responsible for muscular force production, the **thick and thin myofilaments** (Fig. 2.1B). As seen in electron microscopy, the myofilaments are arranged in lengthwise repeating units called **sarcomeres**, which are kept in register within the whole cross-section of a muscle fibre. At its proximal and distal ends, the sarcomere is limited by a plate-like structure, the **Z disk (Z line)**. The thick myofilaments consist of myosin and the thin ones contain actin and the regulatory proteins tropomyosin and troponin (three varieties: C, I, and T). One end of each thin filament is fixed to the Z disk, and the thick myosin filaments occupy a middle position between the actin filaments from opposing Z disks. Each thick filaments is anchored by minute titin threads, connecting its ends to the adjoining Z disks. The A bands seen in polarized light correspond to the portions occupied by thick filaments and the I bands to the intervening sections. Thick myofilaments are about the same length (1.5–1.6 μm) in different vertebrate species, whereas the thin filaments may show systematic differences (e.g. about 0.98 μm or less in frogs, 1.12 μm in cats, and 1.27 μm in humans) (reviewed by Herzog *et al.* 1992).

Contractile force is generated by interactions between the thick and thin myofilaments. Each thick myofilament consists of a braid of many large myosin molecules, each provided with a moveable arm-like sideways extension or 'head', also called a 'cross-bridge' (seen as short 'hairs' in the schematic representation in Fig. 2.1B). When a muscle fibre is activated there is a repeated cyclical interaction between the thick and thin myofilaments, giving rise to the contractile force (**sliding filament mechanism** of muscle contraction) (for further details, see section 2.5.3).

Inside each muscle fibre, the myofilaments of the sarcomeres are surrounded by mitochondria and by a complex vesicular system containing accumulated Ca^{2+} ions (**sarcoplasmic reticulum (SR)**) (Fig. 2.1B). Furthermore, for each sarcomere along the fibre, there are thin tube-like invaginations of the surface membrane (**T tubules**) which make repeated close contacts with the SR inside the muscle fibre (points of contact, **triads**). These structures play an essential role for activating the contractile machinery of the muscle fibre (**excitation–contraction coupling**) (see section 2.5.3). The cytoplasm of muscle fibres is often referred to as **sarcoplasm**, and the muscle fibre surface membrane is frequently called the **sarcolemma**.

2.2.4. Peripheral nerves

Peripheral nerves are bundles of multiple nerve fibres connecting the CNS with various peripheral structures. Each nerve contains many separate 'wires' of different diameters (i.e. **axons** of neurones), each being connected to a separate site in the periphery. In addition to the axons, the nerve contains connective tissue for structural stability and protection, blood vessels for energy supply and waste removal, and a very important class of specialized supporting entities, the **Schwann cells**. In the periphery, Schwann cells have functions similar to those of the oligodendroglia cells inside the CNS. All peripheral axons, whether myelinated or not, are covered with Schwann cells. Within a given portion of the nerve, several small axons may be enveloped by a single Schwann cell. Around larger axons (diameter >1–2 μm) Schwann cells provide an insulating layer of **myelin**, which consists of multiple layers of Schwann cell membrane deposited in a dense spiral around the axon. The myelin sheath is briefly interrupted at the transition between consecutive Schwann cells along the myelinated fibre. Only at these sites, the **nodes of Ranvier**, is the axonal membrane in direct contact with the extracellular fluid. For myelinated axons, diameters are generally given as the outside dimensions of the myelin sheaths. For circular fibres, the diameter of the axon itself is usually about 60 per cent of the outside myelin diameter (outside and inside perimeters are proportional (Gillespie and Stein 1983)), which is the optimal ratio for the conduction of nerve impulses (Rushton 1951). For reasons to be explained later (section 2.4.3), thick axons conduct messages (action potentials) more rapidly than thin axons.

2.3. Muscle innervation

2.3.1. Muscle nerves: afferent and efferent components

Nerves to muscles contain both sensory fibres conveying messages from the muscle to the CNS (**afferent**) and motor fibres (MN axons) conducting outward-directed commands from the CNS to the muscle fibres (**efferent**). Typically, there are about as many myelinated afferents as efferents in a muscle nerve (Table 2.1). In addition, there are often many more unmyelinated than myelinated muscle afferents (Mitchell and Schmidt 1983). For body regions below the neck, the afferent axons belong to neurones with cell bodies in

Table 2.1 Numbers of efferent and afferent myelinated fibres in muscle nerves (cat)

Muscle	Motor%	Alpha%	Alpha	Gamma	I aff	II aff	III aff	Spindles
GM	60	62	280	170	145	80	75	71
Sol	60	57	155	115	90	65	25	56
Ten	50	50	20	20	10	20	10	15
TA	45	59	200	140	165	160	115	64
PerL	70	54	95	80	35	25	15	11
PerB&T	40	53	85	75	105	85	50	31

Composition of muscle nerves in hindlimbs of adult cat. Motor fibres (alpha and gamma) counted and measured after degeneration of afferent fibres, following extirpation of dorsal root ganglia. Afferent fibres (types I, II and III) counted and measured after degeneration of motor fibres, following section of ventral roots. All counts concern myelinated fibres only. Motor fibres showed a bimodal distribution and afferent fibres showed a trimodal distribution, and diameters are ranked such that alpha > gamma motor fibres (see Fig.5.2(a)), and I > II > III for afferent fibres. The precise diameter range for each mode group varied somewhat between the nerves.

Abbreviations: GM, medial gastrocnemius; Sol, soleus; Ten, tenuissimus; TA, tibialis anterior; PerL, peroneus longus; PerB&T, peroneus brevis and peroneus tertius; Motor%, percentage (given to nearest 5%) of all axons that belonged to MNs (i.e. alpha and gamma); Alpha%, percentage of motor axons that belonged to the alpha group; Alpha and Gamma, number of motor axons in the mode groups of the largest and smallest fibres, respectively; I aff, II aff, and III aff, number of afferents belonging to the mode groups of the largest, intermediate, and smallest fibres, respectively; Spindles, number of muscle spindles.

Data from Boyd and Davey 1968.

the **dorsal root ganglia**, accumulations of cells just outside the spinal cord. Their central processes enter the dorsal side of the spinal cord via the **dorsal roots**. The spinal MNs have their cell bodies in the spinal cord (Fig.1.1A) and their axons travel towards the periphery via the **ventral roots**, emerging at the ventral side of the spinal cord (i.e. the side towards abdomen). Within the spinal cord, MNs lie in the ventral portion (**ventral horn**) of the H-shaped grey matter (Figs 1.1A, 5.1B, 5.1C, and 5.2C). MNs innervating a single muscle are said to form the **MN pool** for that muscle (Fig. 5.2D). MN pools of different muscles have, to some extent, different topographical positions in both the longitudinal and transverse directions. Dorsal and ventral root filaments leave the spinal cord continuously all along its length. These filaments are bundled into segmental roots as they exit through the space between adjoining vertebrae; the roots are named and numbered after the vertebral segments, as categorized into cervical, thoracic, lumbar, and sacral divisions. The precise number of segments is somewhat species dependent; for example, cats have seven and humans have five lumbar segments. Motor axons destined for a given muscle often emerge through two or three adjoining ventral roots before being combined into a single nerve. For muscles of the head and part of the neck, afferent and efferent fibres emerge from the brainstem via cranial nerves; there are no afferent and efferent brainstem roots.

2.3.2. **Afferent muscle innervation; muscle spindles**

Fibre sizes do not occur randomly within a muscle nerve; the distribution is typically clearly bimodal for efferent myelinated fibres (Fig.5.2A) and somewhat less distinctly trimodal for the afferents (Table 2.1). Based on such differences in axonal diameter (originally measured in cats), the muscle afferents are subdivided into four functional groups, referred to as **type I** (thickest), type **II**, type **III**, and type **IV** (or type **C**, non-myelinated) (Table 2.1). The two thickest (and fastest) categories are mainly connected to sensory structures for the measurement of changes in muscle length (**muscle spindles, group Ia and II** afferents) and muscle force (**Golgi tendon organs, group Ib** affererents). The two **thinnest categories** of muscle afferents have less well defined functions. Some are high-threshold mechanoceptive fibres reacting to, for instance, muscle pressure. Others are nociceptive, giving rise to sensations of pain and reacting to very strong stretch or to chemicals emerging following tissue damage. Still others are probably chemoceptive in different ways, reacting to metabolicallly evoked changes in extracellular fluid composition during intense and long-lasting contractions.

The most complex sensory structure inside skeletal muscles is the **muscle spindle**. Typically, there are tens to a few hundreds of these organs inside each muscle (Table 2.1). Each muscle spindle consists of a bundle of several types of specialized thin and weak '**intrafusal**' muscle fibres, which are used for regulating the response range and sensitivity of the muscle spindle. The 'normal' skeletal muscle fibres are sometimes also referred to as '**extrafusal**' fibres in order to distinguish them from the very specialized fibres of muscle spindles. Unless otherwise specified, all references to muscle fibres in this book concern the extrafusal variety.

Two types of sensory axons (mechanosensitive afferents of types Ia and II) are attached to central portions of the intrafusal muscle fibres. Stretching these muscle fibres will activate the sensory axons such that they deliver action potentials travelling into the CNS via the dorsal roots. The afferents from muscle spindles are unique in that they have direct monosynaptic connections with MNs (valid for both Ia and II affterents), particularly with those innervating their own muscle. In addition they have many other connections within the CNS.

2.3.3. Efferent muscle innervation; motor units

The two size groups of motor axons (Fig. 5.2A) are:

(1) the thick group of **skeletomotor** or **alpha axons**, which primarily innervate the extrafusal skeletal muscle fibres, but sometimes additionally send collaterals to the intrafusal fibres of muscle spindles (then sometimes called 'beta' axons);

(2) the thin group of **fusimotor** or **gamma axons**, which exclusively innervate the intra-fusal muscle fibres of spindles.

The terms alpha and gamma originally referred to different axon sizes within the peripheral nerves (Erlanger and Gasser 1937). However, in MN contexts (including the rest of this book) these terms are used as synonyms for the physiological terms skeleto-motor and fusimotor, also when dealing with central portions of the respective MNs. Activating gamma axons will cause the intrafusal muscle fibres to contract. These fibres are very thin and weak, they have a compliant central portion, and their contractions add no significant force to the muscle as a whole. However, intrafusal contractions do have a dramatic effect on the sensory functions of the muscle spindle (Matthews 1981).

In the hindlimb muscles of the cat, there is typically very little overlap between the sizes of the skeletomotor and fusimotor axons (Fig. 5.2A). The 'beta' axons do not repres-ent a separate size category; large as well as smaller alpha axons may give collaterals to muscle spindles (i.e. qualify as 'beta' axons). However, fast and slow beta axons may have different effects on the discharge of muscle spindle afferents (Jami *et al.* 1982a).

The ventral roots of the human spinal cord contain, in total, about 200 000 axons on each side (Blinkov and Glezer 1968). Some of these are preganglionic axons destined for sympathetic ganglia. Thus, for body portions served by the spinal cord (i.e. roughly below the head), about 600 muscles are innervated by a total of perhaps 300 000 alpha plus gamma MNs; on average, each muscle is controlled by a whole team of MNs (MN pool). About 50–60 per cent of these MNs are of the alpha type, innervating skele-tal muscle fibres (i.e. a total of about 165 000 alpha MNs); (Table 2.1). This innervation is organized such that, in adult mammals, each single twitch muscle fibre normally receives an axonal connection from only one MN, a neuromuscular junction (Fig. 4.1). However, each MN typically sends axonal branches to a large number of muscle fibres. A MN (or a motor axon) with all the muscle fibres it innervates is referred to as a **motor unit**, and the muscle fibres of a motor unit are collectively called a **muscle unit**.

When a MN is activated it normally causes all its muscle fibres to contract. Thus muscle units are the smallest fractions of a muscle that the CNS can activate. Within a single muscle, the muscle units vary a great deal in maximum contractile force, partly depending on the variation in the constituent number of muscle fibres per unit. Within a muscle, fibres belonging to different units are widely intermingled (see Fig. 3.10D).

2.4. Physiology of peripheral axons

An activated MN sends electrical signals (**action potentials**) along its axon. Following a chemical intermediate step at the neuromuscular junction (a chemical synapse), similar electrical signals appear in the muscle fibres and this leads, ultimately, to activation of their contractile mechanisms. These processes depend on the properties of the respective cell membranes.

2.4.1. Passive electrical membrane and cell properties

The thin lipid membranes of living cells are normally relatively impermeable to water and to ions and compounds in aqueous solution. The cell membrane separates intra- and extracellular solutions of various ions, and the inside of a resting cell is at a more negative electrical potential than the outside (**resting membrane potential**). Positive and negative charges will attract each other across the thin separating membrane, i.e. the cell membrane has the properties of an electrical capacitance. This capacitance is generally assumed to be ~1 $\mu F/cm^2$.

The limited ionic permeability of cell membranes implies that they have a high electrical resistance (i.e. a low electrical conductance, the inverse of resistance). The membrane resistance may vary considerably depending on the type and density of particular kinds of protein (ion channels) that are inserted into the membrane. For some of these channels, the conductance for specific ions may be directly altered (**directly gated**) either by a change in the membrane potential (**voltage-gated channels**) or by the temporary binding of chemical compounds to the channel (**ligand-gated channels**). Directly gated ion channels provide the basic mechanisms for major types of neuronal signalling (action potentials, rapid postsynaptic potentials). Also, without any activation of gated ion channels, ions may pass across the 'passive' membrane at a limited number of non-gated leakage channels. Thus resting or 'passive' membranes have a characteristic basic conductivity (or resistivity) which determines how easily the membrane potential can be altered by currents in accordance with Ohm's law, i.e. the voltage change equals the product of current intensity and electrical resistance: $V = R \times I$. The passive electrical membrane properties provide the starting conditions for electrophysiological signalling.

Electrically, a passive cell membrane has characteristics similar to a simple electrical circuit with a resistor (R) and a capacitor (C) coupled in parallel (RC circuit) (Fig. 2.2A). A sudden step of current applied across this circuit (i.e. between the inside and

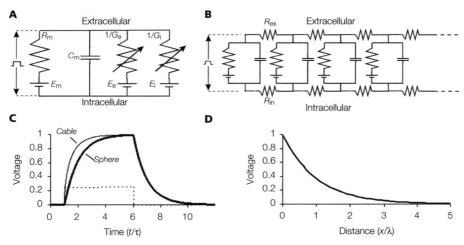

Figure 2.2 Passive membrane properties. (**A**) Electronic model representing the passive electrical properties of a cell membrane: R_m, resistance of unit membrane; C_m, capacitance per unit membrane; E_m, battery representing the mechanisms underlying the resting membrane potential. The model also includes two synaptic sites with a variable excitatory (G_e) and inhibitory (G_i) conductance and batteries corresponding to the respective equilibrium potentials for the postsynaptic current (E_e and E_i). (**B**) A similar membrane model for an elongated cellular structure (e.g. axon, dendrite, muscle fibre; 'leaky cable') consisting of elements like those in (**A**) interconnected with intra- and extracellular resistances (R_{in}, R_{ex}), i.e. conducting paths through the intra- and extracellular fluid ($R_{ex} \ll R_{in}$). (**C**) In a model like that of (**A**), a current step (broken line, timing indication only) causes a gradual rise and fall of voltage with an exponential time course (thick line) related to $e^{-t/\tau}$, where t is the time from the beginning or end of the current pulse and τ is the membrane time constant. Voltage is given relative to the final steady-state value, and time relative to the membrane time constant. The thin line indicates the faster voltage time course for an infinite cable (as in (**B**)) with the same membrane time constant (only the rising portion of this transient is shown). (**D**) A current step applied to one end of an infinite cable (as in (**B**)) will cause a voltage shift showing an exponential decline with distance. In this graph, only steady-state voltages are considered. The voltage shift is largest at the point of current injection, and declines with distance in proportion to $e^{-x/\lambda}$, where x is the distance and λ is the space constant for the cable. In (**D**), voltages are given relative to the value at the site of current injection, and distances relative to the space constant λ. In an infinite dendrite, λ is proportional to $\sqrt{R_m\,d}$, and input resistance to $\sqrt{R_m/d^3}$ (d is diameter). For further information and equations, see Jack et al. (1975) and Rall et al. (1992).

outside of a cell) will cause a gradually increasing potential shift. Similarly, after the sudden cessation of the current step, the potential will gradually return to its resting level (Fig. 2.2c, thick line). For a simple RC circuit these voltage transients have an exponential time course. The time taken for the voltage to shift to within 37 per cent (i.e. 1/e) of the final value corresponds to the **time constant** of the membrane (symbol Greek letter tau: τ_m). The value of the membrane time constant depends on the product R x C, with R equal to the specific membrane resistance (i.e. resistance of 1 cm^2 of membrane), and C equal to the specific membrane capacitance (i.e. capacitance of 1 cm^2 of membrane). Adult MNs often have a membrane time constant of about 5–10 ms (Table 6–1). Thus, in such a cell even a very brief current pulse across the membrane (e.g. caused by synaptic activation) will produce a membrane potential shift lasting several ms.

Axons and muscle fibres are long tube-like structures with less than perfect insulation, i.e. they have properties similar to the 'leaky cables' known from classical telephone and telegraph engineering (see electronic model in Fig. 2.2B). In such a structure, there is a practical limit to how far useful electrical signals can spread without some kind of amplification. Consider an experiment in which current is injected into an axon or muscle fibre through a microelectrode and the voltage effects of this current are measured at different distances with another electrode. In a passive cable (i.e. no voltage-gated ion channels are active), the recorded potential shift across the membrane will be progressively smaller at progressively greater distances from the injecting electrode. This longitudinal voltage drop is partly of a conventional kind, taking place according to Ohm's law for currents flowing across an electrical resistance, in this case the resistive lengthwise core of the cable. For a given length of cable, the core resistance is directly proportional to the cross-sectional area of the cable. Thus the resistive drop of potential will be greater for thin than for thicker cables or axons. Part of the voltage drop along a passive axon is caused by current leakage across the membrane. This drop will be greater for membranes with a high specific resting conductance than for those with less leaky properties.

For a uniform and infinite cable (e.g. a very long axon) with current injected at one point, an exponential relation is found between the recorded voltage change and the distance from the injection site (Fig. 2.2D). The distance at which the potential shift has fallen to about 37 per cent of its starting value (i.e. to 1/e) is called the **characteristic length** or **space constant** of the cable (symbol Greek letter lambda (λ)). Thus λ gives a measure of how effectively changes in potential can spread within passive tube-like structures such as muscle fibres, axons, and dendrites.

2.4.2. Ion channels and the resting membrane potential

The cell membrane is provided with a large number of different kinds of protein, spanning across it from inside to outside. Some of the transmembrane proteins are ion channels (see above), and others provide mechanisms for an active energy-demanding transport of ions or other substances across the membrane ('pumps'). One of the most ubiquitous and important of these latter cell mechanisms is the **Na–K pump**, which uses biochemical energy (ATP) for the active transport of Na$^+$ ions out of the cell and K$^+$ ions towards the inside (reviewed by Clausen 2003). As a result, the intracellular fluid of living cells normally has a relatively low concentration of Na$^+$ ions and a high concentration of K$^+$ ions.

In the resting state, passive diffusion across the membrane is easier for K$^+$ ions (many open K$^+$ channels, including the so-called 'leak' channels) than for the Na$^+$ ions (few open Na$^+$ channels). Because of the concentration gradients maintained by the Na–K pump, K$^+$ ions will tend to diffuse out of the cell. Because of the low resting conductance for Na$^+$ ions, this exit of K$^+$ ions cannot be compensated by a corresponding entry of Na$^+$ ions and a lack of positive charge will develop on the inside, i.e. a negative 'membrane potential'. At a certain level of transmembrane potential difference, an equilibrium will exist between the outward flow of K$^+$ ions according to their concentration gradient and the inward flow according to the electrical gradient (K$^+$ ions attracted by intracellular negative charge). For a given ion, this **equilibrium potential** (E_{ion}) can be calculated from the concentration gradient across the membrane using the Nernst equation. With general constants inserted and using logarithms to base 10, this equation simplifies to

$$E_{ion} = (T/z) \times 0.198 \times \log ([X]_e/[X]_i) \qquad (2.1)$$

where E_{ion} is in mV, z is the valence of the ion (sign according to ionic charge), T is the absolute temperature, and $[X]_e$ and $[X]_i$ are the external and internal concentrations of ion X. If the resting membrane were only permeable to K$^+$ ions, the resting membrane potential would be equal to E_K, the equilibrium potential for K$^+$. In practice, some leakage for other positive and negative ions also exists and the resting membrane potential is somewhat less negative than E_K. In MNs the resting membrane potential is typically about −70 mV.

The existence of a negative resting membrane potential and an inward-directed concentration gradient for Na$^+$ ions is of great importance for the life-sustaining mechanisms of cells in general. For instance, it provides the driving force for various kinds of **secondary active transport** across the membrane (e.g. inward glucose transport; outward Ca^{2+} transport). In addition, the negative resting potential and the Na$^+$ and K$^+$ concentration gradients provide the necessary conditions for the types of electrical signalling used by neurones and muscle fibres—action potentials and postsynaptic potentials.

2.4.3. Conduction of action potentials in axons

Messages are transmitted along peripheral (and most central) axons and twitch muscle fibres by **action potentials**, travelling waves of altered membrane potential (reviewed by Hille 2001). In suitable cells, this phenomenon can be elicited by depolarization, i.e. by making the inside of the cell less negative (see Fig. 4.2A). This can be done experimentally by inserting the sharp tip of a microelectrode through the membrane and injecting an appropriate amount and polarity of current. For instance, in motor axons of rats (Carp *et al.* 2003), an applied shift of membrane potential from its resting level of about −64 mV to a threshold level of about −52 mV will give rise to a very rapid and self-sustained further shift of membrane potential up to a peak at about +7 mV and a subsequent rapid decline back towards resting level. In a mammalian myelinated axon this whole event is over within about 0.5−1 ms.

Once an action potential has been elicited, it will **propagate** along the axon or muscle fibre. This propagation (conduction) takes place because, once it has been elicited, the action potential itself serves as an electrical stimulus for neighbouring membrane regions. These regions will themselves generate action potentials, which will stimulate regions even further away, and so on (cf. the falling of a series of dominoes). The 'active' conduction, caused by a recurring local generation of action potentials, gives this signalling procedure distinct advantages and disadvantages. An important advantage is that, as long as local conditions support its renewed generation, the message will not attenuate with distance. An important limitation of the procedure concerns its 'all-or-nothing' character; the shape and size of the action potential arriving at its destination depends on the membrane properties at this particular site; it tells us nothing about the action potential shape or size at its point of departure (cf. falling dominoes; the last domino to fall tells us nothing about the weight or shape of the initial domino in the row). Thus messages mediated by action potentials can only be modulated by changing when and how often they appear (e.g. by altering their repetition frequency).

The speed of action potential conduction along motor axons reaches maximum values of about 60–80 m/s in rats or humans and 120 m/s in cats, i.e. overlapping with the speeds of very fast cars and slow aeroplanes. It should be noted that the speed of conduction of action potentials is much slower than the speed of electrical current pulses in metal conductors and computer chips. There are two factors of importance which together determine the efficiency of the process of active action potential conduction by repeated self-stimulation.

1 Conduction becomes faster if the passive spread of current along the axon becomes more time and space efficient. For instance, a high conduction speed is promoted by the long space constant and very short membrane time constant of myelinated axons.

2 Conduction becomes slower if the action potential has a less rapid rising phase or a higher threshold. For instance, owing to the temperature-dependent kinetics of voltage-gated Na^+ channels, action potential and conduction speed decrease with cooling.

Because of their brief action potential durations, peripheral motor nerve fibres can typically conduct spikes at discharge rates exceeding 1000 Hz, i.e. spike frequencies considerably higher than those needed for the control of muscle force (cf. Fig. 3.7). In the long unbranched sections of peripheral motor nerve fibres, the safety margin for conduction is typically very high, i.e. messages will normally not become blocked or distorted on their way from the soma-dendrite region of MNs to their intramuscular target regions. However, inside the muscle conduction block is thought to take place more easily at branching points, at which there may be an expansion of the membrane area ahead of the spike and hence an increased electrical load. The possible occurrence of such branch blocks has attracted attention in the context of discussions concerning fatigue and post-tetanic potentiation (see Chapter 9) (Luscher *et al.* 1979, 1983; Sieck and Prakash 1995).

The high conduction velocity of motor axons, compared with muscle fibres, is mainly caused by the fact that these axons are provided with an electrically insulating layer of **myelin** (high internode resistance and low capacitance). Because of this insulation, myelinated fibres have a long characteristic length and a very short membrane time constant. This means that once an action potential emerges at one site in an axon it will rapidly cause a suprathreshold amount of depolarization several millimetres away. Because of their low internal core resistance, large myelinated fibres have a longer λ and a higher conduction velocity than thinner myelinated fibres. At 37°C, the conduction velocity (m/s) of a myelinated axon tends to be about five to six times its external diameter (Hursh 1938; Boyd and Davey 1968; see Jack 1975 for a discussion).

In normal adult nerves, internodal distances are directly proportional to axonal diameter and conduction velocity. However, they do not show a very strong causal relationship with conduction velocity. In regenerated nerves, axonal conduction velocity is still proportional to axonal diameter (Sanders and Whitteridge 1948), but all axons now have the same brief internodal distance (Vizoso and Young 1948). In some textbooks, long internodal distances are said to be crucial for the high conduction speed of myelinated nerve fibres: action potentials are said to jump from node to node, and the further they jump the faster conduction occurs. This view is misleading. In a fast myelinated 20 μm fibre of the cat, for instance, an axonal action potential may last about 0.5 ms and travel at a speed of about 120 m/s. This means that, at any one time, about 60 mm of axon will be covered by different phases of the same action potential. In this type of nerve, internodal distances are typically about 2.6 mm (i.e. about 130 times the fibre diameter) (Hursh 1938; Waxman 1972). Thus, in this case, the single action potential simultaneously covers the membrane of about 23 nodes of Ranvier.

The diameter of peripheral axons is not always constant from beginning to end, but there may be some tapering towards the periphery associated with lower conduction velocities. In addition, it should be realized that axons might run in a zigzag inside a nerve at its 'resting' length (see Clough *et al.* 1968a, discussion), allowing for the possibility that nerves may become considerably stretched during motor behaviour. Thus, although this has not been carefully quantified, peripheral axons might be substantially longer than the nerves themselves. Such factors may be (partly) responsible for the unexpected observation that motor axonal conduction velocity, as calculated from spike latencies and conduction distances along peripheral nerves, tends to be lower close to the spinal cord than at levels about halfway towards the targets (Clough *et al.* 1968a), i.e. there is both a proximal and a distal region of apparent slowing-down, possibly due to different mechanisms.

The conduction of peripheral axons may be blocked by pressure applied to the nerve fibres (Gasser and Erlanger 1929) as well as by interference with the blood supply to the nerve (Lindstrom and Brismar 1991); both mechanisms may play a role when an arm or leg has 'gone to sleep' due to a non-optimal body position of some kind. Fortunately, these incidental conduction blocks are usually reversible. Large-diameter axons are more sensitive than small-diameter ones to the block produced by pressure applied directly to the nerve. Therefore pressure block has been an important tool for analysing differences in function between axons of different diameter, for example for studying the functions of alpha versus gamma axons (Leksell 1945).

2.4.4. Voltage gated ion-channels and action potential generation in axons

The basic ionic currents and the permeability changes responsible for the action potential were first measured for the giant axon of the squid using voltage clamp techniques (Hodgkin and Huxley 1952; reviewed by Hille 2001). These investigations resulted in the famous Hodgkin–Huxley equation system which summarizes empirical findings concerning the voltage and time dependence of the Na^+ and K^+ conductances underlying action potentials in the squid giant axon. For these voltage-gated Na^+ channels, depolarization has a dual effect.

1. First the channels are rapidly opened, allowing Na^+ ions to move across the membrane (**Na^+ conductance activation**).

2. More slowly, the depolarization causes the same channels to close, decreasing the Na^+ current (**Na^+ conductance inactivation**).

For the dominant type of axonal voltage-gated K^+ conductance, the depolarization-induced opening of the channels happens more slowly than the opening of Na^+ channels. Furthermore, these particular 'delayed rectifier' K^+ channels show hardly any voltage-dependent inactivation.

If the membrane potential is made more positive than its resting value (i.e. depolarized) up to just above the action potential **threshold** (often at about -50 to -60 mV), the following sequence of events takes place:

- some Na^+ channels open up (increased Na^+ conductance)
- hence more Na^+ ions flow into the cell, which makes the membrane potential more positive
- hence, more Na^+ channels open up
- hence, more Na^+ ions flow in, which makes membrane potential more positive
- and so on.

In this way, the rapidly rising phase of the action potential emerges. However, the Na^+ conductance soon begins to decrease again due to a voltage-gated inactivation of these channels. At about the same time, an increasing number of K^+ channels open up, leading to an efflux of K^+ ions (outward concentration gradient). Together, the decreasing Na^+ current and the increasing K^+ current cause a rapid return of the membrane potential towards its resting level (falling phase of the action potential). Because of the inactivation of the Na^+ conductance, no new action potential can be generated before the preceding one is more or less over (**absolute refractory period**). Owing to the relatively slow disappearance of the inactivation of Na^+ conductance and of the activation of the K^+

current (and sometimes the presence of long-lasting conductance changes associated with after-potentials, see below), action potentials are less easily generated and may look smaller and wider for some period soon after the end of the preceding one (**relative refractory period**).

Following the voltage clamp measurements on squid axons, equivalent techniques were used to study the much thinner peripheral myelinated nerve fibres in vertebrates (clawed toad, *Xenopus laevis* (Frankenhaeuser and Huxley 1964); rabbit (Chiu *et al.* 1979)). The action potential in myelinated nerve fibres is also generated by a voltage-dependent Na^+ channel which is both rapidly activated (opened) and, with a slower time constant, subsequently inactivated (closed) by depolarization. Amphibian nodes of Ranvier also possess voltage-gated K^+ channels with properties similar to those of the 'delayed rectifier' channels of squid axons; these channels show little inactivation and they are activated with a slower time constant than that for the Na^+ channel (Frankenhaeuser and Huxley 1964). However, there are marked quantitative differences between squid axons (and unmyelinated axons in general) and myelinated mammalian axons with regard to the intramembrane distribution of the various channels and their relative importance.

In myelinated nerve fibres, most of the membrane is covered by the myelin. Action potential generation is restricted to the few micrometres of bare membrane at the nodes of Ranvier, separated by internodes, often of length 1–2 mm. There is an extremely high concentration of the voltage-gated Na^+ channels within the small patches of nodal membrane. There is also a high nodal concentration of K^+-selective but voltage-insensitive 'leakage' channels (Hille 1967), producing a high resting conductance at the node. As the total input capacitance is also very low, because of the myelin sheath, medullated fibres have a very brief membrane time constant, often of the order of 0.1–0.4 ms. Thus, even in the absence of an increased K^+ current, the action potential of a myelinated nerve will be quickly terminated once the Na^+ current becomes inactivated. In mammalian nodes of Ranvier the voltage-dependent increase in K^+ conductance is also barely detectable (Chiu *et al.* 1979). Various types of voltage-dependent K^+ channels are indeed present in such nerve fibres, but the fast-reacting variety of these channels is mainly localized within the paranodal regions which are normally covered with myelin (Roper and Schwarz 1989) (cf. central axons (Rasband and Shrager 2000)). In various diseases (e.g. polyneuritis and other auto-immune afflictions, multiple sclerosis), the myelin may be damaged and lost from several internodes of the individual peripheral nerve fibres. This will cause a drastic increase in axonal input capacitance without any corresponding increase in the number of available Na^+ channels for the generation of action potentials (very few Na^+ channels in the membrane of the internodes). Hence a demyelinization of motor axons may cause a block of action potential conduction along the axon, resulting in motor paralysis.

The voltage-gated Na^+ channels of mammalian myelinated axons are specifically blocked by extracellular application of the poison tetrodotoxin (TTX). The voltage-gated K^+ channels may be blocked using tetraethyl ammonium (TEA) or Cs^+ in the extracellular fluid. Interestingly, in mammalian non-myelinated nerve fibres (Schomburg and Steffens 2002) and denervated muscle fibres (Sellin and Thesleff 1980), action potentials are generated using voltage-gated Na^+ channels of other isoforms which are TTX insensitive (for other examples, see Yoshida 1994).

2.4.5. After-potentials in axons

There are several reports describing a complex sequence of post-spike changes of excitability in mammalian axons, sometimes lasting up to 100 ms following a single spike (Bergmans 1970). However, few publications have described direct recordings of the corresponding kinds of post-spike after-potentials. Voltage clamp studies of voltage-dependent ion channels in axons have usually concentrated on fast processes and the classical equation systems derived from such measurements do not include processes for generating after-potentials (e.g. Hodgkin and Huxley 1952; Frankenhaeuser and Huxley 1964; Chiu *et al.* 1979).

2.4.6. Transport mechanisms in axons and the use of tracing substances

If the axon of a neurone is transected, its peripheral portions will die (Wallerian degeneration). Axons are continuously supplied with molecules synthesized in the soma of the neurone. Part of this material is used for a steadily ongoing replacement of essential molecules in membranes and in the cytoplasm. Molecular supplies are moved towards the periphery, often enclosed in membranous vesicles, using **kinesin** molecules as carriers and motors (Schwartz and De Camilli 2000; Almenar-Queralt and Goldstein 2001; Hirokawa and Takemura 2005). Kinesins are structurally related to myosin and there are several isoforms, specialized for the attachment to different cargoes. Furthermore, there are differentiations enabling a choice between different destinations (e.g. axon vs. dendrites). The energy-requiring movement of the kinesins takes place along microtubuli, and different kinds of supplies are being moved at very different mean speeds. Much of the orthograde transport (central to peripheral) of vesicular material and various organelles takes place at relatively high speeds up to about 400 mm/day (**'fast'** transport), and other substances, including cytoskeleton molecules, move with different phases of **slow** transport (about 0.1–4 mm/day). In addition, material is also transported along the microtubuli in a retrograde direction, from the periphery towards the cell body. This retrograde transport is relatively fast (up to about 200 mm/day) and uses other molecular motors (dyneins; Almenar-Queralt and Goldstein 2001; Hirokawa and Takemura 2005). Both types of molecular motor also have important tasks in all cells during mitosis (e.g. Alberts *et al.* 2002).

Like axons, dendrites also do not survive without being in continuity with the trophic centre of the neurone, the cell body. Various substances and organelles are actively transported along the dendrites, towards the periphery as well as towards the cell body. Speeds and mechanisms seem similar to those in axons, which have been better studied.

The axonal transport mechanisms are not only essential for the functions of neurones, but they are also of practical importance in neuroanatomical research. The origin and destination of nerve fibres can be analysed using orthograde or retrograde transport of tracing substances. Thus the positions of MN cell bodies within the CNS can be visualized by injecting a suitable tracer substance into a target muscle. After waiting an appropriate time for the retrograde transport, the spinal cord or brainstem is removed and and consecutive serial sections are stained for the tracer. The tracer most frequently used is horseradish peroxidase (HRP), a large enzymatic protein obtained from the horseradish plant. These molecules are readily taken up via endocytosis into the intramuscular nerve endings. HRP which has been combined with wheat germ protein (wheat germ agglutinated HRP (W-HRP)) can even be used for the retrograde tracing of cells across synaptic connections. Thus injecting W-HRP into a muscle allows visualization of the positions of cell bodies of the target MNs as well as the sites of some of the interneurones which are synaptically connected to them (Harrison *et al.* 1984).

2.5. Muscle electrophysiology and excitation–contraction coupling

2.5.1. Neuromuscular transmission and muscle fibre action potentials

As early as 1844, Claude Bernard noted that the stimulation of a muscle nerve caused no contraction after application of the toxin curare, and that this was true although the muscle fibres remained electrically excitable (see Black 1999). Thus signals from nerves did not continue directly into the muscles; curare blocks the chemical intermediate step in neuromuscular transmission.

The functional contact between a MN axon and a muscle fibre is called the **neuromuscular junction** (NMJ). The specialized membrane region under the motor nerve ending is referred to as the **motor endplate** (sometimes this term is also used for the whole NMJ). The NMJ is one of the best known and earliest investigated examples of a **chemical synapse**, i.e. a neuronal connection in which an axonal action potential causes the presynaptic nerve ending to release a transmitter substance that influences the postsynaptic cell (the muscle fibre). In the NMJ, the transmitter is acetylcholine (ACh). At the muscle membrane it binds to ligand-gated ion channels, the ACh receptors (AChRs). This leads to a transient increase of membrane conductance for Na^+ and K^+ ions (and some Ca^{2+} ions) which evokes a transient depolarizing response in the muscle fibre—the endplate potential (EPP). Normally, the EPP is large enough to discharge an action potential in the muscle fibre. This action potential conducts along the muscle fibre and triggers the chain of processes that cause the muscle fibre to contract. Curare blocks neuromuscular transmission by binding to the AChRs, thereby preventing the ACh molecules from doing so. Further details about the NMJ and neuromuscular transmission are given in Chapter 4.

2.5.2. **Electromyography (EMG)**

Each time a MN is activated and fires an action potential, action potentials appear in all its muscle fibres. A single motor unit comprises many muscle fibres, and the sum of the almost synchronous action potentials of such a group of fibres (the 'compound' action potential) is easily recorded extracellularly with a needle or a pair of fine wires inserted into the muscle (**motor unit action potential (MUAP)**). The identification of single units is easy in weak contractions but becomes increasingly complex as more units take part in the discharge. One of the great advantages with these EMG methods is that they can be applied to recordings in awake humans or animals with relatively little discomfort. Each MUAP corresponds to one action potential in the corresponding MN. Thus EMG recordings offer the unique possibility of studying the activity of single MNs during normal motor behaviour. No other central neurone is equally accessible. Using coarse surface EMG electrodes, fixed to the skin above the target muscle, one can typically record from many or all the motor units of the target muscle simultaneously, thus obtaining a measure of the degree of total muscle activation. For examples of EMG, see unit recordings in Figures 8.1B and 8.1C and a mass recording in Figure 9.1B.

2.5.3. **Excitation–contraction coupling and contractile events in muscle fibres**

Following the emergence of a propagating sarcolemmal action potential in a muscle fibre, the following events take place.

(1) For each sarcomere along the fibre, the sarcolemmal action potential elicits action-potential-like events (**T spikes**) propagating down the T tubuli (Fig. 2.1B).

(2) When reaching the various T-SR connections (triads), T spikes cause the release of Ca^{2+} ions from the SR into the sarcoplasm.

(3) Released Ca^{2+} ions spread by diffusion and reversibly attach themselves to **troponin C** molecules of the thin myofilaments.

(4) As long as the Ca^{2+} ions remain attached to troponin C, another protein of the thin myofilament (**tropomyosin**) is shifted aside, allowing interactions between thin and thick myofilaments.

(5) Actin molecules of the thin myofilaments become attached to myosin cross-bridges of thick myofilaments.

(6) Myosin cross-bridges undergo a conformational change such that the attached actin filament is pulled towards the centre of the sarcomere.

(7) Following this cross-bridge movement, actin and myosin become detached by a process requiring the hydrolysis of adenosine triphosphate (ATP); this step is mediated by the enzyme myosin ATPase which constitutes part of the myosin molecule.

(8) The detached cross-bridge reverts to its starting conformation, and steps (5)–(8) repeat for as long as sarcoplasmic Ca^{2+} concentration is high enough for an effective binding to troponin C.

(9) After the end of the T spike, sarcoplasmic Ca^{2+} concentration decreases again because of the continuous active transport of Ca^{2+} ions from the sarcoplasm into the SR (process requiring hydrolysis of ATP). (**SR-Ca^{2+} pump**).

(10) Because of the decreased sarcoplasmic Ca^{2+} concentration, troponin molecules lose their Ca^{2+} ions and tropomyosin resumes its resting position which prohibits further interactions between actin and myosin, i.e. the generation of contractile force will stop.

Interestingly, ATP is not only needed for providing the energy driving the cross-bridge cycle, but its presence is also required in the passive muscle (i.e. at low levels of sarcoplasmic Ca^{2+}). If sarcoplasmic ATP concentrations approach zero, as happens after death, myosin and actin filaments will remain attached to each other and the muscle becomes stiff; this is the state of **rigor mortis**. Fortunately, in the living body rigor mortis does not occur after a bout of hard physical activity because mechanisms are present that depress and stop contractions from taking place before energy supplies are depleted (see Chapter 9).

2.6. **Muscle metabolism**

Like many energy-requiring processes in the body, the mechanical work of muscle is paid for with the energy that is released by the splitting (hydrolysis) of ATP (equation (2.2)). Muscle tissue is exceptional in the wide range of its energy requirements; a contracting muscle may need 60–100 times more ATP per unit time than its requirements at rest. Hence many of the biochemical specializations of muscle have to do with the need for a rapid mobilization of metabolic energy, i.e. ultimately of ATP.

Considering the great importance of ATP, the intracellular stores of this molecule are typically relatively modest in living cells, including muscle; the normal level at rest is about 2–8 mmol/l. Mobilizing energy from ATP involves the reaction

$$ATP + H_2O \rightleftarrows ADP + H^+ + P_i + \text{'energy'} \tag{2.2}$$

where ADP is **adenosine diphosphate** and P_i is **inorganic phosphate**. The most rapid mechanism for replenishing ATP in a muscle fibre is to regenerate it from ADP and **phosphocreatine** (PCr) in the reaction:

$$PCr + ADP + H^+ \rightleftarrows Cr + ATP. \tag{2.3}$$

This reaction goes from left to right or vice versa, depending on the substrate concentrations, and the process is extremely fast. Creatine is synthesized in the liver and taken up from the circulation by muscle fibres. The phosphorylation of creatine using ATP is catalysed by the enzyme **creatine kinase**. At rest about 80 per cent of the muscle fibre creatine content is present as PCr, at a molar concentration about five times that of ATP. Generating PCr costs ATP, and new ATP ultimately has to be made using metabolic energy. One method of doing this is to use the complex reactions of anaerobic glycolysis, starting with glucose (or with glycosyl units derived from stored chains of glycogen):

$$\text{glucose} + 2ADP + 2P_i \rightleftharpoons 2\text{lactate} + 2ATP + 2H_2O \qquad (2.4)$$

Much of the lactate (**lactic acid**) may come out of the cell across the membrane and emerge in the circulation. An increase of lactate in blood and, correspondingly, an increased acidification (more H^+ ions) are well-known consequences of intense muscle activity, i.e. signs that the metabolic needs of the musculature were greater than could be immediately fulfilled using oxidative metabolism.

Circulation may be partly occluded in strong contractions, making the availability of glycogen stores and anaerobic ATP production important. In addition, the presence and anaerobic use of intramuscular glycogen stores is important because of its rapidity in initiating metabolic ATP production soon after the start of rapid movements. However, the total energy stores that can be mobilized inside muscles in the absence of oxygen would be sufficient for only about 60 s of relatively strenuous physical exercise (stores of ATP, PCr, and energy from glycolysis, as used at a power output equivalent to 80 per cent Vo_2max (Jones *et al.* 2004)). Glycogen stores are clearly only adequate (but essential) for covering transient peaks of energy needs. Long-lasting and intense physical activity may indeed deplete much of the normal glycogen store (cf. Fig. 3.10D). The replenishment of these stores is relatively slow (days).

With sufficient oxygen, lactate is converted into pyruvate which enters the mitochondria and is further broken down in the tricarboxylic acid cycle of aerobic metabolism (Krebs cycle). This series of reactions yields another 36 molecules of ATP per molecule of glucose, i.e. an enormous increase compared with the yield of the initial anaerobic steps. In the long term, oxidative carbohydrate metabolism and the circulatory provision of fuel (glucose) remain absolutely essential. However, these metabolic processes are relatively slow, requiring several minutes for a substantial energy production.

In the presence of suff<!-- -->cient amounts of oxygen, ATP may also be generated by the metabolism of fat (fatty acids) which is an important fuel for low-level tonic contractions of muscle. There is no anaerobic pathway for ATP generation from fat. Furthermore, the maximum speed of oxidative energy production from fat is only about 50 per cent of that for carbohydrates. Further details and references concerning muscle biochemistry and metabolism can be found in several textbooks and monographs (e.g. Jones *et al.* 2004).

2.7. **Specializations of muscle fibre and motor unit properties**

Muscles produce movements by the generation of repeated transient shortening contractions and, in addition, almost all muscles are also used for more continuous 'postural' tasks (i.e. for the stabilization of joints, often near-isometric contractions) and for transient 'braking' tasks (in lengthening contractions). These different types of motor task are associated with different mechanical, metabolic, and circulatory conditions, and different muscle fibres have specialized accordingly.

Table 2.2 Classification of motor units and their muscle fibres

Physiological motor unit type			
Traditional simple classification	Slow	————Fast————	
'Burke-classification'	S	FR	Fint/FF
Cytochemical fibre type			
mATPase histochemistry	I	IIa	IIb (IIbd, IIbm)
MHC isoform	I	IIa	IIx (=IId), IIb
mATPase/MHC & metabol. enz.	SO	FOG	FG
Physiological characteristics			
Force-sag*	0	+	+
Isometric twitch speed*	+	++	++
Fatigue index (%)*	>75	>75	25–75/0–25
Maximum tetanic force	+	++	+++
Recruitment hierarchy	1	2	3
Amount of daily activity	+++	++	+

Simplified summary of major terminologies and characteristics of motor unit types in mammalian limb muscles.

Abbreviations: mATPase, myofibrillar ATPase; MHC, myosin heavy chain; metabol. enz., activity of metabolic enzymes (oxidative, glycolytic).

* Properties used for physiological classification.

'Speed' has been categorized using different criteria in different investigations (e.g. aspects of twitch speed, or 'sag' behaviour in partly fused contractions). Fatigue index according to Burke *et al.* (1973); a high index indicates a great resistance to fatigue. Use of the intermediate category 'Fint' is rather variable across different investigations; sometimes only the three main categories have been used (i.e. S, FR, FF). The MHC type of the most fatiguable fibre category is species dependent (e.g. rats have both IIx and IIb fibres, whereas humans only have IIx). Further information and references are given in the text.

Individual muscle fibres and units may differ considerably in contractile characteristics, such as speed and gradation properties, within the same muscle, and they may also show large differences in their sensitivity to fatigue and in various biochemical/histochemical aspects (for further details, see Chapters 3 and 9). Most of these characteristics show a continuous variation across a wide range. However, it has been customary and useful to subdivide muscle fibres and units into 'slow' and (one or several) 'fast' categories (Table 2.2); the classification terminology presented in Table 2.2 will be used repeatedly in the rest of this book. Classification methods, neuromuscular specializations, and further details concerning muscle contractions are extensively discussed in Chapter 3.

2.8. **CNS control of motor behaviour**

Much of the CNS is directly or indirectly engaged in the programming and control of motor behaviour. These processes largely fall outside the scope of the present book, which is focused on the properties and functions of the output interface rather than on motor physiology in general. However, as a background to discussions on how the activity of MNs and MN pools are managed by various synaptic systems (Chapter 7), a brief and selective overview is given below.

2.8.1. **Hierarchies in the motor system: interspecies comparisons**

In primitive chordates, such as the Amphioxiformes, the whole CNS is dominated by the spinal cord and there is only a small non-segmental cranial extension similar to a brainstem. Initially, the spinal cord obviously had to regulate much of the (then simple) motor behaviour on its own.

Things are considerably more complex in the phylogenetically oldest versions of true vertebrates (e.g. various kinds of fish-like creatures); the brainstem has become further developed and there are now two extra masses of nerve cells connected to it—the cerebellum and the forebrain, including a forerunner of our basal ganglia. Interestingly, neither of these new portions have direct connections to the spinal cord. Commands to MNs for the whole-body coordination of motor behaviour are issued from the brainstem, and it is apparently helped in this intricate task by the two specialist 'consulting centres', the cerebellum and the forebrain. However, much may also still be regulated by the spinal cord itself (e.g. simple swimming behaviour). In these submammalian species, major connections from the brainstem to the spinal cord come from various parts of the reticular formation and from neuronal accumulations ('nuclei') associated with the processing of information from the organs of equilibrium (vestibular nuclei, connected to labyrinths in terrestrial animals).

The general setup of the brain remained roughly the same (with great differences in many details) until the appearance of mammals, the first and only vertebrates with a sizeable cerebral cortex. A rudimentary cerebral cortex is present in reptiles; birds enlarged their very capable brains by further developments of the basal ganglia. In mammals, the cerebral cortex largely assumed control of the rest and became massively connected to most of the the phylogenetically 'older' parts of the system. Thus in mammals there are very-large-scale bidirectional connections between the cerebral cortex, on the one hand, and the cerebellum, the basal ganglia, and the brainstem, on the other. The cerebral cortex apparently makes use of older networks for motor control besides adding its own. This cortical control of other parts of the CNS has developed so far that the cerebral cortex even sends its own descending fibre systems, the corticospinal tract (also referred to as the 'pyramidal' tract), directly into the spinal cord. In humans, large lesions of the cortical motor command system (e.g. after a stroke) leads, at least for some time, to an almost complete paralysis of the corresponding parts of the body. These dominating and strong motor effects of the cerebral cortex in humans have even led neurologists to describe the output neurones of the motor cortex as the 'upper motoneurones'. In order to avoid confusion, this term will not be used in the present book; all 'motoneurones' (MNs) mentioned in the present discourse are cells with axons innervating muscle fibres.

One consequence of the way in which the brain developed, with new systems becoming superimposed on older ones, seems to be that many functions tend to be regulated in parallel by several alternative circuits. This is important to keep in mind when analysing brain functions; many functions have multiple channels of command and control.

Furthermore, also in the mammalian CNS, interneuronal circuitry of the spinal cord remains important for the organization and transmission of messages to MNs; most descending fibres from the brain and most types of afferents influence MNs via various sets of spinal interneurones. Monosynaptic inputs to MNs from descending fibres exist for systems that seem important for mediating rapid corrective signals (e.g. some of the input from vestibulospinal and reticulospinal fibres) and for other systems that might need to bypass the primitive intraspinal networks for creating 'new' types of motor coordination (e.g. for some of input from the corticospinal system in primates, but not in cats) (reviewed by Lemon and Griffiths 2005).

2.8.2. Complexity of motor control: feedforward and feedback

When walking around in a furnished room in daylight, one can see all the obstacles and easily avoid bumping into them. However, controlling these movements is not a simple and straightforward affair of first looking and then moving accordingly. On the contrary, the process is extremely complex and the minute conscious portion of it covers only the 'highest' levels of motor planning (e.g. 'Now I want to go to this chair and sit down'). This plan is then somehow translated into a detailed motor program for activating the right sets of muscles with appropriate forces and timing sequences for walking in the correct direction. All this programming takes place far below the level of consciousness; one is not even introspectively aware of the existence or contractions of individual muscles (unless they are painful or clearly visible). Furthermore, walking towards the chair is not, at each instance, under immmediate visual control because it takes an appreciable time to analyse visual images; visual reaction times are often about 150–200 ms. Thus, within the next visual reaction time one is literally running blind, i.e. for the immediate future of at least about 150–200 ms all movements have to be predicted and preprogrammed (often referred to as 'feedforward').

One popular view in classical neurophysiology was that movements were largely composed of chains of reflexes, each involving a peripheral feedback loop. According to modern views, most movement patterns are preprogrammed, and peripheral feedback is mainly needed for planning what to do and for the online and post hoc corrections of feedforward programs. The term motor **reflex** is used for a stereotyped motor response to some kind of (typically peripheral) stimulation. The stimulation can be physiological (e.g. muscle stretch) or, under appropriate experimental circumstances, electrical. Two major classes of such reflexes have been extensively studied.

1 Those having their main role in the **correction of motor behaviour**. This includes so-called proprioceptive reflexes evoked via muscle afferents (muscle spindles, Golgi tendon organs) and many (often complex) reactions to various kinds of skin stimulation.

2 Those reactions which in themselves represent **simple kinds of motor behaviour**, often of a protective kind (and hence rapid and stereotyped). An important example in this group is the 'withdrawal reflex', for example the rapid withdrawal of a hand or

foot on a painful stimulus (largely analogous to the 'flexion reflex'). A well-known protective reflex of the eye is the 'blink reflex'—the reflective closure of the eye lids when the cornea is touched.

The best studied 'corrective' reflex loop is the one involving muscle spindles and their fast-conducting Ia afferents (see section 2.3.2). These afferents have monosynaptic excitatory connections to MNs (see Fig. 7.2A), mainly to those of the muscle housing the muscle spindle. The muscle spindle afferents are activated by muscle stretch, which will therefore give rise to reflex excitation in the MNs of the stretched muscle (see Fig. 7.4D). If these MNs are sufficiently excitable (e.g. because of background excitation from other sources), they will be discharged by maintained muscle stretch, giving rise to a tonic **stretch reflex** (e.g. easily evoked in extensor muscles of decerebrate animals) (see Fig. 8.1A).

In addition to the Ia effects on homonymous MNs (i.e. MNs of the spindle-containing muscle), monosynaptic excitation from Ia afferents is typically also distributed to MNs of various synergistic muscles acting on the same and/or neighbouring joints. Furthermore, the Ia afferents excite many other kinds of cells, including segmental interneurones that cause inhibition of MNs innervating antagonistic muscles (disynaptic **reciprocal inhibition**). Other control systems may facilitate or supress this latter interneuronal link, thus enabling or disabling reciprocal inhibition. In addition to the Renshaw cells (see Chapter 8, section 8.5), the neurones mediating reciprocal Ia inhibition are among the best-known interneurones within the spinal cord (e.g. Fig. 7.2D (Hultborn *et al.* 1968, 1971; Jankowska and Roberts 1972).

Chapter 3

Muscle unit properties
and specializations

3.1. General issues

It is difficult to understand the functions (and functional specializations) of a class of
nerve cells if one does not know the properties and functions of its target cells. For
instance, different target cells may require different ranges of impulse frequencies and/or
durations of discharge if they are to fulfil their physiological function adequately. For
central neurones, it is often exceedingly difficult to identify individual target cells and to
determine their functional requirements. For spinal MNs, this is relatively easy because
the main target cells, the skeletal muscle fibres, are readily accessible for experimental
measurements and, in addition, have well-defined functions, the production of contractile force and shortening. Measurements have shown that single muscles are typically
composed of units with highly differentiated functional properties. Such variations in
target cell properties have to be taken into acount in the analysis of MN characteristics.
Combined measurements of MNs and their muscle fibres have demonstrated how
closely the functional properties of neurones may be linked to those of their target cells
(see Chapter 6, section 6.9, Chapter 7, section 7.6, and Chapter 8, section 8.2). This chapter deals with the functional differentiation of major cellular components within skeletal
muscles (muscle fibres, motor axons). Neuromuscular transmission will be treated separately in Chapter 4.

3.2. Muscle heterogeneity: early observations and
the progress of insights

As early as the nineteenth century it was noticed that some limb muscles were unusually
red in colour and contracted more slowly than others (Ranvier 1874; Needham 1926). In
older physiological literature the main distinction with regard to contractile speed concerned whole slow versus fast muscles, and the associated biochemical differences were
often indicated by the terms red versus white. Only much later, after it became technically
possible to investigate muscles physiologically at the level of single units and fibres, did it
become evident that almost all mammalian muscles are of a mixed composition and that
the classical slow or red limb muscles (e.g. soleus, crureus) are not muscles of a distinct
type but rather cases with an unusually high percentage of slow units. Differences in red-
ness are also seen when muscles are bloodless; the red colour of slow limb muscles

reflects cell components associated with energy metabolism (cytochromes, myoglobin) and not characteristics of the contractile machinery itself. Accordingly, some muscles may indeed be 'red' without being 'slow' (Creed *et al.* 1932). Furthermore, slow muscles apparently work normally also when not containing myoglobin (e.g. depigmented muscles of gene knockout mice lacking myoglobin (Garry *et al.* 1998)). Myoglobin concentrations are high in seals, which have particular needs for storing oxygen (Reed *et al.* 1994).

The first recordings of contractions from single motor units were published around 1930 (Denny-Brown 1929; Eccles and Sherrington 1930), and were observations of the most easily activated single units in weak reflex contractions. Systematic studies of intramuscular unit populations were not reported until the 1960s, when new techniques were employed for the isolation of individual units, such as stimulation of single motor axons after ventral root splitting (Bessou *et al.* 1963; McPhedran *et al.* 1965a, b) or stimulation of single MNs during intracellular recording (Devanandan *et al.* 1965; Burke 1968b). Population studies performed with such techniques made it clear that individual muscles are also physiologically heterogeneous (see also Gordon and Phillips 1953). This had been suggested by muscle histologists much earlier (Grützner 1883, cited by Needham 1926), and new investigations using modern histochemical techniques proved it to be true for various cytochemical muscle fibre characteristics (Stein and Padykula 1962; Romanul 1964; Brooke and Kaiser 1970; Guth and Samaha 1970). Soon, both types of study were combined. In one type of approach, single muscle fibres were isolated by dissection and their physiological and cytochemical properties were measured (Smith and Lannergren 1968). A somewhat analogous single-fibre approach has recently been successfully applied to fibre fragments from needle biopsies (Larsson and Salviati 1992). Alternatively, and more commonly, contractile properties were measured for single muscle units, and the fibres were labelled for subsequent histological/histochemical analysis using glycogen-depletion techniques (see Fig. 3.10D) (Edström and Kugelberg 1968).

As will be extensively discussed below, mammalian muscle units and fibres are usually classified into three or more functional categories (Table 2.2). Physiological unit properties are used for a Burke-type classification into slow (type S) and various fast (FR, Fint, FF) categories. Histochemical properties form the basis for largely corresponding categories of slow type I (or SO) fibres and fast type II fibres with various subgroups (e.g. IIa, IIx, IIb; alternatively FOG, FG).

3.3. **Contractile properties**

3.3.1. **Muscle unit force**

3.3.1.1. Twitch versus tetanic contraction

A single sarcolemmal action potential will elicit a transient rise of contractile force, referred to as a **twitch** (Fig. 3.1A,C). The twitch lasts much longer than the muscle fibre action potential; however, it is too short for most types of motor behaviour. Longer-lasting contractions may, of course, be obtained by activating the muscle with a train of repeated action potentials (Fig. 3.1B,D). At low rates single twitches will simply follow each other.

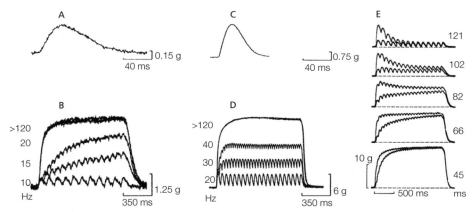

Figure 3.1 Force gradation in single muscle units. (**A**)–(**D**) Isometric contractions from (**A**), (**B**) a slow-twitch and (**c**), (**D**) a fast-twitch muscle unit from the same cat peroneus longus muscle. Upper records show the single twitch. Lower records show superimposed responses to repetitive stimuli at rates indicated to the left of each record. In both units, about the same force-response was produced by stimulation at 120.5 Hz and 151.5 Hz. respectively (both responses included in each record). (Reproduced with permission, from Kernell *et al.* 1983b.). (**E**) Effects of a short initial interval on reponses to longer-interval stimulus trains. Records from a type S muscle unit in cat medial gastrocnemius muscle. A series of photographically superimposed responses during stimulus trains with basic pulse intervals given in milliseconds on the right. At each basic stimulus pulse interval, the larger response resulted from insertion of an extra pulse 10 ms after the first pulse in the basic train. (Reproduced with permission, from Burke *et al.* 1976.)

At stimulation intervals shorter than the twitch duration, the twitches partly fuse and the peak force becomes increased. At sufficiently high rates of activation, separate twitches are no longer visible; the contraction is 'fused'. This process saturates; at a certain activation rate a maximum tetanic contraction is attained and a further increase in rate will not lead to any increase in contractile force. Such a saturation would, of course, be expected to appear if sufficient Ca^{2+} is released to occupy all the available troponin C receptors (Chapter 2, section 2.5.3).

Forces of motor units and whole muscles are sometimes judged from recordings of twitch contractions caused by single-pulse electrical stimulation of the muscle nerve. The peak amplitude of a non-potentiated twitch is often about 10–30 per cent of the maximal tetanic contractile force caused by repetitive stimulation at a sufficiently high pulse frequency. Relative sizes of twitches differ between muscles, and twitches are readily influenced by preceding activity (see section 3.3.4). Therefore comparisons between units or muscle fibres with regard to their force-generating capacity should preferably be done using maximal tetanic contractions (P_0).

The relative peak amplitude of a twitch, i.e. the twitch versus tetanus ratio (**TwTet ratio**) depends on a combination of different factors, including the spatial extent to which the muscle fibres are activated by a single action potential (Gonzalez-Serratos 1975), the level of myosin light-chain phosphorylation (Sweeney *et al.* 1993), the duration of the 'active state' (Ca^{2+} binding to troponin C), and the series elasticity (for further discussion of these latter factors, see Close 1965). The physiological relevance of a high versus a low TwTet ratio varies with activation rate. At slow rates of repetitive activation, with twitches barely fused, a low TwTet ratio means that the unit delivers relatively little of its possible force. At higher rates and a greater degrees of fusion, the TwTet ratio has a smaller influence on force and may be of little significance for contractions greater than 50–70 per cent of P_0 (see Fig. 11.3C).

3.3.1.2. Maximum tetanic force

Muscle unit recordings are almost always made under isometric conditions, and force comparisons are typically done with muscle length set to a level providing a maximum force production (see below). Among the units of individual limb muscles, the maximum tetanic force usually varies by factors of 20 or greater, and in several muscles the force may be more than 100 times greater for the strongest units than for the weakest units (e.g. cat hindlimb muscles in Table 1 of McDonagh *et al.* (1980a)). Within a given muscle, the distribution of unit forces is often skewed, with many weak units and progressively smaller numbers of stronger ones (for functions simulating this distribution, see Fuglevand *et al.* (1993) and Enoka and Fuglevand (2001)). In a maximally activated muscle or muscle unit, the force of a tetanic contraction reflects the sum of the forces delivered by all the activated fibres. For a given muscle unit, the maximal force depends on the following main factors:

- the current relative length of the muscle fibres (**force–length relation**) (Fig. 3.2)
- the ongoing length changes of the muscle fibres (**force–velocity relation**) (Fig. 3.3)
- the number of muscle fibres in the unit (**innervation ratio**) (Table 3.1)
- the mean cross-sectional area of these muscle fibres (Table 3.1, Fig. 3.4)
- the **specific tension** of these fibres, i.e. the force per cm^2 cross-section area (partly dependent on the packing density of myofibrils within the muscle fibres) (Tables 3.1 and 3.2)
- the alignment of the fibres versus the direction of whole-muscle force (i.e. **pennation angle**) (Fig. 2.1A).

3.3.1.3. Force–length relation

Owing to the nature of the sliding-filament mechanism for muscle contraction (see Fig. 2.1B), sarcomeres are maximally effective in producing contractile force only over a limited range of lengths (Fig. 3.2). With a maximum degree of activation, the largest force will be obtained for sarcomere lengths giving a complete overlap between the thin myofilaments and the cross-bridge-carrying regions of the thick myofilaments, without an overlap between opposing ends of the thin filaments. No force is produced if a muscle is extended so much that thick and thin filaments show no overlap (Gordon *et al.* 1966). On the other hand, at sarcomere lengths shorter than twice the thin filament plus the Z disk (about 2.34 μm in cats (Herzog *et al.* 1992)) forces also decrease, possibly because of

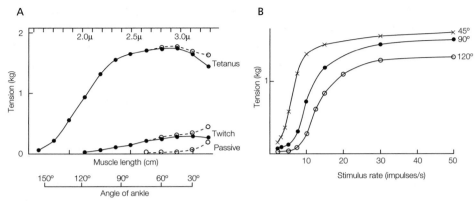

Figure 3.2 Effects of muscle length on force and its gradation. (**A**) Isometric contractile force versus muscle length for soleus muscle of cat hindlimb. Separate curves are shown for maximum tetanic contractions (50 Hz stimulation), twitch contractions (single-pulse stimulation) and passive force (i.e. unstimulated muscle). Tetanic and twitch forces are shown with (broken lines) and without (continuous lines) contributions from the passive force. In the body, the maximum soleus length corresponds to an ankle angle of about 30°. Upper scale: calculated sarcomere lengths. (**B**) Tension–frequency relations at lengths corresponding to the indicated ankle angles. (Reproduced with permission, from Rack and Westbury 1969.)

changes in the geometrical relationships between the various myofilaments. This decrease of force with decreased length often becomes even steeper at sarcomere lengths shorter than the length of the thick myofilament (1.6 μm). In addition to mechanical interference between myofilaments and Z disks, short muscle lengths are also disadvantageous for force production because of less effective excitation–contraction coupling processes (Stephenson and Williams 1982). Under maximum activation, human sarcomeres are expected to give a maximum force at a length of about 2.6–2.8 μm, and 50 per cent or more of the maximum force might be produced over sarcomere lengths of 1.5–3.5 μm (Walker and Schrodt 1974; Herzog *et al.* 1992).

For single muscle fibres, the relation between the absolute end-to-end length and maximum force will depend on the number of sarcomeres coupled in series; the greater the number of sarcomeres, the longer will the fibre be and the wider its possible range of absolute working lengths. Under normal conditions, tendons and joints will limit the possible length changes of muscles. Muscles are also protected by intramuscular connective tissue which counteracts a potentially dangerous degree of hyper-extension. Furthermore, at lengths exceeding those giving a maximum tetanic force, the titin filaments of the sarcomeres are no longer slack but resist further lengthening. In non-activated 'passive' muscle, extension of the titin filaments and the intramuscular connective tissue produces a rapid increase in muscle tension for lengths approaching and exceeding the normal maximum working length (Fig. 3.2A); hence the sum of passive and active forces often shows an increase with length over much of the right-hand declining portion of the active force–length relation.

In many cases, although there are exceptions (Lieber *et al.* 1994), muscles have their main working lengths within the range of a positive active force–length slope (e.g. Fig. 3.2A). The optimum length may vary by several millimetres for different units within the same muscle. For instance, in the cat peroneus longus muscle, the optimum length for twitch tension is longer for single units than for the muscle as a whole (i.e. for all units together), and this deviation is even greater for slow-twitch than for fast-twitch units (the difference may be related to differences in unitary force production and stretching of elastic elements (Filippi and Troiani 1994)). In many measurements of muscle unit properties, muscle length has been set to the same standardized value for all units, often the optimal length for a whole muscle twitch (Kernell *et al.* 1983a) or a corresponding level of passive tension (Burke *et al.* 1973). In a few investigations, the optimal length has been set separately for each muscle unit before the measurements of its mechanical properties (Reinking *et al.* 1975).

3.3.1.4. Effects of ongoing length changes on force: the force–velocity relation

When stimulated at a constant spike frequency, muscles show an inverse relationship between force and the velocity of shortening: the faster the shortening, the weaker the force. This relationship has the non-linear shape seen in Figure 3.3A–C. For lengthening contractions, the relation between force and velocity is usually less steep (left portion of Fig. 3.3A), and the forces are substantially greater than under isometric conditions. Velocity aspects of the force–velocity relation will be commented upon further below (section 3.3.2.1). Muscle unit forces are almost always measured in isometric contractions.

3.3.1.5. Differences in innervation ratio

There are large differences in mean innervation ratio between different muscles. For whole muscles, the mean ratio can simply be calculated by dividing the total number of muscle fibres by the total number of skeletomotor axons. Such calculations have resulted in innervation ratios of about 5–10 muscle fibres per MN in the tiny external eye muscles (Blinkov and Glezer 1968, p.118) and about 580 muscle fibres per MN for the alpha MNs of large human leg muscles like the medial gastrocnemius (Buchthal and Schmalbruch 1980). Direct observations of the number of fibres per muscle unit can be done using the technique of glycogen depletion (see Fig. 3.10D). However, some fibres may fail to become depleted and, because of the complexities of muscle architecture, only some of the fibre profiles are typically visible in a single muscle cross-section (cf. Fig. 2.1A). For these reasons, it is often likely that directly determined fibre numbers are underestimates. Careful direct measurements typically indicate that, within single muscles, a difference in innervation ratio is the most important single factor reponsible for systematic differences in unit tetanic force (Table 3.1) (Bodine *et al.* 1987; Kanda and Hashizume 1992; Totosy de Zepetnek *et al.* 1992; Rafuse *et al.* 1997; Enoka and Fuglevand 2001). However, systematic differences in fibre diameter and in specific tension are also clearly of importance (Table 3.1).

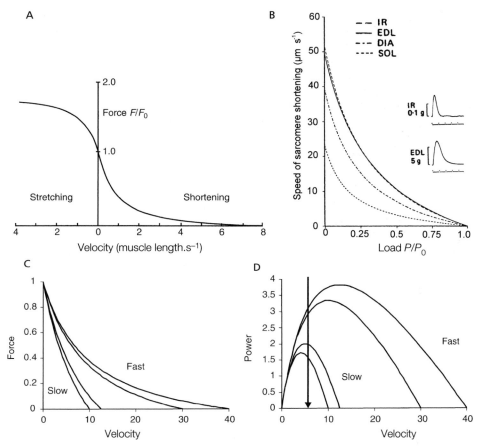

Figure 3.3 Effects of shortening and lengthening velocity on force. (**A**) Force–velocity relation for mouse hindlimb muscle (soleus), for lengthening (left) and shortening (right) contractions at 26°C. Forces (F/F_0) are given relative to the maximum tetanic force at zero velocity (F_0). (**B**) Concentric contractions of muscles of different speed (mouse). Sarcomere shortening velocity (μm/s) versus force (isotonic load, normalized versus maximum tetanic force at zero velocity P_0) for inferior rectus (IR) (moving the eye), extensor digitorum longus (EDL) (fast hindlimb muscle), diaphragm (DIA) (respiration), and soleus (SOL) (slow hindlimb muscle). All recordings were made at about 35°C. The inset shows isometric twitches for IR and EDL muscles recorded at optimum length for isometric tetanic force. Note that IR and EDL have almost the same force–velocity relation although the twitches last about twice as long for EDL. (**C**), (**D**) Schematic representation of the different (**C**) force–velocity and (**D**) power–velocity relations for slow versus fast muscle fibres of human limb muscles. In each case, the pair of curves show conditions at a lower and higher temperature (warm for upper curve of pair). The vertical arrow in (**D**) shows the characteristic shortening velocity of leg muscles during cycling. Note that, at this velocity, warming effects are more significant for the slow than for the fast muscle fibres. All values are in arbitrary units. ((**A**), (**C**), and (**D**) reproduced with permission, from Jones *et al.* 2004; (**B**) reproduced with permission, from Luff 1981.)

Table 3.1 Average innervation ratios and contractile properties of different muscle unit types

	Absolute values			Relative values		
	S	FR	FF	S	FR	FF
Cat TA						
Tet force (mN)	40	100.7	222.8	1	2.52	5.57
Fibre number	93.3	197.3	266	1	2.11	2.85
Fibre X-area (μm^2)	2484	2431	3331	1	0.98	1.34
Calc spec tension (N/cm^2)	17.2	21.1	24.9	1	1.23	1.45
Rat GM						
Tet force (mN)	15	100	201	1	6.67	13.40
Fibre number	66	154	271	1	2.33	4.11
Fibre area (μm^2)	1983	2648	3489	1	1.34	1.76
Calc spec tension (N/cm^2)	16.7	21.4	25.1	1	1.28	1.50

Examples from combined measurements of muscle unit anatomy (using glycogen depletion) and physiology (electrical activation of single muscle units) in hindlimb muscles.

Abbreviations: TA, tibialis anterior muscle; GM, gastrocnemius medialis muscle; Tet force, maximal tetanic force; X-area, cross-sectional area; spec tension, specific tension (i.e. maximum tetanic force per unit cross-sectional area).

Data for cat TA (11 depleted units) from Bodine *et al.* (1987), and data for rat GM (29 depleted units) from Kanda and Hashizume (1992).

3.3.1.6. Differences in muscle fibre diameter

Within a given muscle, fast muscle fibres (mATPase type II) usually have larger mean diameters than the slow fibres (type I). This is true for the majority of muscles although, in both humans (Fig. 3.4A) and rats (Fig. 3.4B–D), some muscles exist in which these differences are non-existent or even reversed. Furthermore, as is apparent for the rat data in Figure 3.4B–D, fast fibre sizes tend to vary such that IIa < IIx < IIb. These differences are similar in direction to those seen in maximum tetanic force between different types of muscle units (Tables 3.1 and 3.3), i.e. the force differences are often partly caused by differences in fibre size. It is striking that, in rats as well as humans, there is a very wide range of variation in mean fibre size between different muscles, and that this variation takes place, in a parallel manner, for fibres of different types (significant positive correlations for all panels of Fig. 3.4). The graphs in Figure 3.4 concern the mean fibre sizes per muscle for each plotted category. However, it is important to realize that there are often large variations in fibre size within single units (e.g. cat tibialis anterior, two- to eightfold variation in cross-sectional area (Bodine *et al.* 1987; see also Edström and Kugelberg 1968; Kanda and Hashizume 1992; Totosy de Zepetnek *et al.* 1992)). Thus, in addition to MN- and activity-associated factors (see Chapter 11), there must also be other causes for differences in muscle fibre size.

3.3.1.7. Differences in specific tension

For whole mammalian muscles studied at body temperature, average values for specific tension tend to be around 10–25 N/cm^2, as measured for maximum tetanic contractions

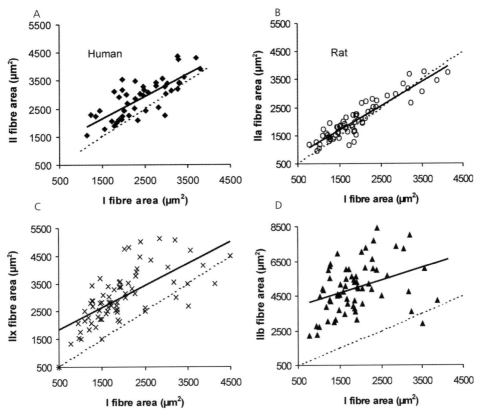

Figure 3.4 Systematic variations in mean size for different types of muscle fibre. (**A**) Mean cross-sectional areas of type II fibres plotted versus those for type I fibres in 47 different human muscles (male subjects). Linear regression line calculated by the method of least squares. Correlation coefficient 0.77 ($P < 0.001$). Broken line drawn for $y = x$. (**B**)–(**D**) Similar plots for data from rat muscles with type II fibres separated into (**B**) type IIa, (**C**) type IIx, and (**D**) type IIb. The correlation coefficients were 0.92 ($n = 65$), 0.67 ($n = 67$), and 0.36 ($n = 66$), respectively (all statistically significant, $P < 0.01$). Calculations and plots based on data from Polgar *et al.* (1973) for (**A**), and from Delp and Duan (1996) for (**B**)—(**D**).

and taking muscle architecture into account, i.e. effects of pennate muscle structures (cf. Fig. 2.1A). In glycogen-depleted and carefully reconstructed muscle units, direct comparisons have been made between the maximum tetanic force and the number and cross-sectional areas of the muscle fibres. In such muscles, slow units tend to have a smaller specific tension than fast units (Table 3.1) (see also Chamberlain and Lewis 1989; Totosy de Zepetnek *et al.* 1992; Rafuse *et al.* 1997). Qualitatively similar results have often been obtained from *in vitro* measurements on skinned fibres (Table 3.2), although in some such cases no significant differences were found (cat soleus versus medial gastrocnemius) (Lucas *et al.* 1987).

Table 3.2 Direct (*in vitro*) measurements of specific tension in single skinned fibres

Animal	MHC-I	MHC-IIa	MHC-IIx	MHC-IIb
Absolute values for specific tension at 12°C (kN/m²)				
Rat	68 ± 4	111 ± 15	95 ± 11	99 ± 10
Rabbit	85 ± 15		106 ± 12	
Human	64 ± 4	84 ± 3	98 ± 5	
Relative values versus type I fibres				
Rat	1	1.63	1.40	1.46
Rabbit	1		1.25	
Human	1	1.31	1.53	

Abbreviation: MHC, myosin heavy chain with indicated isoform (cf. Table 3.4).

Data from those summarized in Table 1 of Reggiani *et al.* (2000).

3.3.1.8. Differences in pennation angle

Within a given muscle, pennation angles often tend to be relatively similar for all fibres. In human limb muscles, mean pennation angles generally vary from 0° up to about 20° (often between 5° and 15°) (Wickiewicz *et al.* 1983; Friederich and Brand 1990) . This implies that the effective force in the main pulling direction of the muscle tendon might be reduced by as much as 6 per cent due to high pennation angles (cos 20° = 0.94), i.e. this factor has typically only a minor influence on effective muscle force.

Large pennation angles are characteristic of muscles in which a high force capacity is combined with a modest total volume, i.e. large numbers of short fibres are contracting in parallel. For instance, in the rat gastrocnemius medialis, fibre lengths are about one-third of that for the whole muscle and pennation angles are about 16° (Wang and Kernell 2000). In such a muscle, individual fibres would exert a 4 per cent greater effective force if their directions were precisely aligned with that of the whole muscle (cos 16° = 0.96). However, a roughly parallel-fibred gastrocnemius muscle with fibres three times longer and a third fewer (i.e. same volume) would exert a maximum force of only 0.33/0.94 = 0.35 of that for the pennate muscle. Thus, at the level of whole muscles, pennate architecture very effectively favours a high force output per unit muscle volume.

3.3.2. Speed

In discussions about muscle and motor unit specializations, terms related to contractile 'speed' are ubiquitous. However, it should be realized that 'speed' is a complex concept in muscle physiology, with components reflecting different characteristics which are often covarying but may conceivably be rather independently controlled. In discussions of muscle 'speed' it should always be made clear which kind of measurements are meant. There are two major categories of 'speed', referred to here as 'shortening speed' and 'isometric speed' (or 'twitch speed', i.e. speed of force changes as seen in isometric contractions).

It should be stressed that the muscles and fibres discussed in this book are generally of the variety capable of twitches. In the literature some confusion is possible regarding the term 'slow', which is sometimes applied to muscles and fibres of the non-twitch kind (also sometimes referred to as 'tonic'). In mammals, non-twitch fibres exist only in muscle spindles and, together with twitch fibres, in some highly specialized cranial muscles associated with sensory functions (muscles of the middle ear; external eye muscles). Non-twitch skeletal muscle fibres are more common in birds and amphibians, for instance, and their properties are very different from those of slow-twitch fibres. For instance, they do not generate action potentials, they have a multiple innervation and a slow shortening velocity, and relatively high activation rates may be needed to elicit their maximum force (Hess 1970; Lännergren 1975).

3.3.2.1. Shortening speed: velocity of length changes

This is the dominating interpretation of 'contractile speed' in everyday language; the difference between a fast and a slow movement can readily be seen, whereas differences in the time course of force development are less directly observable. With regard to concentric contractions, a major complexity lies in the inverse relationship between shortening velocity and force (Fig. 3.3A–C). Results of such measurements are typically plotted on a force–velocity graph and fitted with a line according to Hill's equation, first proposed in 1938 (see comments in Hill 1970):

$$(P + a)V = b(P_0 - P) \tag{3.1}$$

where P is force, P_0 is the maximum isometric force at zero velocity, V is the velocity of shortening, and a and b are constants. With a force–velocity relation according to Hill's equation, the maximum mechanical power (i.e. shortening speed × force) will be obtained at a velocity of about 60–70 per cent maximum (Fig. 3.3D).

For speed comparisons between muscles and muscle fibres, estimates are often used of the **maximum unloaded shortening velocity** (V_{max}), which is calculated from the fitted line of force–velocity plots by extrapolation to zero force. Alternatively, the 'slack method' (Edman 1979) can be used to estimate the maximum unloaded shortening velocity in muscles or single muscle fibres (Bottinelli *et al.* 1994). In this method, the two ends of the muscle (fibre) are kept at a distance short enough to let the muscle be slack (i.e. no passive tension). Then the muscle is activated with tetanic stimulation and the latency is measured from the start of stimulation to the appearance of force. The shorter the setting of muscle length (i.e. the greater the slack), the longer is this latency. The increase of latency versus the change of slack length gives a measure of the maximum unloaded velocity of shortening, often referred to as V_0 in these measurements (Edman 1979).

Force–velocity relations may be markedly different between different muscles (Fig. 3.3B,C). Experimental determinations of maximum unloaded shortening speed are most easily made for whole muscles or, after a dissection, for single muscle fibres (often done for 'skinned' fibre portions from biopsies). Measurements of shortening velocity for

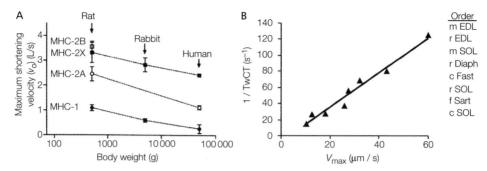

Figure 3.5 Muscle speed for different types of myosin in different animal species. (**A**) Maximum shortening velocity V_0 at 12°C in sets of muscle fibres containing different isoforms of myosin heavy chain (MHC). V_0 is plotted versus average body weight of the animal species to which the fibres belong. L/s, fibre lengths per second. (Reproduced with permission, from Reggiani *et al.* 2000.) (**B**) Inverse value of isometric twitch contraction time 1/TwCT (s^{-1}) plotted versus the maximum velocity of sarcomere shortening (μm/s) for different muscles and animal species. Abbreviations: m, mouse; r, rat; c cat; f, frog; EDL, extensor digitorum longus (fast muscle); SOL, soleus (slow muscle); Diaph, diaphragm; Sart, sartorius. All measurements done at about 35–37°C except those for the frog (20–22°C). Linear regression line. Data from Close (1965), in which references to the sources for the various measurements can be found.

muscle units *in situ* are difficult and uncertain because of the large mass of passive muscle tissue lying around the actively contracting fibres. However, measurements have been performed for such cases, with corrections attempted for the effects of the passive tissue (Devasahayam and Sandercock 1992; see also Petit *et al.* 1993).

Differences in maximum unloaded shortening speed between different muscle fibres depends strongly on their myosin composition (Fig. 3.5A), and one of the important factors is the rate of cross-bridge interactions which is associated with the rate at which energy can be extracted by hydrolysis of ATP (Chapter 2, section 2.6). In comparisons of different types of muscle fibre, the maximum speed of unloaded shortening is highly correlated with the enzymatic activity of the myosin ATPase; the more rapidly this enzyme can split ATP, the faster is the maximum contractile shortening speed (Barany 1967). This has also been seen in measurements on single fibres with different myosin compositions (Reggiani *et al.* 2000). As slowly shortening fibres split ATP more slowly (i.e. have slower cross-bridge kinetics), they also use less energy per unit time for the maintenance of isometric force (Crow and Kushmerick 1982).

3.3.2.2. Isometric speed: time course of isometric force changes

In studies of the contractions of single muscle units, measurements of force are typically done while the length of the muscle is kept constant (isometric contractions). In such recordings, differences in contractile speed between fast and slow muscles (or muscle units or fibres) are often judged from measurements of the time course of the twitch force (Fig. 3.1A,C). Compared with fast muscles, the twitch of a slow muscle typically takes longer to reach its peak (**twitch contraction time** (TwCT)) and also shows a more

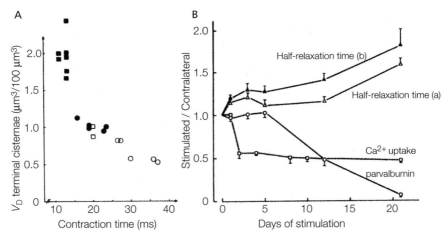

Figure 3.6 Muscle fibre properties of importance for 'isometric speed'. (**A**) Relation between dimensions of sarcoplasmic reticulum (mean volume density of terminal cisternae, electron micro-scopic measurements) and isometric twitch contraction time of muscle units with different types of muscle fibre in rat soleus (open circles, type I; filled circles, type II and 'hybrid') and tibialis anterior (open squares, type I; filled squares, type II). Fibre types determined using mATPase histo-chemistry. (Reproduced with permission, from Kugelberg and Thornell 1983.) (**B**) Time course of changes in twitch time half-relaxation time and parameters of importance for Ca^{2+} homeostasis (Ca^{2+} uptake by sarcoplasmic reticulum, content of Ca^{2+} buffer parvalbumin) in chronically stim-ulated fast-twitch muscles of rabbits (10 Hz during about 50 per cent of total time). The two curves of the half-relaxation time relate to measurements taken (a) before and (b) immediately after a 5 Hz stimulus train lasting for 25 s. All measurements are given relative to values for con-tralateral control muscles. Means ± SE. (Reproduced with permission, from Klug *et al*. 1988.)

prolonged phase of relaxation from twitch peak to 50 per cent peak force (**twitch half-relaxation time** (TwHRT)) and has a longer duration from beginning to end (**total duration** (TwDur)). These aspects of 'isometric speed' are mainly dependent on factors other than those underlying the speed of shortening. Interestingly, although both aspects of speed tend to be highly correlated in comparisons between muscles (e.g. Fig. 3.5B), assessments of maximal shortening speed in single motor units have shown a poor corre-lation with the time course of the isometric twitch (rat soleus, Devasahayam and Sandercock 1992; cat lumbrical, Petit *et al.* 1993).

The duration of force rise during a twitch (TwCT) will partly reflect the time course of the 'active state', i.e. roughly the time course of the rise and fall of Ca^{2+} binding to troponin C. It will also be influenced by the extent and speed of internal sarcomere shortening which generates the external force change by stretching the tendon; however, the relative importance of this 'shortening' factor is uncertain. Systematic variations in TwCT also occur within groups of motor units that all have fibres with the same slow myosin. In such cases, TwCT is correlated to the properties and dimensions of the sarcoplasmic reticulum (SR); a greater Ca^{2+} uptake (Brody 1976) and larger SR terminal cisternae (Fig. 3.6A (Kugelberg and Thornell 1983) correspond to a briefer (faster) TwCT.

Of course, the speed of twitch relaxation will be influenced by the fall of Ca^{2+} binding to troponin C following the brief period of spike-generated Ca^{2+} release. The properties of the SR and the presence and concentration of Ca^{2+} buffering molecules are also of importance for this parameter (cf. Fig. 3.6B). In addition, it has been suggested that differences in the speed of relaxation might partially reflect differences in the rates of cross-bridge detachment (myosin–actin 'stickiness') (Jones *et al.* 2004).

The shortening velocity would be expected to be more important for the maximum rate of rise of isometric tetanic force than for the time course of an isometric twitch; the required degree of internal muscle shortening would be much greater in the tetanic contraction. However, the maximum rate of rise of force would also depend on the speed of Ca^{2+} release and the efficiency of its binding to troponin C at the onset of contraction. Interestingly, both the maximum shortening speed and the maximum rate of rise of isometric tetanic force require much higher stimulation rates than those needed to maintain maximum tetanic force (Buller and Lewis 1965c); for various model calculations concerning factors that influence twitch time course, see Stein *et al.* (1988), Fitts *et al.* (1991), Zandwijk *et al.* (1996), Campbell *et al.* (2001), and Phillips *et al.* (2004).

An interesting example of a dissociation between shortening velocity and isometric speed is given by comparisons between limb muscles and external eye muscles in the mouse. Compared with a fast leg muscle (extensor digitorum longus (EDL)), an external eye muscle (inferior rectus (IR)) has a much briefer twitch although both muscles have sarcomeres with practically the same force–velocity relation (Fig. 3.3B) (Luff 1981); for shortening velocities of external eye muscles, see also Asmussen *et al.* (1994). Other examples of 'speed dissociation' include:

- different temperature sensitivities for shortening speed and isometric twitch speed (Ranatunga 1982)
- changes in opposite directions of twitch speed and maximum shortening speed after immobilization of rat soleus (Witzmann *et al.* 1982)
- changes in myosin composition but not of isometric twitch speed after immobilization of rabbit tibialis anterior (Pattullo *et al.* 1992)
- changes in opposite directions of twitch speed and maximum rate of tetanic force increase after 2 weeks of motor nerve paralysis (St-Pierre and Gardiner 1985)
- non-parallel changes in twitch speed and maximum shortening velocity after chronic stimulation (Eken and Gundersen 1988; Sutherland *et al.* 2003)
- during chronic stimulation of rabbits, different time courses are found for the prolongation of isometric twitches (Fig. 3.6 B) (Klug *et al.* 1988) versus the rise in slow MHC-I myosin (Pette 2002).

Examples of isometric twitch speed in units of cat hindlimb muscles are given in Table 3.3. There is a very large variation of mean TwCT for slow units in these different muscles (34–76 ms). Furthermore, in most muscles that have been investigated, there is a

Table 3.3 Unit populations in cat hindlimb muscles

	S	FR	Fint	FF
Peroneus tertius				
%MU	23	42	15	20
TwCT (ms)	34	27	25	26
Tet (g)	1.3	7.8	26	39.1
%force	2.0	21.4	25.5	51.1
Gastrocnemius medialis				
%MU	30	16	19	35
TwCT (ms)	76	32	29	28
Tet (g)	3.6	16.9	23.8	38.3
%force	5.0	12.5	20.8	61.7
Plantaris				
%MU	52	13	14	22
TwCT (ms)	50	25	22	21
Tet (g)	3.9	17.6	23.3	39.5
%force	12.5	14.1	20.1	53.4
First superficial lumbrical muscle				
%MU	64	17	13	6
TwCT (ms)	46	25	22	18
Tet (g)	1.4	6.3	9.9	16
%force	21.3	25.4	30.5	22.8

Mean properties and distribution of different categories of single muscle units in cat hindlimb muscles. In this investigation, very large samples of units were collected from each individual muscle.

Abbreviations: %MU, percentage of all muscle units found for this muscle; TwCT, mean twitch contraction time (i.e. time from onset to peak); Tet, mean maximal tetanic force per unit; %force, relative contribution of respective unit type to total maximal muscle force (calculated from %MU and Tet).

Data from Emonet-Denand *et al*. (1988).

continuous distribution of muscle unit twitch speed (e.g. Figs. 3.7 and 3.9). In resting muscles there is usually a marked degree of covariation between the speed of isometric force increase (TwCT), the speed of relaxation (TwHRT), and the total twitch duration (TwDur). However, even the TwCT and TwHRT measures may become dissociated under certain circumstances.

Not only muscle force but also isometric twitch speed depends on muscle length. In general, twitches are slower for long than for shorter muscle lengths (Rack and Westbury 1969). The length dependence of isometric speed probably largely reflects the effects of muscle length on the excitation–contraction coupling mechanisms (Stephenson and Williams 1982).

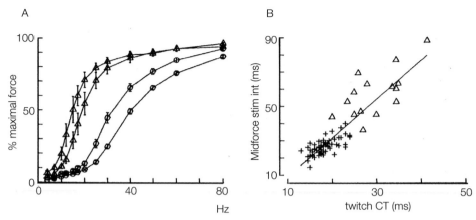

Figure 3.7 Rate gradation of force in muscle units of different twitch speed. Units from cat peroneus longus muscle. Separate symbols for units classified as fast ((**A**) circles, (**B**) crosses) and
slow (triangles), respectively, using the 'sag' criterion. (**A**) Average tension–frequency curves (*T–f*
curves) for four groups of units. As regarded at the level of half-maximum force the curves represent, from left to right, units with a twitch contraction time (TwCT) of >30 ms, 25–30 ms,
20–24.9 ms, and <20 ms respectively. Force data refer to values for mean tension during the
last half of 1 s stimulus bursts at the rates (in Hz) given along the *x*-axis (cf. Fig. 3.1(**B**), (**D**)).
Before calculation of the average *T–f* curves the force values for each unit were expressed as a
percentage of the maximum tetanic force of the unit. Vertical bars give ± SE. (**B**) Plot of stimulus
interval giving 50 per cent of maximum force (midforce stimulation interval (ms)) versus TwCT
($r = 0.89$, $n = 77$, $P < 0.001$). (Reproduced with permission, from Kernell *et al.* 1983b.)

3.3.3. **Spike frequency and isometric force (tension-frequency relation)**

The relation between contractile tension and activation frequency (*T-f* relation) is
S-shaped with a steep middle region covering a limited range of stimulation rates
(Fig. 3.7A) (Cooper and Eccles 1930). There is usually an obvious relationship between
the rates needed for an effective gradation of isometric force and the time course of the
isometric twitch: the slower the twitch, the slower the range of gradation rates (Fig. 3.7)
(Cooper and Eccles 1930; Kernell *et al.* 1983b; Botterman *et al.* 1986; Thomas *et al.* 1991a;
McNulty *et al.* 2000). The process of partial twitch 'fusion' starts at stimulation intervals
about equal to the duration of the twitch (Fig. 3.1B,D). The stimulation rate (or interval)
required for half-maximum force is a commonly used measure of the 'speed' of the *T–f*
relation (Fig. 3.7B) (Buller *et al.* 1960a; Kernell *et al.* 1983b; Thomas *et al.* 1991a; McNulty
et al. 2000). This interval (Int50) is often about 1–2 times the twitch contraction time,
and the precise relationship may vary somewhat between units of different muscles
(Kernell *et al.* 1983b). For instance, Int50/TwCT averaged about 1.3–1.9 for peroneus longus
of the cat hindlimb (Kernell *et al.* 1983b), about 1.1–1.2 for the flexor carpi radialis of the cat
forelimb (Botterman *et al.* 1986), and about 1.4–1.7 for human finger muscles (Fuglevand
et al. 1999). The *T–f* relation is, in itself, a physiologically relevant expression of isometric

muscle speed ('encoding speed'), presumably largely reflecting the intramuscular Ca^{2+} kinetics (reviewed by Binder-Macleod 1992).

The sigmoid T—f relation is often (and most easily) measured at the peaks of partially fused twitches. However, with regard to the force control during motor behaviour, it is more correct to determine the mean tension, i.e. the force $\times$ time area (as in Fig. 3.7). When many different units are simultaneously activated at low rates, but asynchronously with each other, each unit contributes its force $\times$ time area and only minor variations of total muscle force are seen despite the markedly unfused contractions of each individual unit. Furthermore, at submaximal force levels, mean force generation is more effective with an asynchronously distributed unit activation than with synchronous stimulation (Rack and Westbury 1969; Wise et al. 2001). It should be remembered that, in single units and in synchronously stimulated whole muscles, the stimulation rate needed for generating a maximum tetanic force may be substantially higher than the minimum needed for a contraction to look 'fused'.

In accordance with the behaviour of isometric twitches, the T–f curve is also length dependent, shifting to the right as a muscle is shortened (Fig. 3.2B) (Rack and Westbury 1969; Brown et al. 1999).

3.3.4. **After-effects of activity**

In this chapter, the after-effects of activity will primarily be discussed from the point of view of how units differ in their properties within single muscles, and how such differences can be used for unit categorization. However, after-effects of activity are also important in their own right, comprising events on several different timescales. Such problems and the mechanisms concerned will be dealt with in more detail in Chapters 9 and 11.

3.3.4.1. **Short-term contractile after-effects: 'sag' and 'catch-like' properties**

The force profile obtained at the onset of partly fused contractions is generally markely different for slow- and fast-twitch units of limb muscles (e.g. Fig. 3.1B,D). In typical slow-twitch units, a progressive growth is seen for a number of consecutive twitches until, finally, a relatively steady force is attained. In typical fast-twitch units, the first (or first few) twitch(es) may be relatively large, after which there is a dip ('sag') followed by a plateau. At their extremes, these are distinct reactions (Burke et al. 1973). However, there is also a wide range of intermediate cases: the 'sag' property is not an all-or-nothing behaviour (Kernell et al. 1983a; see also Carp et al. 1999). Furthermore, the relationship of the 'sag' property to muscle 'speed' is not unambiguous; in external eye muscles, which have a very high twitch speed, partly fused contractions show no sag (Barmack et al. 1971; Asmussen and Gaunitz 1981b). The precise mechanisms underlying the 'sag' property are still obscure. It is interesting to note that increased Ca^{2+} buffering seems to produce an increased 'sag' (Johnson et al. 1999).

In slow-twitch units in particular, the initial force profile of a partly fused contraction looks markedly different for a constant stimulation frequency than for a burst with a shorter first interval (Fig. 3.1E); in the latter case, force is rapidly increased to a level which is otherwise only gradually attained. This has been termed 'catch-like' behaviour (Burke *et al.* 1976; reviewed by Binder-Macleod and Kesar 2005) by analogy with the true 'catch' contraction of clam muscles, which is physiologically very different (Hoyle 1983).

3.3.4.2. Fatigue

In this book the term 'fatigue' is used purely descriptively to indicate a reversible decrease in output (e.g. force) for a given input (e.g. stimulation pattern). All muscles show fatigue if activated strongly enough during a suffiently long period of time.

   Motor units in the same muscle may show large differences in their fatigue sensitivity (Burke 1981). Many stimulation protocols have been used for testing units (or muscles or muscle fibres) with regard to such properties. The most widely used are variations of the protocol originally introduced by Burke and his colleagues for comparing muscle units of the cat's hindlimb (Burke *et al.* 1973): 40 Hz bursts of 0.33 s repeated once a second for at least 2 min (Burke-type fatigue test) (Fig. 3.8). Typically, a 'fatigue index' is calculated, indicating the relative force production after 2 min of such stimulation. Thus, somewhat paradoxically, a high 'fatigue index' signifies a great resistance to fatigue. In cat's hindlimb muscle units such tests are highly effective for discriminating between different units; the fatigue index varies from <0.1 to 1 (or <10 to 100 per cent) (Fig. 3.9A,C). Among the motor units of a single cat muscle, the Burke-type fatigue index is often more or less bimodally distributed, although intermediate cases may be relatively common (cf. Fig. 3–9C, Table 3.3). In human muscles, few units are as fatiguable as the FF units of cat or rat muscles when tested with the same kind of Burke test (Fig. 3.9B: thenar muscles (Thomas *et al.* 1991b); finger muscles (Fuglevand *et al.* 1999)).

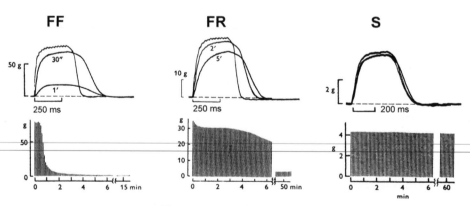

Figure 3.8 Reactions of different categories of muscle units in Burke-type fatigue test. Isometric force recordings from type FF, FR, and S units of cat gastrocnemius muscles. Test stimulation given in 0.33 s bursts of 40 Hz, repeated once per second. Upper row: forces of burst contractions obtained initially and at various later times during the test (FF at 30 sec and 1 min; FR at 2 and 5 min; S at 2 and 60 min). Lower row: peak amplitudes of burst contractions plotted versus time during the fatigue tests. (Reproduced with permission, from Burke *et al.* 1973.)

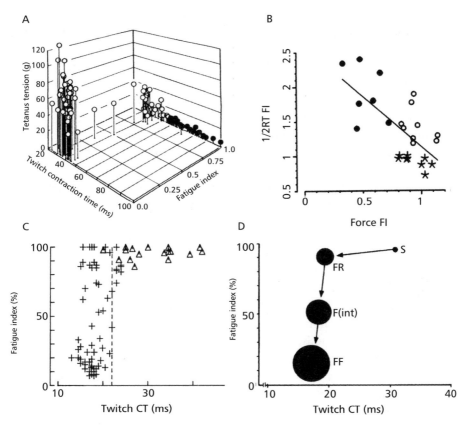

Figure 3.9 Covariation between contractile properties among normal muscle units. (**A**) From cat gastrocnemius medialis muscle. Three-dimensional plot of maximum tetanic force (g, *y*-axis) versus twitch contraction time (TwCT) (ms, *x*-axis) versus fatigue index (high value for high fatigue resistance) (*z*-axis). Filled symbols for units without 'force-sag'. (Reproduced with permission, from Burke *et al*. 1973.) (**B**) From human thenar muscles. Plot of fatigue index for half-relaxation time after burst stimulation (1/2RTFI) versus force fatigue index (Force FI) in Burke-type fatigue test with 40 Hz bursts. Fatigue indices are relative values of half-relaxation time and force after 2 min versus those recorded at the start of the test. Mean values for maximum tetanic force were 118 ± 33 mN (mean ± SD) for units labelled with filled circles, 92 ± 35 mN for open circles, and 53 ± 33 mN for asterisks. (Reproduced with permission, from Thomas *et al*. 1991b.) (**c**),(**D**) From cat peroneus longus muscle. Plot of fatigue index (per cent) versus TwCT (ms). In (**c**) all individual values are shown, and in (**D**) mean values are plotted for the same muscle units after classification into categories S, FR, F(int), and FF, respectively, according to the criteria of Burke *et al*. (1973). In (**c**), crosses and triangles refer to units classified as fast and slow using the 'sag' criterion (triangles, no sag). The vertical broken line is drawn through TwCT of 22 ms. In (**D**), plotted symbols have diameters in direct proportion to the average maximum tetanic tension of the respective group of units (mean value for FF units, 27.9 g). Arrows in (**D**) indicate the expected order of recruitment in most kinds of contractions. (Reproduced with permission, from Kernell *et al*. 1983a (**c**) and Kernell 1986 (**D**).)

A physiologically interesting type of fatigue test was introduced in the 'force-clamp' experiments of Botterman and Cope (1988). Repetitive electrical stimulation was used to produce a submaximal muscle force, and the extent of fatigue could be quantified by measuring how the stimulation rate had to be increased to keep the force constant. Furthermore, fatigue sensitivity could also be quantified by measuring how long the specified submaximal force could be maintained ('endurance time'). Such measurements revealed the existence of large differences in fatigue sensitivity between units that had relatively similar Burke-type fatigue indices.

3.3.4.3. Potentiation

Twitches (but not maximal tetanic contractions) can be increased by a period of preceding 'priming' activity of the same muscle fibres (Brown and von Euler 1938). Purely descriptively, this is often referred to as 'twitch potentiation', and it is often associated with a slowing of the twitches. During and after the repetitive stimulation of a muscle, this phenomenon contributes to a shift of the $T–f$ curve towards lower rates (leftward shift, Fig. 6.8D) (Kernell et al. 1975). Such a shift may be very large if the stimulation rate is continuously shifted first up and then down in a sawtooth pattern ($T–f$ curve hysteresis) (Binder-Macleod and Clamann 1989). Fatigue and potentiation depend on different mechanisms and may be simultaneously present; low rates of activation may show potentiation and, simultaneously, high rates may show fatigue (cf. Fig. 9.4C).

Twitch potentiation is typically greater in fast- than in slow-twitch units (Bagust et al. 1974; Kernell et al. 1975; Jami et al. 1982b; Rankin et al. 1988), although this is not always the case (Burke et al. 1973). Potentiated twitches of some fast units may be up to 50–75 per cent of the maximum tetanic force. In slow units, twitches may even show a post-activity depression instead of a potentiation (e.g. units of the cat soleus muscle (Burke et al. 1974)). Slow muscles and units are generally more stable in their contractile properties than fast muscles and units (less fatigue and less potentiation); this is one of the practical reasons why so much interesting research has been performed on the slow soleus muscle, although it is not very representative of hindlimb muscles in general. For further comments on twitch potentiation, see Chapter 9, section 9.8.1.

3.3.5. Physiological classification of muscle units

Despite the large variation in dimensions between limb muscles of commonly studied experimental mammals (e.g. cat, rat), they are generally similar in their patterns of covariation between various unit properties (Table 2.2, Fig. 3.9A,C). At one end of the spectrum muscle units are slow, weak, and highly fatigue resistant. At the other end they are fast, strong, and fatigue sensitive. In between there are fast units with a range of different fatigue sensitivities. Much of this covariation is continuously graded and concerns properties with (largely) different underlying mechanisms. Thus the 'co-ordinated' patterning of properties is not caused by direct causal links but rather by organizing mechanisms with parallel effects on the various cell properties (partly mediated, for instance, by long-term effects of MN activity patterns (see Chapter 11)). The patterns of covarying contractile properties represent important adaptations to the differences in motor function between various units. In addition, for the physiologist, the systematic covariation of contractile properties simplifies the description of muscle unit populations, which can be viewed as if consisting of a limited number of categories (Table 2.2, Fig. 3.9).

The dominating system and terminology for mammalian muscle unit classification is that introduced by Burke *et al.* (1971b, 1973), separating the units according to their 'speed' and fatigue resistance into fast-twitch fatigue-sensitive (FF), fast-twitch intermediate (Fint), fast-twitch fatigue-resistant (FR), and slow-twitch fatigue-resistant (S) units (Table 2.2). Some issues concerning the classification parameters are dealt with below.

3.3.5.1. 'Slow' versus 'fast'

In most muscles investigated, there is a continuous distribution of isometric twitch speeds (Fig. 3.9A,C), i.e. it is usually not immediately obvious how units should be categorized into different categories of 'speed'. In some earlier studies, a subdivision was made by denoting as 'slow' units whose twitch contraction time exceeded a more or less arbitrarily chosen value in the middle of the distribution. In the classical study by Burke *et al.* (1973), the fast versus slow unit categorization was not done using true speed parameters but rather by comparing units with regard to their contractile 'sag' behaviour (section 3.3.4.1); units were classified as 'fast' if they showed a force sag in a burst with stimulation intervals equal to 1.25 × twitch contraction time. This method of classifying units into slow versus fast categories has since been extensively used. In the original material from cat gastrocnemius medialis (Burke *et al.* 1973), non-sagging units consistently had slower twitches and a different histochemical composition (type I fibres) than the sagging units (type II fibres). However, in other published unit populations, sagging and non-sagging units have sometimes shown wide degrees of overlap in twitch speed (e.g. McDonagh *et al.* 1980b, Fig. 8C).

Taking the usual covariation between twitch speed and the resistance to fatigue into account, one might define units as 'slow' if their twitch is slower than that seen for highly fatiguable units of the same muscle (vertical line in Fig. 3.9C (Kernell and Monster 1982a; Kernell *et al.* 1983a). In experimental material from cat muscles, the 'twitch versus fatigue' analysis and the 'sag' behaviour often lead to unit classifications with only rather minor differences (cf. Fig. 3.9C; Kernell *et al.* 1983a). However, in some animal species and muscles, other testing procedures and/or classification methods have to be used for a 'slow' versus 'fast' unit categorization. For instance, in human thenar units, no sagging behaviour was seen and there was no evident difference in twitch speed between more or less fatiguable units, as tested with the Burke test. In these cases it was suggested that the units should be classified on the basis of their fatigue index and their relative degree of slowing during the fatigue test (Fig. 3.9B) (Thomas *et al.* 1991b). In yet another study of human muscles it was found that units fell into two categories according to their tension–frequency characteristics (interval for 50 per cent maximum force) but not with regard to twitch characteristics (Fuglevand *et al.* 1999). However, this type of bimodality does not seem to occur generally; for instance, it is not obviously present for units of the cat peroneus longus (Fig. 3.7B).

3.3.5.2. 'Fatiguable' versus 'fatigue-resistant'

Methods of classifying units according to their fatigue sensitivity are often based on the fatigue test procedures introduced by Burke *et al.* (1973) for hindlimb muscles of the cat (section 3.3.4.2, Fig. 3.8). Units with a fatigue index of 0–0.25 were originally termed fatigue-sensitive, those with 0.25–0.75 intermediate, and those with 0.75–1 fatigue-resistant. The choice of these limits was inspired by the fact that, in the original material, very few units had fatigue indices in the range 0.25–0.75 (Burke *et al.* 1973). However, units of intermediate fatigue resistance may be relatively common in other muscles (Fig. 3.9B,C, and Table 3.3), i.e. the standardized categories of fatigue resistance are convenient but not self-evident.

The Burke system of classification, including the original stimulation parameters, has been applied to widely different animal species which have muscles of different twitch speed. Test bursts of 40 Hz give little fusion in fast limb muscles of rat or mouse, and a rather high degree of fusion in the much slower homonymous muscles of humans. Despite this, the Burke-type fatigue test allows no human units of the thenar muscles to be classified as 'fatiguable' with a fatigue index of 0.25 or less. More severe tests have sometimes been used to obtain a wider degree of fatigue separation of human units (e.g. human gastrocnemius units, classified into types S, FR and FF (Garnett *et al.* 1979)), and tests with higher stimulation rates have sometimes been employed in studies of rat muscles (Kugelberg and Lindegren 1979).

In a series of partly fused contractions, such as those obtained during a Burke-type fatigue test (Fig. 3.8) (Burke *et al.* 1973), potentiation is often seen as a gradual increase in peak force during the initial 30–60 s ('force potentiation') (Kernell *et al.* 1975, 1983a); in such cases, a fatigue index might be calculated by comparing the largest peak force with that produced by the stimulation bursts 2 min later. In some studies, this potentiating behaviour is avoided by performing the fatigue test after a series of initial tetani causing twitch potentiation (Burke *et al.* 1973). Several alternative algorithms, including cumulative measurements, have been used to calculate a fatigue index from Burke tests of 2–4 min duration (Reinking *et al.* 1975; McDonagh *et al.* 1980b; Kernell *et al.* 1983a).

3.3.6. Contractions of whole muscles versus those of muscle units: summing up

Within a skeletal muscle, there are many connective tissue links between neighbouring muscle fibres, and there will always be a certain degree of friction as the fibres of one unit contract while others are inactive. Hence it is not surprising that muscle unit forces do not sum in a simple linear manner. This non-linearity has been repeatedly analysed (Merton 1954a; Lewis *et al.* 1972; Clamann and Schelhorn 1988; Emonet-Denand *et al.* 1990; Powers and Binder 1991b; Troiani *et al.* 1999; Perreault *et al.* 2003). Generally, the deviations are such that, in weak contractions, a few units activated together deliver more force than the sum of their separate contractions (Powers and Binder 1991b). Most of the studies concern contractions evoked by repetitive stimulation, but the non-linearity of summation seems to be even greater for twitches (Merton 1954a; Lewis *et al.* 1972). The non-linear behaviour becomes less evident if the muscle is subjected to small stretches during the contractions (Powers and Binder 1991b). In strong contractions, produced by many units together, the force additions of individual units are less than their separate contractions (Perreault *et al.* 2003). The deviations from linearity are often around 5–10 per cent or less, although effects as large as 20 per cent have occasionally been noted (Emonet-Denand *et al.* 1987).

3.4. **Cytochemistry**

In this context, only those cytochemical muscle fibre properties that are of importance as a direct correlate to physiology, either for the purpose of fibre classification or in relation to mechanisms underlying contractile muscle unit properties, will be considered. Whenever appropriate, physiological relationships will be briefly mentioned. A full treatment of muscle biochemistry falls far outside the scope of this book (for some basic facts, see Chapter 2, section 2.6). In physiological contexts, the cytochemical classification of muscle fibres is typically based on comparisons between fibres with regard to:

- their contractile components, in particular those related to myosin
- their metabolic properties and provisions, in particular those associated with energy metabolism.

3.4.1. **Myosin**

The thick myofilaments of sarcomeres (Fig. 2.1B) are chains of intertwisted myosin molecules. Each thick myofilament is ~1.5–1.6 μm long and has two symmetrical portions, each containing ~300 myosin molecules (reviewed by Schiaffino and Reggiani 1996; Reggiani *et al.* 2000; Pette 2002). Each myosin molecule has six components: two heavy chains (MHC) and four light chains (MLC), including two 'essential' ('alkaline') and two 'regulatory' MLCs. Each MHC has a globular head and a long tail. The globular head contains the site for actin binding and the catalytic site for ATP hydrolysis, the 'myosin ATPase'. The shaft connecting the head and the tail has one essential and one regulatory MLC wrapped around it. The movable heads of the MHCs constitute the cross-bridges which extend from the side of the thick filaments and which may attach to and pull on the thin myofilaments.

MHC and MLC molecules occur in several variants (isozymes or isoforms) with different functional properties (Table 3.4), and there are many possible combinations of MHC and MLC isoforms. Biochemical techniques may be used for separating the MHC and MLC components from each other, such that the various portions can be further characterized using electrophoretic separation techniques and immunological reactions (see section 3.4.1.2). However, the earliest method available for distinguishing between fibres with different types of myosin was based on myofibrillar ATPase histochemistry.

Table 3.4 Myosin isoforms

A. Myosin heavy-chain (MHC)

MHC type	Occurrence
I = Iβ	slow skm, heart-vm
Iα	extraocular, diaphragm, masticatory skm, heart-am(-vm)
I$_{ton}$	non-twitch skm
IIa	fast skm
IIx = IId	fast skm
IIb	fast skm
exoc = eom = eo	extraocular & laryngeal skm
II$_m$	masticatory skm (carnivores)
emb	developing skm
neo	developing skm

B. Myosin light-chain (MLC)

MLC type	R/E	Occurrence
2s	R	slow skm, heart-vm
2f	R	fast skm
2a	R	heart-am
2m	R	masticatory skm (carnivores)
1sa	E	slow skm
1sb	E	slow skm, heart-vm
1f	E	fast skm
1e/a	E	developing skm, heart-am
3f	E	fast skm

Myosin heavy chain (MHC) and light chain (MLC) isoforms that are commonly encountered in heart and extrafusal muscle fibres of mammals. *Abbreviations: skm*, skeletal muscle fibres; *heart-am*, atrial heart muscle; *heart-vm*, ventricular heart muscle; *R*, regulatory MLC; *E*, essential MLC. Each myosin molecule consists of 2 MHCs, 2 essential MLCs, and 2 regulatory MLCs; very many different combinations occur, including mixtures of "fast" and "slow" varieties (see Text). Note that some isoforms have two or more alternative names; furthermore, MHC names are case-neutral and may use Roman or Arabic numerals (i.e., IIa = IIA = 2a = 2A). For further information, see reviews (Schiaffino and Reggiani 1996; Reggiani *et al.* 2000; Pette and Staron 2000; Gardiner 2001).

3.4.1.1. Myofibrillar ATPase histochemistry

The ATPase function of the MHC portion of myofibrils (mATPase) may be investigated for two different purposes.

1 For analysing differences in the activity of this enzyme at a neutral pH (i.e. under physiological working conditions). Such measurements show a continuum of fibre properties witin a single muscle (van der Laarse *et al.* 1984), presumably covarying with differences in maximum shortening speed of the fibres (see section 3.3.2.1).

2 For ascertaining whether the ATPase function of the MHC portion is still intact after preceding treatment with potentially destructive procedures (e.g. non-neutral pH, paraformaldehyde). These aspects of mATPase histochemistry have led to the discovery that myosins in different kinds of muscle fibres can be distinguished from each other by their different vulnerability profiles.

In the 1960s it was discovered that, if the histochemical procedure for demonstrating mATPase activity was preceded by acid or alkaline preincubation (e.g. pH 4.1 or 10.4), a distinctly bimodal pattern of staining emerged: some fibres were dark (mATPase still active) and others were light (mATPase largely inactivated), with just a few intermediate

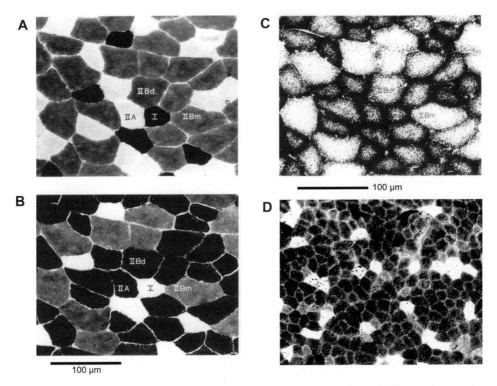

Figure 3.10 Muscle fibre histochemistry. (**A**)–(**C**) Serial cross-sections of rat tibialis anterior muscle (same fibres seen in each section). Stains for myofibrillar ATPase (mATPase) after (**A**) acid preincubation (pH 4.7) and (**B**) after alkaline preincubation plus paraformaldehyde treatment (pH 10.4). In (**C**) fibres are stained for the oxidative enzyme succinate dehydrogenase (SDH). Representative examples of four different fibre types indicated (types I, IIA, IIBd, and IIBm); type IIBd corresponds to IIx. (Reproduced from Lind and Kernell 1991, unpublished.) (**D**) Distribution of muscle fibres belonging to a single muscle unit. Cross-section from part of rat tibialis anterior muscle; PAS staining for demonstration of glycogen content. Prior to the histochemical procedures, the axon of a single motor unit had been stimulated until its glycogen stores had become depleted. The white fibres all belong to this motor unit. Note the presence of many other fibres between those belonging to this single unit. (Reproduced with permission, from Kugelberg 1973.)

cases. Furthermore, fibres that were dark after acid preincubation tended to become light after alkaline treatment, and vice versa. Thus the fibres could be separated into acid-stable type I fibres and alkali-stable type II fibres (Brooke and Kaiser 1970; Guth and Samaha 1970). Combined physiological and histochemical studies (Edström and Kugelberg 1968; Burke *et al.* 1973) showed that, within a given muscle, the fibres of histochemical type I were slow and those of histochemical type II were faster. It should be emphasized that, compared with other classification parameters, these aspects of mATPase histochemistry (and other myosin-based methods) are unique in that they often seem to separate fibres from normal muscles neatly into two categories with almost no borderline cases. With most other histochemical measures and for practically all physiological parameters there is a continuous variation in properties.

Different versions of the mATPase preincubation techniques have been used for a further and more refined myosin-related subdivision of muscle fibres. Intermediate levels of preincubation acidity (e.g. pH of about 4.5–4.7) may give three recognizable degrees of greyness: black I, grey IIb, and white IIa fibres (Fig. 3.10A) (Brooke and Kaiser 1970). However, for these measurements, the optimal setting of the pH for preincubation may be different for different muscles. At least in rats, the IIb category can be further subdivided by pretreatment with paraformaldehyde, producing darker and lighter subcategories of fibres (Fig. 3.10B) (IIx and IIb fibres: Schiaffino *et al.* 1989; Gorza 1990; IIbd and IIbm fibres: Lind and Kernell 1991).

3.4.1.2. Myosin isoforms

A list of the major kinds of myosin isoforms in skeletal muscles is shown in Table 3.4. There are four common types of MHC in limb muscles: types I, IIa, IIx (also called IId) and IIb. In addition, specialized MHC types occur in, for instance, slow non-twitch fibres (not normally present as extrafusal fibres in mammalian limb muscles) and extraocular and masticatory muscles (Table 3.4).

In skeletal muscles of the limbs, there are two types of regulatory and four types of essential MLCs available for combining with the MHCs (regulatory, 2f, 2s; essential, 1sa, 1sb, 1f, and 3f). Many of the theoretically possible combinations between MHCs and MLCs actually exist. In a study of human myosin (Wada *et al.* 1996), MHC-I combined in nine different ways with MLC 1s, 2s, 1f, and 2f, and each of the two fast MHC varieties (IIa and IIx) combined in 11 different ways with MLCs 1s, 2s, 1f, 2f, and 3f. Thus, at least 31 varieties of myosin were observed, taking both MHC and MLC components into account. It should be noted that most of the 'slow' MLCs may also combine with 'fast' MHCs and vice versa; 'slow' and 'fast' are not absolute terms for the MLCs, but rather indicate the statistical probability of finding the respective MLCs in a particular variety of skeletal muscle fibre. MLCs have an influence on the shortening velocity of a fibre. For instance, for fibres with myosin heavy chains of type IIa, IIx, or IIb, the maximum unloaded shortening velocity was proportional to the ratio MLC-3f/MLC-2f (Bottinelli *et al.* 1994).

In normal adult muscle, most muscle fibres are clearly classifiable with regard to their MHC content. Hybrid fibres, containing more than one type of MHC, do occur but normally they constitute a small minority. In this respect, conditions change drastically if muscle fibres are subjected to altered innervation or a changed pattern of daily use (Chapters 10 and 11). For non-hybrid fibres, classification according to mATPase reactions typically corresponds well to the MHC-type classification, although special kinds of preincubation may be needed for separating subgroups of histochemical IIb fibres, if any (Gorza 1990; Lind and Kernell 1991). The presence of different MHC isoforms in single fibres can sometimes be quantified using special types of mATPase histochemistry (Santana Pereira *et al.* 1995), and the mATPase reactions are not influenced by the MLC composition of the fibres (Billeter *et al.* 1981).

For historical reasons, the term 'IIb' has acquired a potentially different meaning in mATPase histochemistry and in MHC immunocytochemistry. In the rat hindlimb, many muscles contain all four main types of MHC, and studies of such muscles have shown that fibres classified as type IIb with the original tripartite mATPase method (Brooke and Kaiser 1970) could indeed be separated into two distinct categories using additional preincubation procedures (Schiaffino *et al.* 1989; Gorza 1990; Lind and Kernell 1991). However, only one of the two new MHC categories that emerged from mATPase-type IIb was given the new name IIx (Schiaffino *et al.* 1986; 1989; Schiaffino and Reggiani 1996), also referred to as IId (Termin *et al.* 1989; Pette and Staron 2000); the other portion of the mATPase-IIb group retained its original name. Thus rat muscle fibres classified as IIb using mATPase methods (which are still extensively used) might correspond to fibres of types IIb, IIx/IId, or both in MHC-immunohistochemistry. In humans, all the histochemical IIb fibres have MHC isozymes of the IIx variety. In this book, the term 'IIb' will be reserved for mATPase-classified fibres (i.e. human muscles still have IIb fibres), and muscle fibres similarly classified using immunological or electrophoretic methods for MHC identification will be termed MHC-IIb (or MHC-IIx).

3.4.2. **Other proteins of importance for contractile functions**

Qualitative cytochemical differences between different physiological types of muscle fibre (e.g. fast versus slow) have also been found for the composition of proteins of importance for excitation–contraction coupling, such as troponin C, I, and T, tropomyosin, and the Ca^{2+} pump molecules of the sarcoplasmic reticulum (cf. Table 11.1) (Schiaffino and Reggiani 1996; Pette and Staron 1997). Because of such qualitative differences, and quantitative differences in the membrane density of the various molecules, slow fibres have a lower Ca^{2+} threshold for activation and fast fibres have a faster removal of released Ca^{2+} ions. The speed of Ca^{2+} removal depends not only on the activity and density of the Ca^{2+} pumps, but also on the presence of effective Ca^{2+} buffering molecules, such as parvalbumin, in the sarcoplasm. In rabbits, for instance, this buffering molecule is present in various fast-twitch muscles but is almost absent in the slow-twitch ones (Leberer and Pette 1986). For single rabbit muscle fibres, much parvalbumin is present in type IIb fibres, less in IIa, and hardly any in fibres of type I (Schmitt and Pette 1991). In knockout mice lacking parvalbumin, twitches of fast-mixed muscles are slower and larger than normal (Schwaller *et al.* 1999). In humans, the twitch of a fast limb muscle is normally even slower than the twitch of a slow rabbit or rat muscle; correspondingly, parvalbumin is lacking in human extrafusal muscle fibres (Fohr *et al.* 1993).

3.4.3. Metabolic enzymes

A very large number of enzymes are involved in energy metabolism in muscle fibres as well as in all living cells (for basic background information, see Chapter 2, section 2:6). In this context the discussion will focus on a few representatives that have been widely used in combined physiological and histo/biochemical studies of muscle. With regard to glucose/glycogen metabolism, these enzymes can be subdivided into two major categories:

- **glycolytic enzymes** used in relation to processes for the anaerobic breakdown of glucose or glycogen fragments into pyruvic or lactic acid (delivers two ATP molecules per glucose fragment)

- **oxidative enzymes** used in the tricarboxylic acid cycle for the subsequent oxidative breakdown of pyruvic acid into CO_2 and water (delivers an additional 36 ATP molecules per glucose fragment).

Many enzymes are involved within each of these categories. However, to a great extent their activities covary within each category. For both the main categories of metabolic enzymes, large and consistent differences exist between different physiological types of muscle fibres. In addition to the enzymes concerned with glucose processing, there are also other important biochemical pathways in energy metabolism (e.g. using fuels like fat, hexoses, amino acids, etc.). For further details on the various enzymes concerned, the reader is referred to biochemical textbooks.

3.4.3.1. Oxidative enzymes

The most commonly used marker enzyme for histochemical/physiological muscle and neuronal studies is succinate dehydrogenase (SDH) (Fig. 3.10c), which is bound to mitochondria and hence is not as diffusable as free cytoplasmic enzymes. Measurements of SDH activity demonstrate that there is a continuous variation in this property between the muscle fibres of a muscle (e.g. Fig. 11.1c,d), including large variations *within* each of the mATPase categories of fibres. The different mATPase types occupy different ranges within the variation of SDH activity, and averages are typically significantly different, although the direction of these differences differs between different mammal species (Reichmann and Pette 1982). For instance, in cat or human, averages of SDH per mATPase type differ such that I > IIa > IIb, and in rat they differ such that IIa > I > IIb (Fig. 3.10c). Morphometric electron microscopy studies have demonstrated that, as expected, SDH activity shows a positive correlation with the relative volume of mitochondria within a fibre. Other commonly studied oxidative enzymes include citrate synthase, malate dehydrogenase, and cytochrome oxidase.

3.4.3.2. Glycolytic anaerobic metabolism

The most commonly used marker enzyme in this group is alpha-glycerol phosphate dehydrogenase (GPD) (Martin *et al.* 1985). Other enzymes in this group include lactic dehydrogenase and phosphorylase. Typically, there is an inverse relationship between the activities of SDH and GPD. For standard fibre types in the rat, GPD activity is typically ranked such that I < IIa < IIx < IIb (Rivero *et al.* 1998).

3.4.4. Fuel supplies

Much of the fuel needed for muscle contractions is continuously delivered via the blood vessels. As might be expected, there are also more capillaries around oxidative muscle fibres (types I and IIa) than around other types (IIb) (Ingjer 1979; Degens *et al.* 1992). There are also functionally important buffer supplies of fuel stored within the fibres themselves: fatty acids in fat droplets and glucose in chains of glycogen. The size of the intramuscular glycogen stores varies considerably depending on the amount of preceding activity (Hultman 1967; Edström and Kugelberg 1968; Kernell *et al.* 1995) and on hormonal levels (e.g. epinephrine) (Bonen *et al.* 1989).

3.4.5. Cytochemical homogeneity of muscle units

In normally innervated adult muscles, fibres that belong to the same motor unit are generally cytochemically similar; their variability is much smaller than that seen across the muscle as a whole (Edström and Kugelberg 1968; Nemeth *et al.* 1981, 1986). Thus they generally have the same type of myosin MHC and mATPase reaction (Unguez *et al.* 1993). However, some differences may occur also within normally innervated units. Thus Larsson (1992) observed that single-unit fibres at different positions within the muscle might differ systematically in metabolic enzyme characteristics (SDH, see above). Furthermore, using immunohistochemistry, even longitudinal heterogeneities in myosin composition can be detected within single fibres (Edman *et al.* 1988). The cytochemical heterogeneity of motor units becomes drastically increased after (self-)reinnervation (Unguez *et al.* 1993, 1995) (see Chapter 10).

3.4.6. Cytochemical classification of muscle fibres

As is apparent from the preceding sections there are two, mutually largely consistent, systems in current use for the cytochemical classification of muscle fibres according to their myosin composition.

◆ Types I, IIa, and IIb, using mATPase histochemistry with preincubation at various pH values (Brooke and Kaiser 1970). In rat muscles, simple extension of these techniques allows the further subdivision of group IIb into subtypes (IIx and IIb (Gorza 1990; Santana Pereira *et al.* 1995); IIbd and IIbm (Lind and Kernell 1991)).

◆ Types MHC-I, MHC-IIa, MHC-IIx = MHC-IId, and MHC-IIb, using immunohistochemical and/or electrophoretic methods for determining the MHC composition of the muscle fibres (Staron and Pette 1990; Schiaffino and Reggiani 1996; Pette and Staron 2000). Such techniques also make it possible to identify various types of hybrid fibres, containing mixtures of different MHC isoforms.

In an alternative approach, fibres are first classified into the two main categories, 'slow' or 'fast' (S, F), using mATPase histochemistry or MHC-immunohistochemistry. The

F fibres are then further subdivided depending on whether they have a high activity for oxidative (O) and/or glycolytic (G) enzymes. This leads to the following tripartite classification.

- ◆ SO, FOG, and FG (Peter *et al.* 1972). On the whole, fibres belonging to these categories correspond to those classified as I, IIa, and IIb according to mATPase histochemistry, but some differences may occur.

Each nomenclature should be reserved for its own specific type of measurement. For instance, the relation between mATPase type and metabolic profile shows characteristic differences between different animal species (Reichmann and Pette 1982).

3.5. **Muscle unit and fibre classification: relationships and predictions**

One of the major reasons for classifying units into discrete groups lies in its predictive power; using a few parameters for the categorization, one might predict relative differences between the groups with regard to many other covarying properties. Thus, taking only physiological parameters into account, there are typically systematic (but continuously graded) differences in maximum tetanic force across the various muscle unit types, generally such that S < FR < Fint < FF (Fig. 3.9A,D, and Table 3.3) (Burke *et al.* 1973; McDonagh *et al.* 1980b; Kernell *et al.* 1983a; Zengel *et al.* 1985). The negative correlation between maximum tetanic force and endurance is also a highly reproducible relationship, which is seen in a wide range of different motor unit populations (Fuglevand *et al.* 1999). Other characteristics may be well related in some muscles but not in others; these include the relationship between isometric twitch speed and various other parameters such as 'sagging' behaviour, maximum force, or endurance (for further discussion, see Fuglevand *et al.* 1999). Thus, from some points of view, the predictive 'power' of particular schemes of muscle unit classification appears highly muscle specific.

An important issue in muscle unit classification concerns the relationships between physiological and histochemical categories of units. One of the problems in this context is that there are no strong and direct causal links between the parameters generally used in these two sets of classifications. In physiological classifications, 'speed' is evaluated from sagging behaviour or twitch speed, neither of which is very directly related to myosin composition. Similarly, differences in fatigue resistance, as measured in Burke tests, are likely to be more directly related to differences in excitation–contraction coupling mechanisms than to metabolic enzyme activities (see Chapter 9, section 9.5). Despite these indirect relationships between the physiological and histochemical classification systems, there is normally a considerable degree of systematic covariation between the two sets of parameters. Thus, on average, the main physiological categories of S, FR, and FF units generally correspond to the histochemical categories of I, IIa, and IIb (or SO, FOG, and FG) fibres (Table 2.2). However, under particular circumstances, these patterns of systematic covariation may become distorted (e.g. relationships between fatigue and metabolic properties after chronic stimulation (cf. Fig. 11.1)). Furthermore, a coarse-grained correspondence may exist between physiological and histochemical parameters without an equivalence in finer details. For instance, myosin composition is causally related to shortening velocity and, as expected, MHC I, IIa, and IIx/IIb fibres also systematically differ in their V_{max} (Fig. 3.5A). With regard to the potential classification parameter isometric twitch speed, S units (type I fibres) are indeed systematically slower than fast units (FR and FF, IIa and IIb fibres). However, there are often no significant differences in twitch speed between the two main categories of fast units and fibres (Fig. 3.9A,C, and Tables 3.3 and 6.1) although their myosin types seem associated with different speeds of shortening (Fig. 3.5A; for temperature effects, see Lionikas *et al.* 2006).

It is important to remember that the parameters used for muscle unit classification are relative and not absolute measures. Thus, with regard to isometric twitch speed, all the commonly investigated mammals have slow-twitch type I fibres and fast-twitch type II fibres. However, for corresponding categories of units and fibres, the absolute twitch speeds (e.g. reciprocal twitch contraction time) and the maximum unloaded shortening velocities are ranked rat > cat > human (Fig. 3.5). Thus smaller animals typically have faster muscles than larger animals. With regard to maximum shortening velocity, these differences depend on quantitatively minor (but important) differences in protein composition between analogous MHCs of the different animal species (Reggiani *et al.* 2000).

3.6. Distribution and topographical organization of fibre types

In a normally innervated muscle containing different cytochemical fibre types (as most muscles do), fibres of the same minority type seldom lie beside each other (even less than by chance) (Grotmol *et al.* 1988; Venema 1988). As a result, in histochemical cross-sections, normal muscles show a 'checker-board' pattern of fibre types (Fig. 3.10) (see Chapter 12 for a discussion of developmental backgrounds). This pattern of fibre type distribution also implies that the fibres of a single motor unit will tend not to lie directly adjacent to each other. Glycogen depletion experiments, mapping the topographical distribution of fibres within single units, have confirmed that this is also the case (Fig. 3.10D) (Rafuse and Gordon 1996a). On the other hand, the fibres of single motor units are typically not distributed randomly across a whole muscle or neuromuscular compartment, but tend to be more restricted in their distribution. The relative position of a unit within a muscle depends, among other things, on its fibre type (fibre type regionalization, see below) and on the intraspinal position of its MN in the spinal cord (see Chapter 5, section 5.4.2).

3.6.1. Differences in unit and fibre type distibution between muscles

There are large systematic differences in fibre type composition between homologous muscles of different mammalian species. Furthermore, within a given animal species, muscles within the same limb vary considerably and systematically in their fibre type composition. Thirdly, different individuals of the same species may display large differences in their fibre type composition.

Among common laboratory species, the relative percentage of type I fibres (i.e. slow muscle fibres) tends to be ranked mouse < rat < cat and rabbit < human. For instance, for the large knee extensor vastus lateralis (which is the most commonly investigated muscle in humans with regard to its histochemistry), the content of type I fibres is about 2 per cent for rats, 27 per cent for cats, and about 40–50 per cent in humans (Ariano *et al.* 1973; Johnson *et al.* 1973; Lexell *et al.* 1983). Larger animals do not necessarily have even greater fractions of slow fibres; in the bull, the vastus lateralis contains only about 20 per cent type I fibres (Totland and Kryvi 1991).

In human limb muscles, the mean percentages of type I fibres may vary from roughly 33 per cent for triceps brachii, 40 per cent for brachioradialis and up to ~80 per cent for the hand muscle adductor pollicis (means for deep and superficial values when both are given) (Johnson *et al.* 1973); however, large differences may occur between different individuals (see below). In the rat, the corresponding range of variation is only from about 2 to 5 per cent type I fibres (Ariano *et al.* 1973). Even in rats and cats, a few specialized muscles are dominated by slow fibres, most notably the deep ankle extensor soleus (one of the heads of triceps surae, the muscle of the Achilles tendon). The percentage of type I fibres for this muscle is ~85 per cent in rats, 100 per cent in cats and rabbits, and ~88 per cent in humans.

Differences between individuals are very evident when comparing the muscles of sport champions versus those of non-sporting persons. For instance, long-distance runners and cyclists typically have comparatively large fractions of non-fatiguable type I fibres in their vastus lateralis muscles (78–80 per cent) (Howald 1982; Baumann *et al.* 1987), which gives them an evident advantage in their sports activities. Such inter-individual differences might depend partly on differences in muscle training (see Chapter 11) and partly on genetic factors. Comparisons of mono- and dizygotic twins have indicated that genetic factors have a strong influence on the myosin-related fibre type composition of the muscles (Komi *et al.* 1977); thus persons who successfuly engage in endurance sports are probably born with a competitive myosin advantage. In contrast, no evidence was found for a strong genetic control of inter-individual differences in the distribution of metabolic enzyme activities within the muscles (Komi *et al.* 1977).

3.6.2. Regionalization of myosin-associated fibre types

Since it became clear that most muscles are of a mixed fibre type composition, it was also noted that the different fibre types (e.g. type I versus type II fibres) often tended to be preferentially distributed to different muscle portions. In large limb muscles of experimental animals (cat, rat), slow fibres were typically found to be more common in deep regions (i.e. far from the limb surface) than in more superficial regions (Gordon and Phillips 1953; Armstrong 1980), and a similar tendency has also been seen in human muscles (Lexell *et al.* 1983). In cats and rats this is very obvious for muscles like gastrocnemius or tibialis anterior, and such distributions are consistent with the fact that the few muscles which are known to be dominated by slow units (i.e. 'slow' muscles or muscle heads, such as soleus) also commonly lie relatively deep within the limb (Creed *et al.*

1932). When using quantitative measures for the direction and extent of fibre type regionalization (Fig. 3.11), this general kind of organization was seen to exist in almost all limb muscles investigated (mouse, rat, rabbit) Wang and (Kernell 2001a, b). Although exceptions occurred, the direction of heterogeneity was such that slow fibres tended to be more common towards the geometrical centre of the limb (Fig. 3.11B,C). Furthermore, this tendency was more marked in muscles lying far from the centre than for those present in the inner limb core (Fig. 3.11D). Most limb muscles have a pennate structure (cf. Fig. 2.1A), and in such cases the length of the whole muscle is greater than the lengths of its constituent muscle fibres. Thus muscle fibres of different types may also be unevenly distributed in a lengthwise direction. In several fast mixed muscles of the rat hindlimb, this lengthwise regionalization was very marked, with slow fibres being more common in proximal than in more distal locations (Wang and Kernell 2000). In rabbit and mouse, lengthwise distributions were less consistently regionalized than in rats (Wang and Kernell 2001a), and little is known about these aspects of intramuscular fibre distribution in other species.

The physiological relevance of the preferential localization of slow fibres to deep muscle regions is still unknown. The resting blood suppply is probably greater for slow than for fast fibres (Reis and Wooten 1976; Ingjer 1979; Degens *et al.* 1992), and it has been suggested that a deep and well-insulated location of these fibres will help to conserve body heat (Loeb 1987). In addition, during intense muscle work, the deep localization of slow fibres would make them particularly sensitive to the effects of the increased muscle temperature, causing an increase in their shortening speed and mechanical power output (Fig. 3.3C,D). Interestingly, at least for shortening speeds seen in human bicycling, the slow fibres might profit more than the fast ones from such temperature effects (Fig. 3.3D, vertical arrow) (Jones *et al.* 2004). However, it must not be forgotten that the accumulation of slow fibres in deep portions of adult regionalized muscles might also be (partly) interpreted as 'vestiges of the original muscle primordium', reflecting topographical aspects of early muscle differentiation (see Chapter 12) (Narusawa *et al.* 1987). In some poikilothermic (cold-blooded) animals, various other patterns of preferential slow-fibre localization have been reported (e.g. hindlimb muscles of turtles (Laidlaw *et al.* 1995)), and a preferentially superficial localization of slow fibres is commonly present for trunk musculature of fish (Rome *et al.* 1988).

3.6.3. **Regionalization of metabolic fibre properties**

Histochemical measurements have demonstrated that, for fibres of the same mATPase type (e.g. subtypes of IIb), the SDH activity is higher in 'red-slow' than in 'white-fast' regions of the same muscle (Lind and Kernell 1991; De Ruiter *et al.* 1995). The opposite pattern is found for glycolytic enzyme activity (GPD) (De Ruiter *et al.* 1995; Kernell and Lind 1995). Thus fast IIb fibres lying close to slow oxidative fibres also tend to become more oxidative in their characteristics. Such local variations in enzyme activity (SDH) have even been observed within single motor units (Larsson 1992).

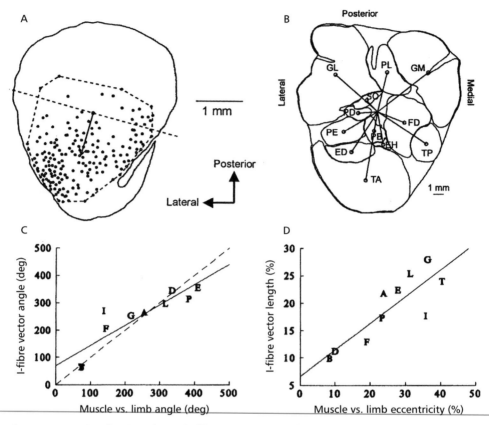

Figure 3.11 Regionalization of muscle fibre types. Muscles from rat hindlimb. (**A**) Digitized version of cross-section of plantaris muscle. Positions of all 'slow' fibres (type I) indicated by dots. The type I fibres were identified by staining for mATPase (cf. Fig. 3.10). An arrow ('type I fibre vector') has been drawn from the centre of mass of the whole muscle section to the centre of mass for all the type I fibre sites (for calculations, see Wang and Kernell 2001b). In addition, a straight broken line has been drawn at right angles to the vector arrow and through the muscle centre (used for other types of distribution analysis). The 'type I fibre region' is enclosed by interrupted lines according to borders calculated using the 'convex hull method'. The 'fold' in the lower-right part of the section represents a tendon sheath. (**B**) Digitized cross-section of whole lower hindlimb through the level in the middle between knee and ankle. Outline and calculated centre of mass (small circle) are shown for each muscle. Lines drawn from the calculated centre of mass for the whole limb cross-section to the centre of mass for each muscle. The length and angle of each such line represent the polar coordinates for the respective muscle, as seen from the limb centre. (**C**), (**D**) Charts showing the relationship between polar muscle coordinates within the limb (**B**) and the direction and extent of type I fibre regionalization within each muscle (**A**). In (**C**), the direction of vector angles of type I fibre regionalization inside individual muscles were plotted versus 'inverse' angle values (i.e. actual value −180°) for the respective polar muscle coordinates. This graph demonstrates that, within individual muscles, type I fibres tended to be accumulated in a direction towards the limb centre. In (**D**), values for relative type I fibre vector length (per cent) are plotted versus the lengths of the corresponding polar muscle

3.6.4. Regionalization within intramuscular fascicles

Muscle fibres are surrounded by sheets of connective tissue, which are important for general muscle structure and muscle fibre protection. Thin sheets surround every single fibre, and somewhat thicker sheets surround small bundles ('fascicles') of fibres. Single fascicles contain fibres of various types, belonging to several different motor units. Within fascicles the distribution of fibre types is non-random; fast fibres are more common along the rim of fascicles than more centrally (human vastus muscle (Sjöström *et al.* 1986, 1992; Pernus and Erzen 1991); horse muscles, more IIB along rim (Grotmol *et al.* 2002)).

3.7. Motor axons and muscle innervation

General axon properties were dealt with in Chapter 2, section 2.4. With regard to electrophysiological characteristics, there are no clear differences between peripheral motor axons and correspondingly large sensory axons.

3.7.1. Distribution of MN axons to muscles and neuromuscular compartments

For almost all kinds of motor behaviour, many muscles are used together. It is even doubtful whether it would be possible, voluntarily, to produce a strong contraction of only a single muscle. However, separate muscles very seldom have obligatory links by being controlled by the same MNs. Only a few examples are known of such arrangements: (a) the first and second superficial lumbrical muscles of the cat's foot share some of their MNs (Emonet-Denand *et al.* 1971); (b) axons of single MNs go to both the left- and right-side eyelid elevator in the monkey (levator palpebrae superioris) (Sekiya *et al.* 1992); (c) some single MNs innervate both the retractor bulbi and the lateral rectus muscle in cat (Gurahian and Goldberg 1987). In case (a), the relation between axonal conduction velocity and muscle unit maximal force is normal (i.e. similar to that of single-muscle MNs) only when adding up the forces from both innervated muscles for each unit. However, puzzlingly, in case (c) the same MN innervates fibres of differing fatigue resistance in retractor bulbi and lateral rectus.

Often the peripheral innervation fields are distinctly different for the MNs of different primary branches of the same muscle nerve (neuromuscular compartments) (English and Letbetter 1982; reviewed by Kernell 1998). This may also be true for compartments with very similar biomechanical functions, i.e. with tendons pulling in the same direction. The compartmental organization of the motoneuronal target tissue is of great interest with regard to the mechanisms for axon guidance and target finding during

Figure 3.11 (Continued)

coordinates (per cent, normalized versus limb equivalent diameter). This graph demonstrates that the tendency for a heterogeneous fibre type distribution was more marked for muscles far from the limb centre than for those more centrally placed. (Reproduced with permission, from Wang and Kernell 2001b.)

neuromuscular development. One might consider neuromuscular compartments as being equivalent to morphologically defined muscles; some muscles consist of several compartments ('submuscles') glued together by connective tissue to give one morphologically identifiable unit. Interestingly, however, from some points of view multicompartmental muscles still seem to behave as single entities. Fibre type regionalization, as described above, takes place within single compartments as well as across muscle regions composed of different compartments. There is still no convincing evidence that neuromuscular compartments with equivalent biomechanical properties are dealt with by the CNS as distinct functional entities (for further details, see Kernell 1998).

3.7.2. Number of peripheral axon terminals

Estimates of the total number of peripheral terminals of single alpha axons have been made in the context of muscle unit studies calculating innervation ratios (Table 3.1). As will be considered further in the next section, a significant correlation is typically found between maximal unit force and axonal conduction velocity, much of which is caused by a correlation between axonal size and the number of peripheral terminals. The branching is associated with an appreciable increase of the summed cross-section area (Zenker and Hohberg 1973).

3.7.3. Axonal conduction velocity in motor units of different maximum force and type

Axons of slow-twitch units tend to be slower than those of fast-twitch units whereas, at least in the cat gastrocnemius, there is often no difference in conduction speed between axons of FR versus FF units (Table 6.1 and Fig. 6.7A, open versus filled circles) (Burke *et al.* 1973; Dum and Kennedy 1980a). Within a given muscle, there is typically a significant positive correlation between axonal conduction velocity and maximum motor unit force; thick and fast-conducting axons tend to have stronger units than axons that are thinner and slower (Bessou *et al.* 1963; Emonet-Denand *et al.* 1988). For muscles from individual animals, such correlations were also seen within the combined little-fatiguable categories of units (S and FR) Emonet-Denand *et al.* 1988). However, for unclear reasons, such correlations were not evident within the category of the fatigue-sensitive FF units (Emonet-Denand *et al.* 1988).

In comparisons between axons with regard to their conduction velocity, it is typically assumed that systematic differences reflect variations in axonal diameter, with large axons being faster than thinner ones. However, the membrane properties also play a role in this context; for instance, slower Na^+ channel kinetics would slow down conduction velocity (cf. slowing effects of cooling on conduction velocity). There are suggestions that such differences in nodal membrane properties might be responsible for some of the differences in axonal conduction velocity between units of the same muscle (Carp *et al.* 2003). Changes in axonal conduction velocity that take place after particular kinds of training might depend on changes in axonal membrane properties (Carp *et al.* 2001).

Axonal size and conduction velocity are important markers of muscle unit characteristics in experiments concerning the ranking order of MN recruitment (see Chapter 8, section 8.2) (Henneman *et al.* 1965; Henneman and Mendell 1981). In this context, it is interesting to note that the muscle unit characteristic which is most directly associated with axonal size is muscle unit innervation ratio and maximum force.

3.7.4. Functional relevance of high conduction velocities of motor axons

Motor alpha axons are one of the fastest types available in the peripheral or central portions of the nervous system. The large size and correspondingly high conduction velocity of these axons is likely to represent part of a biological specialization for promoting high speed in motor behaviour. Fast motor actions may clearly be advantageous for survival, and, in all species, central axons controlling motor behaviour also tend to be the fastest ones available. For instance, various kinds of well-known giant axons (i.e. very fast-conducting) are specialized for mediating flight and avoidance behaviour. This is true for the famous giant axon of the squid (mediating flight reaction by mantle contraction), giant axons in earthworms (withdrawal reactions), and giant Mauthner cells in fish (escape reactions by tail flip). Similarly, the corticospinal 'motor command' axons of the Betz cells are among the largest and fastest nerve fibres inside the CNS of primates. The largest mammalian afferents in peripheral nerves (Ia afferents from muscle spindles and Ib afferents from Golgi tendon organs (cf. Table 2.1)) are those directly used for sensory feedback in motor behaviour.

Even though fast peripheral conduction speeds are likely to be of importance for fast motor reactions, it is less certain whether the different axonal velocities of weak versus strong (or slow versus fast) muscle units are of direct physiological significance. However, it is notable that fast and strong units, which are typically equipped with the most rapid axons, are probably also those contributing most of the power to rapid motor acts such as the limb acceleration in ballistic movements.

Chapter 4

Neuromuscular transmission

4.1. General issues

The subject matter of this chapter is often treated as a subfield of its own, separate from other aspects of MN and muscle unit physiology. Historically this is understandable; the neuromuscular junction (NMJ) is one of the most intensely studied synapses and it was used for much of the early research concerning general principles of chemical synaptic transmission. In addition to its role as a model synapse, the NMJ is a crucial component of the neuromuscular apparatus and its properties should be understood in the light of the functional requirements of this system. General background information and further references can be found in recent reviews (McComas 1996; Kandel and Siegelbaum 2000b; Wood and Slater 2001).

The most thorough studies of neuromuscular transmission in twitch fibres have been performed in frogs and rats, supplemented by observations in many other species including humans. The NMJ is a chemical synapse, using ligand-gated ion channels, and it shares basic characteristics with many chemical synapses inside the CNS. However, compared with most CNS synapses the NMJ is of enormous size, and its main function is to *amplify* the weak currents associated with presynaptic axonal spikes such that action potentials will be safely transmitted in a 1:1 fashion from the nerve terminal to the muscle fibre. This is quite different from the integrative or state-setting functions of central synapses; for most neurones inside the CNS (e.g. for MNs), the discharge of action potentials depends on the summed effects of many of the synapses that are attached to its membrane.

4.2. Morphology and molecular organization

A chemical synapse consists of three portions:

- the presynaptic nerve terminal
- the synaptic cleft(s), i.e. the space between the pre- and postsynaptic membranes, containing the basement membrane
- the postsynaptic membrane just under the presynaptic terminal.

In the NMJ the region under the nerve terminal is referred to as the motor endplate; sometimes this term is used for the whole neuromuscular synapse.

4.2.1. Presynaptic terminal

Inside the target muscle (and, to some extent, in the nerve trunk) (Eccles and Sherrington 1930) each motor axon splits into many terminal branches (Chapter 3, section 3.3.1.5,

Table 3.1). Normally, each adult twitch muscle fibre receives only one NMJ, typically located in the middle between the two ends of the fibre. In mammals, the presynaptic axon terminal splits up into several small 'twigs' when contacting a muscle fibre. The final branches are thin (about 2 μm), unmyelinated, and covered with Schwann cells. Each twig may show several varicosities (boutons) and is situated in a groove or gutter of the postsynaptic membrane. The gutter has many transverse folds with clefts between them (secondary folds) (Fig. 4.1). The contact region tends to be oval or circular in shape. The presynaptic nerve ending is densely packed with small spherical vesicles (**synaptic vesicles**) about 50–60 nm in diameter, containing the neurotransmitter acetylcholine (ACh) (Fig. 4.1). These vesicles are not present in a random array; there are electron-dense guiding structures which lead vesicles towards membrane sites at which their contents can be released by exocytosis. A queue of vesicles waits in front of each release site, and these sites tend to be opposite postsynaptic secondary clefts. In addition to ACh, the vesicles contain ATP and a proteoglycan. As well as the vesicles, the presynaptic terminals contain neurotubuli and many mitochondria. During motor nerve activation, vesicles can be seen that are fusing with the sarcolemma, apparently in the process of exocytosis (seen using EM freeze fracture techniques). In addition to the clear synaptic vesicles, a small number of larger (70–110 nm) dense-core vesicles are also present. Their function is unknown; they may contain neurotrophic substances with an

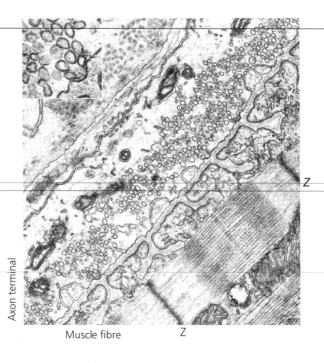

Figure 4.1 Muscle innervation. Electron micrograph of the neuromuscular junction of frog. An axon terminal with synaptic vesicles (left) is separated from muscle fibre (right) by a synaptic cleft with large postsynaptic folds of the muscle membrane. A sarcomere with two Z lines can be seen in the lower right-hand corner. The distance between the Z lines is about 2.8 μm. (Reproduced with permission, from Heuser 1976, added labels.)

Axon terminal

Muscle fibre   Z

Z

influence on muscle (e.g. CGRP) (cf. Chapter 5, section 5.3.5). In frogs, the terminal axonal branches of an individual NMJ are longer and the subterminal membrane folds are less complex than in mammals. Hence, in frogs, the NMJ region is elongated. With regard to major functional properties, there is a great similarity between amphibian and mammalian neuromuscular synapses.

4.2.2. Synaptic clefts and basement membrane

Pre- and postsynaptic membranes are separated by a 'primary' synaptic cleft with a width of about 70 nm. Under the presynaptic terminal, the 'gutter' of the postsynaptic membrane is folded repeatedly into junctional folds. The 'secondary' synaptic clefts extends to a depth of about 0.5–1 μm.

The **basement membrane** (basal lamina), a complex structure of collagen and other fibrils (10–15 nm thick) which completely surrounds the external membrane (plasmalemma) of the whole muscle fibre, extends throughout the central portions of the primary and secondary synaptic clefts. The term sarcolemma is sometimes used as a synonym for plasmalemma (nomenclature used in this book), and sometimes as a synonym for plasmalemma plus basement membrane. In the primary and secondary synaptic clefts, the basement membrane contains ACh esterase (AChE) molecules (reviewed by Rotundo 2003), which are anchored to collagen fibres and are needed for the rapid breakdown and inactivation of released ACh. The junctional AChE molecules have a half-life of about 3 weeks and are partly synthesized by the MN (McComas 1996). However, muscle fibres are also capable of synthesizing AChE, and this synthesis is under the trophic control of the MN and its activity (Lomo *et al.* 1985; Sketelj *et al.* 1992). Recent experimental studies of muscle innervation *in vitro* indicate that both cells contribute; most of the AChE comes from the muscle and a smaller fraction from the MN (Jevsek *et al.* 2004). In the rat, three molecular forms of AChE are found in both fast and slow muscles (globular forms G1 and G4, and asymmetric form A12), and three additional forms are found in slow muscle only (soleus: globular G2, asymmetric A4 and A8) (Lomo *et al.* 1985). In mouse endplates, the density of AChE molecules is about 3000 per μm^2, i.e. much lower than the subterminal density of ACh receptors (see below and Barnard *et al.* 1975).

In addition to AChE and collagen, the basement membrane of the NMJ contains several other proteins including the non-specific **choline esterase** (ChE) which may split different varieties of choline esters; **fibronectin** and **laminin** which link the basement membrane to the plasmalemma, **agrin** and **ACh-receptor inducing activity** (ARIA) which are involved in the formation of the NMJ, and neurotrophic substances like **fibroblast growth factor** (FGF) (McComas 1996; Wood and Slater 2001).

4.2.3. Postsynaptic membrane

Because of the junctional folds, the subterminal membrane area is much expanded, allowing a larger number of ion channels to be present than in a flat membrane. The distribution of ACh receptor molecules (AChRs) can be visualized by irreversible binding to labelled α-bungarotoxin. The crests of the folds are very densely packed with AChRs at a density of about 10 000 per μm^2. Each AChR has two binding sites for ACh; thus the density of ACh binding sites is about 20 000 per μm^2. The depths of the folds contain many voltage-gated Na^+ channels of the type needed for the generation of action potentials. The AChRs at the NMJ are of the 'nicotinic' type, i.e. they can be activated by nicotine and blocked with curare.

4.2.4. **The ACh receptor**

This was the first transmembrane ion channel to be purified, visualized, and analysed as to its molecular composition (reviewed by Kandel and Siegelbaum 2000b; Hille 2001). The whole AChR has a diameter of about 8.5 nm and extends about 6 nm outside the membrane (the membrane thickness is about 3 nm). In adults, the average half-life of junctional AChRs is 8–11 days. Their synthesis is regulated by several muscle fibre nuclei lying in the direct vicinity of the NMJ, and it can be accelerated by two neurotrophic peptides which are released by presynaptic motor axon terminals: **calcitonin gene related peptide** (CGRP) and ARIA. Myonuclei lying outside the NMJ region normally have their AChR genes downregulated, probably mainly via effects of muscle fibre activity (Ca^{2+} initiated cascade). In denervated or inactivated muscle fibres (e.g. block of axonal action potentials with TTX), extrajunctional AChRs will emerge; their appearance can be prevented by chronic electrical activation of the muscle (Lomo and Rosenthal 1972). Normally, the majority of the ACh receptors are localized in the immediate vicinity of the endplate. However, low densities of receptors may also be present at both ends of the muscle fibres, close to the tendinous junctions (i.e. far from the endplate) (Cull-Candy *et al.* 1982). It has been suggested that these AChRs may play a role in repair processes (Bernheim *et al.* 1996).

4.3. **Transmitter release and postsynaptic action**

4.3.1. **Presynaptic ACh metabolism**

ACh is synthesized in the nerve endings from acetate and choline. A key enzyme in ACh synthesis is choline acetyltransferase (ChAT), which is synthesized in the MN soma and transported to the nerve terminals. The terminal contains mechanisms for transmembrane uptake of choline from the extracellular fluid; in this way choline is reused after the extracellular AChE-mediated hydrolysis of ACh. The choline uptake mechanism, and thus the NMJ function, can be blocked with hemicholinium.

4.3.2. **Presynaptic Ca^{2+} channels**

The membrane at each end of a motor axon has more complex electrical properties than that within its intermediate and major conducting portion. Notably, voltage-gated Ca^{2+} channels appear to be almost absent from the conducting portion but play an essential role in the soma-dendrite region (Chapters 6 and 7) and in presynaptic terminals. When an action potential arrives at a presynaptic terminal, voltage-gated Ca^{2+} channels become depolarized, leading to increased Ca^{2+} conductance and an inward-directed Ca^{2+} current; this current constitutes much of the total inward current for the terminal action potential. The Ca^{2+} channels are located at the docking sites for the synaptic vesicles, at presynaptic thickenings referred to as 'active zones'; some of these Ca^{2+} channels are even visible on electron micrographs (as membrane 'particles'). The incoming Ca^{2+} ions will activate exocytosis mechanisms and thus cause the release of ACh from synaptic vesicles. If the inward Ca^{2+} currents of the presynaptic terminal are blocked, action potentials arriving along the axon will cause no release of transmitter. The Ca^{2+} ions which enter the terminal during action potentials are rapidly removed by the various procedures for Ca^{2+} sequestration (e.g. binding to buffers, active transport into membraneous organelles or out of the cell).

4.3.3. **Exocytosis and endocytosis**

In most types of cells that make use of regulated exocytosis for secretion (neurones, various kinds of gland cells), this process is triggered by an increased cytoplasmic concentration of Ca^{2+} ions ('excitation–secretion coupling'). During presynaptic exocytosis at a motor nerve ending, the synaptic vesicles which are close to active sites in the membrane will fuse with the plasmalemma and the whole water-soluble contents of the vesicle will be released into the synaptic cleft. Typically, in mammals, a synaptic NMJ vesicle contains about 5000–10000 molecules of ACh (one ACh 'quantum'). Normally, one presynaptic action potential will cause the exocytosis of about 20–200 of such vesicles within a fraction of a millisecond, i.e. during a time shorter than the total duration of the action potential. Together, the ACh from all these vesicles gives rise to the postsynaptic endplate potential, the EPP (Fig. 4.2(A), (B), (D)). The number of vesicular quanta represented in an EPP is referred to as its **quantal content**.

The processes for eliciting exocytosis take a measurable time. This release delay is responsible for a major part of the **synaptic latency** of a chemical synapse, i.e. the delay between the arrival of a presynaptic action potential and the onset of the resulting postsynaptic potential. The synaptic latency is longer at low than at high temperatures. In mammalian NMJs it is about 0.2 ms at normal body temperature, and in frog NMJs it is about 0.5 ms at room temperature.

During exocytosis, the vesicle membrane fuses with the external cell membrane, i.e. the total presynaptic membrane area would grow if there were no recycling of membrane. This does not happen because there is an approximate balance between exocytosis at the endplate and endocytosis taking place in more proximal membrane regions, close to the synaptic release sites. In the frog, increased endocytosis is already detectable 1 s after ACh release and continues for about the next 90 s (Miller and Heuser 1984). The endocytosis takes place as an invagination of membrane and an associated intracellular trapping of extracellular fluid and molecules in a new cytoplasmic vesicle, which may be transported along the axon towards the MN cell body. Via endocytosis, proteins and other substances, some of which are released by the nearby muscle fibres, will be taken up

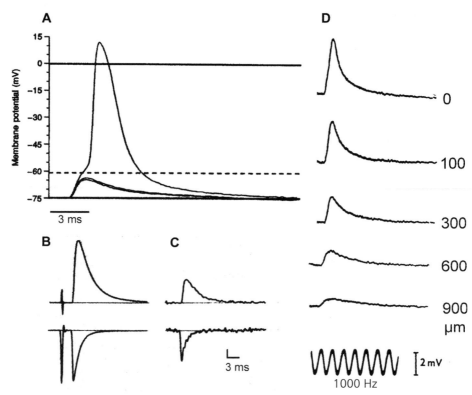

Figure 4.2 Electrophysiology of the neuromuscular junction. (**A**) Determination of the action potential threshold at the NMJ. The amplitude of the endplate potential (EPP) in an isolated rat soleus nerve–muscle preparation has been reduced by blocking many of the acetylcholine receptors (AChRs) with **D**-tubocurarine. Depending on the extent of the block, EPPs are either too small to elicit an action potential (lower trace) or are large enough for reaching the threshold (upper trace). The threshold, defined as the first point of inflection on the rising phase of the action potential (upper trace), is −61 mV in this example. (Reproduced with permission, from Wood and Slater 1995.) (**B**) Average of full-sized EPP and (**c**) spontaneous miniature EPP (mEPP) recorded in the presence of μ-conotoxin, which blocks muscle fibre action potentials without blocking axonal spikes. By using a two-electrode voltage clamp arrangement, the corresponding flows of endplate current were also recorded (downward transients, averages of EPC in (**B**) and of mEPC in (**c**)). The vertical calibration bar represents 4 mV and 30 nA in (**B**), and 0.25 mV and 1 nA in (**c**). The horizontal bar represents 3 ms for all traces. (Reproduced with permission, from Wood and Slater 1997.) (**D**) Spatial decay of EPP in a cat muscle fibre (tenuissimus muscle). Recordings were made at the distances from the endplate indicated (curarized preparation). (Reproduced with permission, from Boyd and Martin 1956.)

by axon terminals of MNs. Hence these processes are potentially important for the communication from muscles to MNs. However, the endocytosis process is not very selective; various molecules which happen to lie in the vicinity, including macromolecules that have no normal roles in animal tissues (e.g. viruses such as rabies, and plant-derived tracing substances such as horseradish peroxidase (HRP)), are taken up.

4.3.4. Spontaneous quantal and non-quantal release

Even in the absence of presynaptic action potentials, the nerve ending releases ACh in vesicular quanta, i.e. there is also a spontaneously occurring exocytosis. For individual NMJs, this release takes place at frequencies ranging from several times per second to several times per minute. Each released vesicle gives rise to a miniature EPP (mEPP) with an amplitude of about 0.5–1 mV (Fig. 4.2(c)). This phenomenon of spontaneous quantal transmitter release, which was first discovered at the motor endplate, is a general property of chemical synapses. The frequency of the vesicular release is (partly) Ca^{2+} dependent and increases with increasing intracellular Ca^{2+} concentration. Thus a very large number of vesicles are released as Ca^{2+} concentration rapidly increases on the arrival of an action potential because of the opening of presynaptic Ca^{2+} channels (see above). The vesicular ACh content has been calculated from comparisons of the sizes of the mEPPs with those of postsynaptic depolarizations caused by known quantities of ACh applied close to the NMJ using microelectrodes (micro-iontophoresis). Comparisons of mEPP and EPP amplitudes are important for determining the quantal content of EPPs.

In addition to the spontaneous quantal release of ACh, as signalled by the appearance of mEPPs, there is also a spontaneous transmembrane 'leakage' of non-vesicular ACh from the axonal cytoplasm (reviewed by Tauc 1982). The physiological function of this leakage is still uncertain.

4.3.5. Postsynaptic effects of released transmitter: endplate currents and potentials

4.3.5.1. Single-channel currents

When harbouring two bound molecules of ACh, the pore at the centre of the AChR opens up to a diameter of about 0.8 nm, allowing K^+ and Na^+ (and some Ca^{2+}) ions to pass through. The ratio of the Na^+ to the K^+ conductance is typically around 1.8. The currents through single ion channels can be monitored using patch clamp techniques with the fine tip of a microelectrode pressing against, and recording from, a small piece of the total membrane; these methods were first used to measure currents through AChR channels of the type seen in neuromuscular junctions (Neher and Sakmann 1976a, b). Such experiments show that the individual channel switches between only two states: open and closed. Once a channel is transiently activated by ACh, the duration of the open state varies randomly and is on average around 1 ms. In the open state, the conductance of the single AChR channel is 30 pS and the equilibrium potential for the resulting current is about 0 mV. This means that, at a membrane potential of −90 mV, the current through the single channel is 2.7 pA, i.e. 17×10^6 ions will pass through the channel every second.

4.3.5.2. Total endplate current

The ACh released by a single action potential may cause a current representing the summed activation of >200000 AChR channels. The sum of the resulting transient currents constitutes the endplate current (EPC), which will give rise to the EPP (Fig. 4.2(B)). The EPC lasts for only a few milliseconds, and it can be recorded using voltage clamp techniques. The EPP typically has a rapid rising phase lasting about 1 ms, and a slower approximately exponential decline of about 10–20 ms (Fig. 4.2). This declining phase is influenced by the passive membrane properties of the muscle fibre, i.e. by its membrane time constant and cable properties which determine the speed at which charge leaks away (cf. Fig. 2.2(c)).

4.3.6. Interruption of postsynaptic ACh effects: actions of acetylcholine esterase

The binding ACh—AChR is quite unstable and following a single presynaptic action potential, the postsynaptic ACh effects are of a very transient nature (cf. brief duration of EPC). Some of the released ACh is rapidly lost by diffusion out of the synaptic cleft and some is hydrolysed by acetylcholine esterase (AChE) before reaching any postsynaptic receptors. However, most of the ACh molecules will bind to an AChR at least once before being hydrolysed. Thereafter, AChE-catalysed hydrolysis is very effective and rapid; most ACh molecules will interact with AChR molecules only once. The supply of AChE is normally in considerable excess of that needed; small changes of AChE concentration have little effect.

4.3.7. Short-term modification of pre- and postsynaptic functions

In the time span of seconds to minutes, the functional properties of the NMJ may be influenced via receptors on the presynaptic terminal, the postsynaptic membrane, or the membrane of the Schwann cells. At one or several of these sites, receptors are present that react to ACh, purinergic and adrenergic agents, nitrous oxide (NO), 5HT, and glutamate (for further details and references, see Wood and Slater 2001). These modifying mechanisms include the following.

- Cholinergic presynaptic receptors which may decrease or increase the spike-evoked release of ACh.

- Purinergic P1 receptors which decrease the spike-evoked ACh release. These receptors may be located on nerve and/or Schwann cell membranes and agonists include ATP, ADP, and adenosine (experiments on rat and frog). P1 receptors are likely to be activated during normal neuromuscular transmission because ATP is co-released with ACh.

- Adrenergic presynaptic $\alpha-$ and β-receptors causing an increase in spike-evoked ACh release. Agonists include norepinephrine and epinephrine. Thus, via these receptors, neuromuscular transmission may become influenced by the effects of stress and physical exercise on the adrenal glands.

- Postsynaptic desensitization, i.e. an effect by ACh itself whereby AChR molecules revert to a state in which they are insensitive to ACh.

Other, less well-defined and more complex, modifying effects have been described (Wood and Slater 2001). The importance of these mechanisms for normal NMJ functions is largely unknown.

4.4. Physiology of neuromuscular spike transmission

4.4.1. Spike response properties of skeletal muscle fibres

The resting membrane potential of normally innervated mammalian muscle fibres is typically around -80 mV (Hicks and McComas 1989), close to the equilibrium potential for K^+ ions. The underlying mechanisms are similar to those of most other cells (see Chapter 2, section 2.4.2). Muscle fibres have complex passive properties because of the presence of the thin inward-directed T tubuli which are open to the surface. These structures help to produce a high membrane capacitance and a correspondingly long membrane time constant (the two components of capacitance: 4.1 and 2.6 $\mu F/cm^2$ surface membrane) (Falk and Fatt 1964). After glycerol treatment, which disrupts the T tubuli, the membrane time constant and capacitance decreased by a factor of about 3 (Gage and Eisenberg 1969).

The action potentials of twitch muscle fibres (Fig. 4.2(A)) depend essentially on the same types of voltage-gated ion-channel mechanisms as those in peripheral nerves (Chapter 2, section 2.4.4), i.e. a rapidly activating and inactivating Na^+ conductance system and a somewhat slower and less inactivating K^+ system. Conduction along the muscle fibres occurs in a fashion similar to that along non-myelinated nerve fibres. However, muscle fibres are much thicker (often about 50 μm or more) than mammalian non-myelinated axons (about 2 μm or less), and their conduction speed is higher (muscle fibres about 5 m/s; non-myelinated axons ≤ 2 m/s).

At the level of the endplate, the voltage threshold for an action potential is relatively low owing to the large accumulation of Na^+ channels in the depths of the junctional folds. For instance, in the extensor digitorum longus of the rat, the depolarization needed to elicit an action potential was about 12 mV close to the NMJ and about 30 mV further away along the fibre (resting membrane potential -75 mV) (Wood and Slater 1995, 2001).

4.4.2. The triggering of single muscle fibre action potentials by EPPs

In the rat NMJ in Fig. 4.2(B), the EPP reached an amplitude of roughly 30 mV in the absence of muscle action potentials. However, according to Fig. 4.2(A), the depolarization needed to elicit an action potential at the NMJ was only about 14 mV. Hence, in this case, the EPP was more than twice as large as would be needed for a spike transmission across the NMJ, i.e. there was a 'safety margin' (or 'safety factor') of about $30/14 = 2.14$ (Wood and Slater 1997). When calculated in this way, mammalian endplates normally show a safety margin of 2–6 or more for single-spike transmission (Wood and Slater 2001, Table 1). However, the safety margin becomes much lower under normal conditions when the NMJ will be activated by repetitive action potentials, sometimes continuously over long periods.

4.4.3. Time- and frequency-dependent effects on neuromuscular transmission

During repetitive activation, the EPP will rapidly decline in size because of a decrease in its quantal content during the initial 20–40 spikes. Thereafter, the EPP declines more slowly with time during the continued repetitive activation. As might be expected, the rapid initial EPP decrease is frequency dependent, being greater for higher stimulation rates. For instance, according to measurements by Kamenskaya *et al.* (1975), EPP size might drop to a plateau of around 0.65 of the single-spike EPP at 1 Hz, 0.45 at 20 Hz, and 0.30 at 40 Hz. Thus, in such a case the single-spike EPP would have to show a safety margin of at least >3 to achieve a 1:1 NMJ transmission at 40 Hz. These data imply that a block of NMJ transmssion might easily appear at (too) high rates of activation. However, under normal conditions, the NMJ properties of muscle fibres appear to be remarkably well adapted to the kind of repetitive activation they will receive from their MNs. Block of NMJ transmission seldom appears to be a factor of importance for fatigue in voluntary contractions (Merton 1954b; Bigland-Ritchie *et al.* 1982; for further discussion, see Chapter 9).

In addition to these processes of time- and frequency-dependent EPP depression, there are also facilitating effects of preceding activation, emerging as tetanic or post-tetanic potentiation of EPP quantal content (Lev-Tov and Fishman 1986); this potentiation might largely depend on changes in intraterminal Ca^{2+} concentration. The underlying processes are of great interest for the general understanding of chemical synapses. However, it is uncertain whether potentiation processes are of any importance for the use of neuromuscular transmission in normal motor behaviour (however, see symptoms in the Lambert–Eaton myasthenic syndrome, section 4.5.2). The activity-dependent potentiation of contractile force, as seen during or after a period of repetitive activation, is typically not reflecting changes in neuromuscular transmission but depends on other, intramuscular, factors (Chapter 3, section 3.3.4.3, and Chapter 9, section 9.8.1).

4.4.4. Neuromuscular transmission for different types of twitch muscle fibres

NMJs of different types of muscle fibre show different degrees of frequency dependence for the initial EPP depression and different degrees of time dependence for the more grad-ual decline subsequently. Interestingly, these differences are such that they serve to adapt the muscle fibres and their NMJ transmission to different physiological tasks. In slow fibres, the time-dependent decline of quantal content is less marked and less rapid than that seen for fast fibres of the same animal (Fig. 4.3) (Gertler and Robbins 1978; Reid *et al.* 1999), allowing terminals in slow (postural) muscles to sustain ACh release during the prolonged firing trains experienced *in vivo* (Bewick *et al.* 2004). These differences are related to the presence of a larger releasable vesicle pool in the slow fibres than in the fast fibres (Reid *et al.* 1999). In contrast, the initial EPP quantal content is greater and the single-spike safety factor is larger in fast fibres than in slow fibres (Gertler and Robbins 1978), which seems appropriate as fast fibres might tend to become activated (briefly) at higher

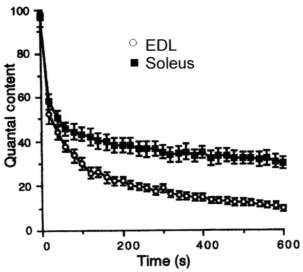

Figure 4.3 Decline of EPPs of slow versus fast muscle during repetitive activation. Isolated nerve–muscle preparations from fast (EDL) and slow (soleus) rat muscles stimulated at 20 Hz for 10 min. The quantal content of EPPs (see text) was plotted versus time (means ± SE). Quantal release during repetitive activity at NMJs was better maintained in slow than in fast rat muscles. (Reproduced with permission, from Reid *et al.* 1999.)

stimulation rates than those encountered by the slower fibres (cf. Chapter 3, section 3:3.3, and Chapter 6, section 6.9.3.4) (Reid *et al.* 1999). Furthermore, the tetanic or post-tetanic potentiation of the EPP quantal content is larger for NMJs in fast muscle units than for those in slow muscle units (Lev-Tov and Fishman 1986).

4.5. **Pathophysiological issues**

4.5.1. **Myasthenia gravis**

In this autoimmune disease (reviewed by Romi *et al.* 2005), the patient's lymphocytes produce antibodies against the AChR proteins of the endplate. As a result, the postsynaptic density of such receptors may decrease dramatically (this can be visualized in biopsy material after staining with labelled α-bungarotoxin) and many of the EPPs will therefore become too small to generate postsynaptic action potentials in the muscle fibres. However, the effects of the few remaining ACh receptors may be considerably increased by letting the released ACh act for a longer time. This is achieved by counteracting the ACh breakdown using an AChE blocker (usually pyridostigmine or neostigmine). The first symptoms of myasthenia gravis are usually found for distal and facial muscles. The affected muscles typically show a marked fatigue when used during longer time periods.

4.5.2. **Lambert–Eaton syndrome**

This is also an autoimmune disease (reviewed by Seneviratne and de Silva 1999), often associated with small carcinomas of the lung. In this case, antibodies appear that are directed against voltage-gated Ca^{2+} channels of the motor axon terminals. As a result, presynaptic action potentials cause subnormal presynaptic Ca^{2+} currents and a subnormal release of ACh quanta. In such cases, the initial reaction during continued exercise is, paradoxically, a temporary increase in force, presumably caused by Ca^{2+} accumulation inside the motor terminals, i.e. an effect of post-tetanic potentiation (see section 4.4.3). The symptoms of the Lambert–Eaton syndrome can be treated with 3,4-diaminopyridine. This drug blocks voltage-gated K^+ channels in the nerve terminals, thereby prolonging the action potential and enhancing the voltage-gated entry of Ca^{2+} into the terminal.

4.5.3. **Endplate blockers used in general surgery**

During certain types of general surgical procedures it is desirable to block NMJ transmission in order to decrease the force of disturbing (reflex) muscle contractions; one can then use lower doses of anaesthetics than would otherwise be possible. The neuromuscular blockers most commonly employed in such situations are modern versions of curare-like drugs (e.g. rocuronium and mivacurium) (Flood 2005) which have a more rapid onset of action. Curare blocks transmission simply by binding to AChR molecules without causing the ion channels to open (competitive block).

Chapter 5

Motoneurones: morphology, cytology, and topographical organization

5.1. General issues

Many aspects of neuronal function depend on structure. The synaptic input to a single nerve cell is partly determined by the extent and directions of its dendrites, and the neuronal output is highly dependent on the distribution of its axon branches. Similarly, at the level of functional neurone populations, topography often seems to be a major organizing principle within the CNS; cells with similar functions tend to lie clustered together. Much of classical neuroanatomy concerns the maps of such clusters and how they are interconnected. We are just starting to understand something about the developmental mechanisms underlying such topographical CNS maps; very early during embryonic development, the topographical position of a cell will often determine its future fate and functional tasks (cf. Chapter 12, section 12.3, Fig. 12.1D).

When analysing the morphological organization of neuronal populations, we would also like to know as much as possible about the functional properties of the various cells involved. For MN pools, this can be done to an extraordinary degree using the techniques of single-cell physiology in combination with various anatomical labelling procedures. Theoretically, MN properties might possibly be deduced from molecular markers of various kinds. This chapter also includes such cytological data, and considers which aspects of MN 'personalities' might be visualized using cytological staining methods in microscopic displays.

5.2. Motoneuronal morphology

MNs of particular muscles can be stained and identified using retrograde tracing techniques (see Chapter 2, section 2.4.6). The most commonly used tracer is HRP, and the completeness of retrograde HRP staining of MN pools can be assessed by comparing counts of stained MNs with counts of efferent fibres in the respective motor nerves (counts done after degeneration of all afferent fibres (cf. Boyd and Davey 1968)). Such comparisons generally indicate that the HRP staining is incomplete to various degrees; completeness has apparently been approached with regard to the number of alpha MNs in only a few cases (e.g. Swett *et al.* 1986). The intraneuronal concentration of retrogradely transported HRP is generally too low to be used for tracing dendrites. However, when applied to single cells in greater quantities, via an intracellular microelectrode, HRP may also provide a very complete labelling of the dendrites and axons of individual

MNs (e.g. Figs. 5.3A, 5.4A, and 8.7A). Cholera toxin subunit B (CTX-B) can be used for retrograde staining of dendrites and dendrite bundles (Gramsbergen *et al.* 1996). For cell body labelling, several other alternative retrograde tracers have been employed, which are useful for multiple labelling experiments (e.g. various fluorescent compounds (Illert *et al.* 1982)).

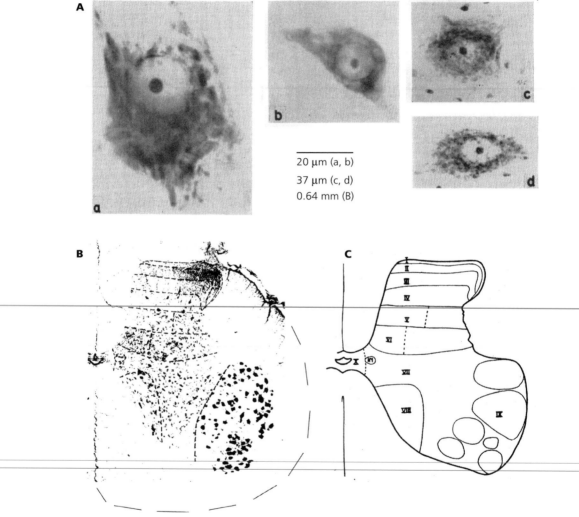

Figure 5.1 Cytoarchitectonic organization of the cat spinal cord. (**A**) Cell bodies from lamina IX of ventral horn (presumed MNs). Nissl stain, toluidine blue (a,b) or gallocyanin (c,d). (Reproduced with permission, from Rexed 1952.) (**B**) Nissl-stained lumbar segment 7, showing sizes and distribution of neuronal cell bodies. Half cross-section shown: dorsal upwards, midline to the left. Broken line, approximate outline of white matter. (**C**) Schematic drawing of lumbar segment 7 with cytoarchitectonic laminas of Rexed numbered I to IX. Lamina IX, which contains the MNs, is shown here as several round regions (one labelled, five unlabelled; cf. panel **B**). (**B**,**C** after Rexed 1954.)

5.2.1. **Cell bodies**

The cell body of a neurone may be only a small portion of its total volume, but this portion governs the rest of the cell as it contains the nucleus and the essential machinery for protein synthesis. Other neuronal portions cannot survive when isolated from the cell body. The cell bodies of spinal MNs lie in the ventral horn of the spinal cord, within lamina IX of Rexed (1952) (data from cat) (Fig. 5.1B,C). Some of the motoneuronal cell bodies are larger than those of most other spinal nerve cells; however, some other types of cell with large somas may also lie in the same spinal region (e.g. 'spinal border cells', relay cells for spinocerebellar tracts) (Cooper and Sherrington 1940). Thus, for motoneuronal counts and other quantitative estimates, a positive identification of MNs using retrograde tracing (see above)is desirable. In cross-sections, shapes of MN somas vary

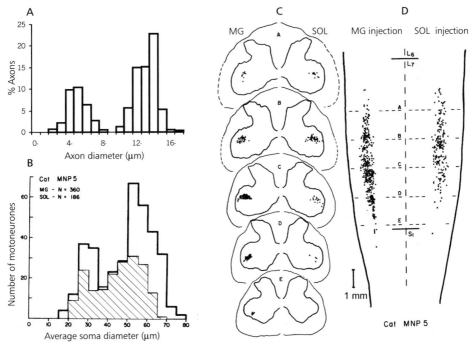

Figure 5.2 Composition and anatomy of MN pools in the cat. (**A**) Distribution of diameters of myelinated axons in nerve of medial gastrocnemius muscle after degeneration of all afferent fibres (replotted from Eccles and Sherrington (1930)). Diameters measured to the outside of the myelin sheaths. (**B**) Distribution of soma mean diameters for labelled MNs of medial gastrocnemius (MG, bold lines) and soleus (SOL, lighter lines, hatched). The MNs had become retrogradely labelled by a preceding intramuscular injection of horseradish peroxidase (HRP). (**C**), (**D**) Intraspinal distribution (dots) of the MG and SOL MNs of panel **B**, as shown in (**C**) a series of cross-sections and (**D**) a dorsal view of the spinal cord outline (white matter–pia boundary in bold lines). The broken lines across the dorsal view of the cord (**D**) denote the rostro-caudal levels at which the cross-section reconstructions (**C**) were made. Each cross-section diagram includes all labelled cells within ±300 μm of the indicated rostro-caudal level. (Reproduced with permission, from Burke *et al*. 1977.)

from rather round to elongated (Fig. 5.1A), and the projected size is typically quantified by measuring its area or, quicker but less precise, by measuring the average of its largest and smallest diameter. For descriptive purposes, it may be convenient to convert the area measurements into 'equivalent diameters', i.e. the diameter of a circle with the measured area (Zwaagstra and Kernell 1981).

For MNs of a given muscle, there is typically a bimodal distribution of the average soma diameters (Fig. 5.2B) . However, this bimodality is usually less distinct than that seen for motor axon sizes (Fig. 5.2A). For instance, in the cat gastrocnemius medialis, the group of smaller cells (mainly gamma or fusimotor neurones) apparently varied between 15 and 35 μm and the group of larger cells (the alpha or skeletomotor neurones) varied mainly between 40 and 75 μm (Fig. 5.2B) (Burke *et al.* 1977). In intracellularly labeled MNs of the cat triceps surae that had been physiologically identified as skeletomotor cells commanding muscle units, mean soma diameters usually exceed about 40 μm (Ulfhake and Kellerth 1982; Cullheim *et al.* 1987a) although smaller diameters have occasionally been observed (30 μm) (Burke *et al.* 1982). In Figure 5.5B many of the presumed alpha MNs were in the size range 30–40 μm although their axonal conduction velocities were in the alpha axon range (60 m/s or more for cat hindlimb) (Zwaagstra and Kernell 1980). The apparent overlap in mean soma diameter between alpha and gamma MNs might partly reflect the 'noisiness' of these size measurements, which are derived from two-dimensional reconstructions (area or mean diameter of projected profile) of three-dimensional structures. In small a careful study of peroneal MNs of cats, Destombes *et al.* (1992) found a bimodal distribution of soma sizes which was consistently correlated with synaptic features; synapses of type C (see Fig. 7.1C) were only present on the larger (alpha) category of MNs. In small rodents, hindlimb MNs are smaller than in the cat; cells identified as gamma MNs had mean diameters of 15–20 μm in mice and 15–35 μm in rats, whereas the total range of MN sizes reached up to 40 μm for mice and 50 μm for rats (all data for MNs of soleus muscle) (Vult von Steyern *et al.* 1999).

5.2.2. Dendrites

The typical alpha MN is a large multipolar neurone with several dendrites emerging from its cell body (Fig. 5.3A). In the lumbosacral cord of the cat, the average alpha MN has about 11–12 dendrites, and the number of dendrites is not correlated with soma size. The stem diameters of the dendrites vary between 0.5 and 19 μm, and trees often extend more than 1 mm from the soma (Fig. 5.3A) (Ulfhake and Kellerth 1981; Zwaagstra and Kernell 1981; Cullheim *et al.* 1987b; 1987a; Kernell and Zwaagstra 1989b). For comparison, in this region the maximum width of the grey matter of the ventral horn is only about 1.5-2 mm (cf. Fig. 5.1C). Many of the transversely directed dendrites have branches protruding into the white matter (Fig. 5.4A). Whether located in grey or white matter, the dendrites are covered with axon terminals from other neurones (for white matter dendrites, see Rose and Richmond (1981)).

Large as well as smaller MN cell bodies all have some thin dendrites with stem diameters of about 2 μm or less. However, the largest dendritic stems are seen in MNs with the

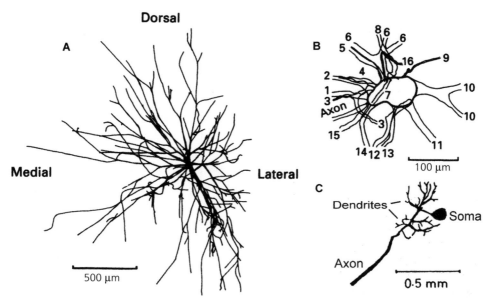

Figures 5.3 Morphology of MNs. (**A**), (**B**) Large alpha MN innervating the medial gastrocnemius muscle of a cat. Labelled by intracellular injection of HRP. (**A**) Dendrites and (**B**) soma reconstructed from serial sections and drawn as projected in a transverse plane through the spinal cord. The drawing in panel **A** represents the extent and direction (but not the diameters) of the many dendritic trees emerging from the MN. (Reproduced with permission, from Kernell and Zwaagstra 1989b.) (**c**) Typical invertebrate neurone, with the dendrites emanating from an initial portion of the axon rather than from the cell body. MN from third thoracic ganglion of cockroach (*Periplaneta americana*) stained by intracellular cobalt injection. (Reproduced with permission, from Tweedle et al. 1973, labels added.)

largest soma diameters. The total area of 'dendritic holes' in the soma membrane is almost directly proportional to soma volume; the sum of the cross-sectional areas of all dendritic stems is, on average, about 3.3 per cent of the total soma area (Zwaagstra and Kernell 1981). Dendrites with thick stems have a larger combined length and a larger total area than those with thinner stems (Fig. 5.4B,C) (Ulfhake and Kellerth 1981). Thus, in comparison with MNs with small cell bodies, those with a large soma area also have a large total dendritic area.

Dendrites typically branch in a binary manner, with one parent having two daughters (although three daughters also occur), and in a cat hindlimb MN each dendrite tends to have about 13–14 terminal branches (Table 5.1). Different dendrites have different shapes, and among lumbosacral cat MNs there is no correlation between dendritic stem diameter and the amount of dendritic area beyond a certain radial distance from the cell body (Fig. 5.4D) (Kernell and Zwaagstra 1989b). Thus, irrespectively of size, some dendrites seem specialized for collecting information close to the cell body ('close' dendrites) and others for obtaining an input from further away ('remote' dendrites). For the few MNs that have so far been measured from this point of view, these shape characteristics

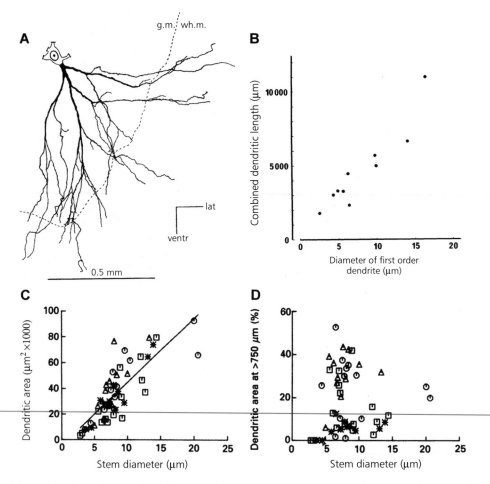

Figure 5.4 Dimensions of dendritic trees. (**A**) Transverse reconstruction of MN dendrite from L7 segment. Broken line: border between grey matter (g.m.) and white matter (wh.m.). (**B**) Evident relationship between combined dendritic length (i.e. sum of lengths of all dendritic segments) versus diameter of dendritic stems (first-order dendrites). (**A** and **B** reproduced with permission, from Ulfhake and Kellerth 1981.) (**C**), (**D**) Plots of (**C**) total dendritic area and (**D**) the percentage of this area that was located at radial distances of more than 750 μm from the cell body versus dendritic stem diameters (Same dendrites in **C** and **D**). Significant correlation in panel **C** ($r = +0.80$, $P < 0.001$), but not in panel **D** ($r = -0.08$, $P \gg 0.5$). (**C** and **D** reproduced with permission, from Kernell and Zwaagstra 1989b). All dendrites were labelled with intracellularly injected HRP and located in the cat lumbosacral spinal cord.

(degree of dendritic 'remoteness') seemed to differ systematically between different MNs of the same muscle (Kernell and Zwaagstra 1989b). Such differences in dendritic architecture might perhaps be related to 'task-associated' differences in motoneuronal activation (see Chapter 8, section 8.2.3 and 8.2.4).

Table 5.1 Mean sizes of MN soma and dendrites

Ref.	MN (species)	Soma diam. (μm)	Soma area (%)	Total MN area (μm^2 × 1000)	No. dendr. stems	Mean stem diam. (μm)	Term. per dendr.	$\Sigma(d^{1.5})/D^{1.5}$
1	GSol (cat)	51.5	1.5	558.7	11.3	6.8	14.2	1.13
2	GSol (cat)	59.3	2.3	488.4	13.0	8.4	13.1	1.19
3	GSol (rat)	35.2	2.7	151	8.0	5.3	14.6	1.11

Examples of data from complete reconstructions of single hindlimb MNs in cat (ref 1, seven cells, Cullheim *et al.* 1987a; ref 2, four cells, Kernell and Zwaagstra 1989b) and rat (ref 3, 13 cells, Chen and Wolpaw 1994). All measurements concern MNs of the triceps surae muscle complex (i.e. gastrocnemius and soleus), and the cells were reconstructed after being intracellularly labelled with HRP.

Abbreviations: diam., mean diameter; soma area (%), relative soma area in relation to total MN area (i.e. membrane area of soma plus dendrites); dendr., dendrite or dendritic; term., terminations; $\Sigma(d^{3/2})/D^{3/2}$, mean value of branch point calculations for dendritic trees, where *d* represents the daughter branch diameters and *D* is the parent diameter (for the relevance of this measurement, see Chapter 6, section 6.4.2). The calculations were performed for measurements taken close to the branching, i.e. dendritic tapering between branch points was here not taken into account. For the cat data, the soma membrane area was calculated from the mean diameter according to the formula for the surface area of a sphere (i.e. πd^2).

Table 5.1 gives examples of the dimensions of soma and dendrites in HRP-stained spinal alpha MNs from various laboratories. As can be seen, the cell body proper is, on average, responsible for less than 3 per cent of the total soma-dendritic area of a MN, i.e. the soma represents a minor portion of the total membrane area that receives the synaptic input from other cells. In comparison with alpha MNs, gamma MNs have dendrites with about the same radial extent, but the number of trees per cell is fewer and the branching pattern is simpler (Ulfhake and Cullheim 1981; Westbury 1982).

The general shape of MNs, a soma with dendrites extending in several directions (Fig. 5.3A), is similar in all vertebrates. However, invertebrates often have central nerve cells (including MNs) of a different morphology, with dendritic trees extending from the axon at some distance from the soma (Fig. 5.3C). These cell bodies are typically devoid of synapses and often are not even electrically excitable. It has been suggested that, in comparison with vertebrate multipolar neurones, the long-term properties of such invertebrate unipolar neurones might be less easily influenced by synaptic signalling (i.e. they may be less 'plastic') (Cohen 1987).

5.2.3. **Dendrite bundles**

The dendritic stems of a motoneuronal cell body emerge in all directions, sometimes without any obvious preference. However, several reports have indicated that elements of dendritic trees are often oriented in longitudinal rather than transverse intraspinal directions (Sterling and Kuypers 1967), sometimes forming distinct dendrite bundles, observed long ago in Golgi-stained preparations (Scheibel and Scheibel 1970). Such bundles also appear among retrogradely labelled MNs of certain muscles (Westerga and Gramsbergen 1992; Gramsbergen *et al*. 1996). The dendrite bundles might reflect a tendency for members of the same group of MNs to collect their incoming synapses from the same intraspinal region. MNs with different muscles and motor functions may show distinct differences in their dendritic topography, for example MNs of trapezius versus neighbouring dorsal neck muscle MNs (Vanner and Rose 1984) and MNs of jaw closers versus openers (Moritani *et al*. 2003).

Gap junctions, characteristic of electrical connections, have been noted between neighbouring dendrites in dendrite bundles (van der Want *et al*. 1998). These junctions might represent remnants of the ubiquitous connections of this kind between neighbouring neurones in embryonic spinal cords, then presumably serving as bridges for molecular communication between the cells (trophic interactions?). It is not known whether the gap junctions are of any importance for the electrophysiological properties of adult mammalian MNs with dendrite bundles (cf. effects of axotomy on gap junctions but not on electrical coupling, as seen from the soma (Chang *et al*. 2000)). Normally, discharges of mammalian limb MNs are not strongly synchronized, and little direct evidence has been found for an effective electrical coupling between different individual MNs in the mammalian spinal cord. Only weak and shortlasting interactions have been observed (Nelson 1966; Gogan *et al*. 1977); however, such effects might partly have reflected the influence of extracellular field potentials. Direct electrotonic interactions seem more prominent between MNs of external eye muscles (Gogan *et al*. 1974).

5.2.4. **Central axons and their collaterals**

The single axon of a MN generally takes off from the soma. Axons of most lumbosacral cat MNs give off one to five collaterals before leaving the spinal cord (Cullheim and Kellerth 1978b). These collaterals and their targets are further described in Chapter 8, section 8.5.1. Some classes of MNs lack axon collaterals (e.g. MNs of short plantar muscles (Cullheim and Kellerth 1978b)). Peripheral (motor) axons have been dealt with in Chapter 2, section 2.4 and Chapter 3, section 3.7.

5.2.5. **Central motoneurone morphology versus target type**

As one might intuitively expect, there is a positive correlation between axonal size or conduction velocity and soma size (e.g. mean diameter (Fig. 5.5A)) (Cullheim 1978; Kernell and Zwaagstra 1981). Thus, large MNs indeed tend to have large axons. This means that, on average, one would expect MNs of slow units to have a smaller soma than those of fast units (Chapter 3, section 3.7.3). Such differences in mean size have been noted when comparing MNs of fast and slow heads of triceps surae (Fig. 5.2B) (Burke *et al*. 1977; Ulfhake and Kellerth 1982), but when compared within the same muscle the degree of overlap between soma sizes of F and S MNs may be very large and a significant difference is not always found (Burke *et al*. 1982; Ulfhake and Kellerth 1982). However, when the size of the dendrites is also taken into account, as indicated by the number and diameters

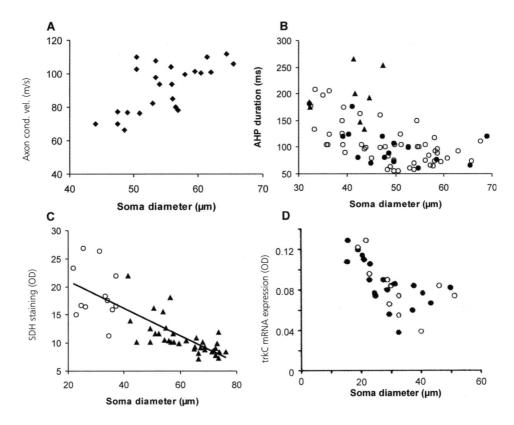

Figure 5.5 MN properties with relation to MN soma size. (**A**) Axonal conduction velocity (m/s) versus mean diameter of MN cell bodies in cat spinal cord ($r = +0.673$, $n = 24$, $P < 0.001$). MNs of cat sciatic nerve labelled with intracellularly injected HRP. (Reproduced with permission, from Cullheim 1978.) (**B**) Duration of afterhyperpolarization (AHP) versus diameter of cell body for eight MNs of the soleus muscle (filled triangles), 16 MNs of the triceps surae (filled circles), and 52 MNs of other cat hindlimb nerves (open circles). All cells had axonal conduction velocities exceeding 60 m/s. (After Zwaagstra and Kernell 1980.) (**C**) Staining intensity for succinate dehydrogenase (SDH, measured as optical density (OD), %)) versus soma diameter for neurones from ventral horn regions corresponding to the MN pools for cat peroneal muscles. Regression line calculated by the method of least squares for all values of the plot ($r = -0.80$, $P < 0.001$). Filled triangles, presumed alpha MNs ($>40\ \mu m$); open circles, possibly (largely) gamma MNs ($<40\ \mu m$). (Data from Donselaar *et al.* 1986.) (**D**) Level of expression of mRNA (non-radioactive *in situ* hybridization) for neurotrophin trkC receptor versus mean soma diameter in rat MNs innervating the slow soleus (filled circles) or the fast extensor digitorum longus (open circles). The MNs were identified, in adjacent serial sections, by retrograde labelling with HRP injected into the respective muscles. Levels of mRNA expression were quantified using measurements of optical density (OD) in juxtanuclear regions of cytoplasm. There was significant negative correlation between the level of trkC receptor mRNA expression and the soma diameter ($r = -0.73$, $n = 30$, $P < 0.001$). (Reproduced with permission, from Copray and Kernell 2000.)

of the dendritic stems, FF and FR MNs turn out to be significantly larger than the S MNs (Burke *et al.* 1982; Ulfhake and Kellerth 1982). In such comparisons of calculated total surface area, FF MNs may even be significantly larger than the FR MNs even though these two types of MN have nearly the same soma size (Burke *et al.* 1982; Ulfhake and Kellerth 1982) and axonal conduction velocity (Burke *et al.* 1973; Kernell and Monster 1981; Zengel *et al.* 1985). Furthermore, dendrite bundles are characteristic of MNs of muscles with pronounced postural tasks, which have a high percentage of type I fibres (e.g. rat soleus but not tibialis anterior) (Westerga and Gramsbergen 1992; Gramsbergen *et al.* 1996). Physiologically, the relative 'slowness' of a MN is indicated by the duration of its post-spike after-hyperpolarization (AHP) (Chapter 6, sections 6.9.3.2 and 6.9.3.3). When using this criterion, 'slow' MNs with long-lasting AHPs tend to be small whereas 'fast ' MNs may have widely varying sizes (Fig. 5.5B) (Zwaagstra and Kernell 1980).

5.3. **Motoneuronal cytology and cell biology**

Of course, MNs share basic biochemical properties with many central neurones of other types. In this section, special attention will be given to biochemical *differences* between different kinds of MNs, or between MNs and other neurones.

5.3.1. **Energy metabolism, protein synthesis, and related enzymes**

Like most neurones, MNs have a very active energy metabolism, which is needed for the maintenance of various ionic transmembrane concentration gradients (including Na^+, K^+, Cl^-, Ca^{2+}) and the resting membrane potential, for the generation of action potentials, for synaptic functions, and for their high level of protein synthesis (Attwell and Iadecola 2002). Among neurones in general, large differences are known to exist in their provisions for oxidative metabolism, with more active neurones tending to have higher activities of key enzymes such as succinate dehydrogenase (SDH) or cytochrome oxidase (COX). Among spinal MNs, differences exist in their activity for oxidative enzymes, and such differences are present across populations of alpha MNs that innervate the same muscle or muscle group (Campa and Engel 1970b, 1973; Sickles and Oblak 1984; Donselaar *et al.* 1986; Chalmers and Edgerton 1989; Ishihara *et al.* 1995). Large ventral horn cells within the alpha MN size range tend to have a consistently low oxidative enzyme activity whereas in small alpha MNs the activity may be high or low (e.g. SDH measurements (Fig. 5.5C)). The activity of oxidative enzymes tends to be even higher for gamma MNs (i.e. the very smallest MNs) than for MNs in the alpha size range. As might be expected, small MNs with a high SDH activity also have a high density of mitochondria (Ishihara *et al.* 1997a). Surprisingly, in MNs of the zebra fish the ratio of COX to SDH is systematically different for fast and slow MNs (high for fast, lower for slow MNs) (van Raamsdonk *et al.* 1987).

No relation between MN size and SDH activity was found for muscles which were almost completely composed of fast-type IIb fibres (rat bulbocavernosus or levator ani) (Ishihara *et al.* 1997b). Thus the differences in oxidative enzyme activity might be less closely related to neuronal size as such than to the motor tasks of the various MNs. The differences in SDH activity might be (partly) related to the fact that the small MNs of slow muscle units are active during longer accumulated periods per day than are larger MNs of faster units (Chapter 8, section 8.2.5). Differences in the relative level of protein synthesis may be less important as causes for differences in oxidative enzymes, because these differences tend to be more marked for dendritic than somatic regions (Wong-Riley 1989).

Unfortunately, differences in SDH activity are too imprecise to be used as a reliable indicator of MN type. There is still no good cytochemical marker available for this purpose. However, statistically, there are other cytochemical differences between fast and slow (large and small) MNs. For instance, enzymes involved in anaerobic metabolism apparently vary in a manner reciprocal to that for oxidative enzymes (e.g. measurements of phosphorylase activity) (Campa and Engel 1970a, 1973; Sickles and McLendon 1983). These aspects have been less well investigated and their functional relevance is intriguing; in contrast with muscle fibres, neurones (including MNs) store very little glycogen or other substrates that might be used for anaerobic energy production. Neurones are very sensitive to blocking of their oxidative metabolism, for example by restricting their oxygen supply. However, these sensitivities are markedly different for different classes of neurones: some nerve cells become irreversibly damaged already after a few minutes whereas others may survive for much longer periods of time. In the spinal cord, MNs are less sensitive to ischaemia than many of the surrounding interneurones (Gelfan and Tarlov 1963), perhaps partly because of their provision for anaerobic metabolism (Campa and Engel 1970a). Anoxia has been used as an experimental tool for the local 'denervation' of spinal MNs (Gelfan and Tarlov 1963).

5.3.2. Calcium ion homeostasis

Calcium ions play an important role in intracellular signalling, and therefore it is important to keep the resting cytoplasmic Ca^{2+} concentration low (normally at 10^{-7} M or less). Several mechanisms are used in parallel for the sequestration of Ca^{2+} ions.

1 Some Ca^{2+} ions are actively pumped out of the cell by energy-requiring transmembrane transport mechanisms, using ATP. Such transport can take place across the surface membrane (plasma membrane calcium-dependent ATPase (PMCA)) or across membranes of the endoplasmic reticulum (sarcoplasmic/endoplasmic reticulum calcium ATPase (SERCA)). Little or no reactivity was found when applying available antibodies against PMCA or SERCA2, to rat spinal MNs (Kernell et al. 1999).

2 Some Ca^{2+} ions are transported out of the cell by a transmembrane Na^+–Ca^{2+} exchange mechanism, with the influx of Na^+ ions 'driving' the efflux of Ca^{2+}. The molecular nature of this mechanism is still uncertain in spinal MNs. Little or no reactivity was found in MNs when applying antibodies against Na^+–Ca^{2+} exchange protein (Kernell et al. 1999).

3 Some Ca^{2+} ions are removed from the cytoplasm by being bound to buffering substances and/or being sequestered into various intracellular membrane compartments. In this context, mitochondria play an important role. Sequestration into

intracellular compartments means that, if required for signalling purposes, Ca^{2+} ions may also undergo rapid intracellular release. In rats, a high reactivity was found in spinal MNs of all sizes for antibodies to the buffer calreticulin (Copray *et al.* 1996), which is probably mainly used for Ca^{2+} binding in intracellular stores. Little or no reactivity was observed for antibodies to parvalbumin, calbindin-28K, or calsequestrin (Kernell *et al.* 1999). Parvalbumin is known to be present in certain specialized kinds of MN, such as those of external eye muscles (Alexianu *et al.* 1994). In general, the Ca^{2+} buffering of spinal MNs is kept at a low and potentially dangerous level (Lips and Keller 1998; Palecek *et al.* 1999).

5.3.3. Transmitter biochemistry

All vertebrate MNs are cholinergic. Hence MNs necessarily contain the enzymes needed for the synthesis of ACh. An important enzyme in this context is choline acetyl transferase (ChAT). Few cholinergic neurones apart from the MNs exist in the spinal cord. Thus ChAT staining is often used as a means of MN identification. The acetylcholine esterase (AChE) that is present at a neuromuscular synapse (Chapter 4, section 4.3.6) is apparently mainly synthesized in the muscle fibre and partly in the MN (Jevsek *et al.* 2004). There are several different globular and asymmetric isoforms. Like all enzymes, ChAT and AChE are proteins; they are synthesized in the cell body and transported to the nerve terminals along the axon. Thus, in (immuno-)histochemistry not only the axon terminals but also the soma and the axon have the characteristic staining properties of a cholinergic cell, demonstrating the presence of ChAT and AChE. The AChE staining in axons has been reported to be less marked for nerves of a slow muscle (soleus) than for those of faster (mixed) muscles (Gruber and Zenker 1978), and similar differences have been reported for slow (small) versus fast (large) MNs in the monkey (Odutola 1972). However, no such differences were observed for hindlimb MNs in the rat (comparison of MNs of fast extensor digitorum longus with those of slow soleus (Kernell *et al.* 1999)).

5.3.4. Neurotrophic factors

Many years ago, Levi-Montalcini and her colleagues discovered and characterized **nerve growth factor** (NGF), a peptide with dramatic effects in promoting the growth of sensory and autonomic neurones. Subsequently, several other biochemically related molecules belonging to the same family of **neurotrophins** have been discovered (reviewed by Lewin and Barde 1996): **brain-derived neurotrophic factor** (BDNF, NT2) and **neurotrophins 3, 4** and **5** (NT3, NT4, NT5). NT4 and NT5 are practically identical and treated as one entity. These various neurotrophins act on neurones via two kinds of membrane receptors: p75, a low-affinity receptor for all the neurotrophins, and tyrosine-kinase linked receptors (trk) which are specific for different neurotrophins (trk-A for NGF, trk-B for BDNF and NT4/5, and trk-C for NT3). Many of the neurotrophins have a bidirectional role in relation to the MNs; they may derive from external sources and affect MNs via membrane receptors and/or they may be synthesized and secreted by the MNs themselves, having effects on various target cells.

The neurotrophins and their receptors play important roles, both during MN development and in adults, promoting cell survival and mediating various cellular interactions including 'trophic functions' (see Chapter 11, section 11.4.6). Because of their low concentrations, these peptides might be difficult to visualize directly using immunohistochemistry. The expression of their mRNA can be shown using the very sensitive technique of *in situ* hybridization. Interestingly, such studies demonstrate that there is differential expression across individual MN pools with regard to many of these molecules. The functional significance of most of these differences is still unknown. Although neighbouring individual MNs may differ very much in their mRNA expression for BDNF, NT3, NT4/5, and trk-B receptors (Buck *et al.* 2000; Copray and Kernell 2000), no consistent differences have been found between the MNs of different soma size or between cells of predominantly fast versus slow muscles (rat extensor digitorum longus versus soleus) (Copray and Kernell 2000). mRNA expression for the trk-C receptor was significantly higher for small (presumed gamma MNs) than for larger cells (Fig. 5.5D) (Copray and Kernell 2000; Simon *et al.* 2002). The trk-C receptor is specific for NT3, which is a neurotrophin with a high concentration in intrafusal muscle fibres (Copray and Brouwer 1994), i.e. structures innervated by gamma MNs. A differential expression of trk-C mRNA has also been observed for alpha MNs; the expression was then greater for MNs of a fast muscle (extensor digitorum longus) than for those of a slow muscle (soleus) (Simon *et al.* 2002). The low-affinity receptor p75 and its mRNA are normally not expressed in adult spinal MNs, but only during early embryonic development or under pathological conditions (Copray *et al.* 2003).

5.3.5. Other trophic and/or signalling substances

MNs exert trophic effects on other cells using substances that are synthesized in the MNs themselves. In addition to the neurotrophins (see above), a well-known representative of this group is the **calcitonin gene related peptide** (CGRP). As shown in immunohistochemistry, this peptide and its mRNA are differently expressed for individual MNs in the same pool and, although the variability is large in all MN pools, CGRP-like reactivity is more often lacking in MNs with small and slow muscle units than in those with large and fast units (Piehl *et al.* 1993). However, the variability is great within predominantly slow as well as within predominantly fast MN pools (Piehl *et al.* 1993; Kernell *et al.* 1999), and no significant correlations were found versus the staining for AChE or SDH (Kernell *et al.* 1999). Expression of CGRP increases after axotomy (Caldero *et al.* 1992; Piehl *et al.* 1993), probably while the neurone is sending out new collaterals from its axon (Tarabal *et al.* 1996). In the motor nerve terminals, CGRP is stored in large dense core vesicles (Matteoli *et al.* 1988), and there is evidence indicating that it is released by nerve impulses (Sala *et al.* 1995). In muscle fibres, CGRP has been shown to induce AChR expression (Fontaine *et al.* 1986) and to modify the properties of existing AChR channels (Eusebi *et al.* 1988; Mulle *et al.* 1988; Lu *et al.* 1993).

Other MN-derived substances with a 'trophic' effect on neuromuscular junctions include Agrin and ARIA (see Chapter 4, section 4.2.2). Furthermore, MNs apparently secrete several other substances with long-term effects on muscle properties, including compounds with an anti-atrophic effect (see Chapter 11, section 11.3.6.1).

5.3.6. Homeobox and other differentiation genes and their products

The main identifying (and defining) property of MNs is that their axons leave the CNS and innervate skeletal muscle fibres. During embryonic development, the choice of peripheral targets is regulated by a separate class of organizing genes belonging to the homeobox family. This class of genes was first studied in the fruit fly (*Drosophila*), and it has analogous body-field organizing tasks in widely different animal species, including mammals (Alberts *et al.* 2002).

During initial stages of development (and often later on as well), particular transcription factors of the homeodomain family, such as Islet-1, are expressed in MNs of both the muscular and vegetative systems (i.e. preganglionic autonomic cells). This makes Islet-1 and other homeodomain transcription factors important tools for the cytochemical identification of MNs within the CNS (for further comments on homeobox genes and their functions, see Chapter 12, section 12.4). Vult von Steyern *et al.* (1999) found expression of both Islet-1 and HB9 in adult rat MNs; the staining intensity was variable but no unique combination of expression was found per MN type (slow versus fast hindlimb muscle, alpha versus gamma MNs).

5.4. Motoneurone populations innervating different muscles and muscle fibres

5.4.1. Muscle identity and the intraspinal distribution of motoneurone cell bodies

When classical methods of neuroanatomy, such as Nissl staining (Fig. 5.1A,B), are used, cell bodies are by far the most easily visualized portion of a neurone. The soma represents only a tiny (but biochemically essential) portion of the synaptically receptive surface of a MN (Fig. 5.3 and Table 5.1). However, the cell body will generally be rather centrally placed within the 'receptive field' of a MN (Cullheim *et al.* 1987b), i.e. maps of cell body distributions also show roughly how the total soma-dendritic fields are localized for the respective MNs. The topographical organization of MNs is of interest from a very general and functional point of view because, during embryonic development, the position of a MN determines its future innervation target and central connections and hence its motor functions (see Chapter 12, section 12.6).

In the spinal cord, MN cell bodies occupy a substantial portion of the ventral horn of the grey matter (lamina IX according to Rexed (1952)) (Fig. 5.1C). There is a continuous string of motor cells throughout the whole length of the cord. This string becomes thicker at the cervical and lumbar widening of the cord (**intumescence**), i.e. for the regions innervating the extremities. In experimental animals, the oldest method for the differential labelling of MNs innervating different muscles was based on the changes visible by light microscopy that occur in MN cell bodies after transection of their axon

(**chromatolysis**) (Chapter 10, section 10.2.1). These methods were used in several laboratories, and a particularly useful and detailed map of lumbosacral MNs of the cat was
produced by Romanes (1951), demonstrating the relative intraspinal positions for MNs
innervating different limb muscles. His results were largely confirmed and expanded by
later investigators using modern retrograde tracing techniques (Fig. 5.2C,D). One of the
most extensive studies of this type is that by Vanderhorst and Holstege (1997b). There
are characteristic lengthwise as well as transverse differences in the positions of MNs
belonging to different muscles. Many MN pools are longer than one spinal segment;
hence their axons emerge through two or three adjacent ventral roots. Because of
changes in the absolute position of the spinal cord in relation to the vertebrae, the precise
exit roots may vary by ±1 vertebral segment between animals; the MN pool position
versus the cord intumescence is more reproducible (Vanderhorst and Holstege 1997b).
The relative positions of MNs destined for different limb muscles have been mapped for
various vertebrate species, for example chick (Landmesser 1978), mouse (McHanwell
and Biscoe 1981), and rat (Nicolopoulos-Stournaras and Iles 1983).

In the transverse plane (cross-sections) MNs of proximal muscles (e.g. gluteus) tend to
lie ventral to more distal ones (e.g. intrinsic foot muscles), and MNs of anterior muscles
(e.g. tibialis anterior) lie lateral to more posterior ones (e.g. triceps surae). Axial muscles
of the trunk lie in the most medial corner of the ventral horn (not represented in the low
lumbar segment of Fig. 5.1). Within each of such rather coarse groupings, there is no
clear difference in transverse localization of MNs belonging to different muscles.
However, within each such group, the transverse range of possible variation is very
limited, being less than the total dendritic width of a single cell (cf. Figs 5.1B and 5.2C
compared with Fig. 5.3A). The extent of the MN pools in the lengthwise direction is
much greater and differences are more clearly observable, and the MNs of close synergists may also show reproducible differences (with, typically, a substantial overlap) in
their cranio-caudal extent. Thus, for instance, within triceps surae the MNs of gastrocnemius lateralis occur up to much more rostral levels than those of gastrocnemius
medialis or soleus.

The topographical organization for cranial MNs is rather different; these cells are not
localized within a continuous rostro-caudal motor column but occur in discrete cell
accumulations (**nuclei**), separately for each cranial nerve. Within each cranial nucleus,
MNs of different muscles or muscle groups typically have topographicaly distinct localizations. Examples include the MNs of the facial muscles (cranial nerve VII: rat (Martin
et al. 1977; Aldskogius and Thomander 1986); rat and rabbit (Furutani *et al.* 2004)) and
the hypoglossal MNs innervating the tongue (cranial nerve XII (Uemura *et al.* 1979;
McClung and Goldberg 1999)). A highly specialized group of MNs are those of muscles
moving the eyes. These **extraocular MNs** are collected into the oculomotor (cranial
nerve III), trochlear (cranial nerve IV) and abducens (cranial nerve VI) nuclei in the
brainstem, and many studies have been made of their topographical organization in
different species. Interestingly, some of the extraocular muscles may be (partly or
completely) innervated by contralateral MNs (superior rectus, superior oblique)
(Akagi 1978; Glicksman 1980; Augustine *et al.* 1981; Murphy *et al.* 1986; Evinger *et al.* 1987).

The eyelid muscle (levator palpebrae superioris) may have an ipsilateral, contralateral, or bilateral innervation: cat, bilateral (Akagi 1978); rat, bilateral (Glicksman 1980); baboon, ipsilateral (Augustine *et al.* 1981); guinea pig, contralateral (Gomez Segade and Labandeira Garcia 1983; Evinger *et al.* 1987).

5.4.2. Intraspinal sites of MN cell bodies versus intramuscular sites of their muscle units

In most of cases which have been carefully investigated, a relationship has been found between the cranio-caudal position of MNs within the spinal cord and the position of their muscle fibres within the target muscle; examples include cat medial gastrocnemius (Swett *et al.* 1970), rat gluteus maximus (Brown and Booth 1983), rat biceps brachii and pectoralis minor (Bennett and Lavidis 1984), cat tibialis anterior (Iliya and Dum 1984), cat peroneus longus (Fig. 5.6) (Donselaar *et al.* 1985), cat lateral gastrocnemius (Weeks and English 1985), rat diaphragm and serratus anterior (Laskowski and Sanes 1987), and rat extensor digitorum longus (Balice-Gordon and Thompson 1988). Because of the variety of techniques used and muscles studied, it is still too early for a conclusion to be drawn as to the precise general rules for these correspondences, partly because muscle

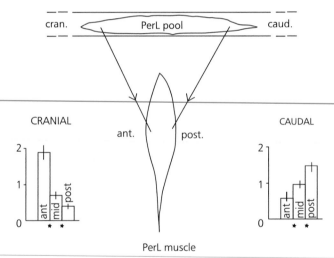

Figure 5.6 Intraspinal position of MNs versus intramuscular sites of innervation. Relevant ventral roots were subdivided into rostro-caudally distinct subfilaments. In each cat, one subfilament was chosen for stimulation to exhaust its muscle fibres of glycogen. Insets show normalized data indicating the relative numbers of depleted fibres in different muscle portions (anterior, middle, posterior) after stimulation of cranial (left) and caudal (right) ventral root filaments, respectively. Bars are means ± S.E. ($n = 9$ muscle sections per bar), and asterisks indicate the presence of statistically significant differences between adjoining mean values (*t* test, $P < 0.05$). The results demonstrate that cranial MNs preferentially innervated anterior PerL portions, and vice versa. (Insets reproduced with permission, from Donselaar *et al.* 1985.) (Reproduced with permission, from Kernell 1992.)

architecture and the lengthwise distribution of the muscle fibres have not yet been included in these considerations. Some muscles may not show the cord versus muscle kind of topographical correspondence (e.g. cat tensor fasciae latae (Gordon *et al.* 1991a); rabbit soleus muscle (Cramer and Van-Essen 1995)). In the latter case the authors suggested that the absence of a cord–muscle topography might be related to the absence of neuromuscular partitioning (see Chapter 3, section 3.7.1). However, in the rat lateral gastrocnemius Bennett and Ho (1988) found a topographical relationship between spinal cord and muscle for the MNs of a single compartment.

5.4.3. Intraspinal position of MN cell bodies innervating different muscle fibre types

As described in Chapter 3, section 3.6.2, muscles are generally more or less regionalized with regard to the topographical distribution of different muscle fibre types. If this regionalization occurred along the same axis as the relationship between MN soma position and intramuscular unit position (see above), MNs of different muscle unit types would, of course, be expected to be differentially located in the cord. Such cases have been described (Grow *et al.* 1996). Typically, however, consistent relationships of this kind are rare. Within individual hindlimb MN pools of the cat spinal cord, no strong and generally reproducible relationship was found for cranio-caudal position versus soma size (plantaris and gastrocnemius medialis) (Clamann and Kukulka 1977), and MNs of different sizes and muscle unit properties were very widely intermingled at all levels of the pool (peroneus longus) (Kernell *et al.* 1985).

5.5. Pathophysiological issue: vulnerability of large versus small motoneurones

Statistically speaking, alpha MNs of different sizes often tend to innervate different types of muscle fibres, although with a variable degree of overlap (see section 5.2.5), and they show a number of appropriate differences in their functional properties and normal behaviour (see Chapter 6, section 6.9, and Chapter 8, section 8.2). Hence it is of general physiological interest that, in several different contexts, alpha MNs of varying sizes also show a differential vulnerability, almost always such that large MNs are more easily killed than the smaller ones. This has been reported for poliomyelitis (Chapter 10, section 10.6.2; see also Hodes 1949; Hodes *et al.* 1949), motoneurone disease (amyotrophic lateral sclerosis) (Chapter 6, section 6.10; see also Sobue *et al.* 1983), spinal cord injury (Thomas and Grumbles 2005; Thomas and Zijdewind 2006), and normal ageing (Chapter 12, section 12.12; see also Hashizume *et al.* 1988). It is not known whether the greater vulnerability of large MNs has something to do with their particular physiological tasks (e.g. stress caused by the maintenance of many axon terminals and target cells) and/or with the soma size itself (e.g. smaller membrane area relative to cell volume and thus possibly more difficult removal of undesirable ions and substances) and/or with yet other factors.

Chapter 6

Motoneurones: electrophysiology

6.1. General issues

Spinal MNs were among the first central neurones to be investigated with intracellular microelectrodes (Brock *et al.* 1952; Eccles 1957) and, compared with other types of nerve cell, much is known about their activation properties and the manner in which these characteristics are matched to those of the innervated target cells, the various types of skeletal muscle fibres. Unless specified otherwise, the findings summarized below concern spinal MNs from the adult cat, as studied using sharp microelectrodes.

6.2. Motoneurone action potentials: regional differences in excitability

In anaesthetized animals, good intracellular recordings from the soma of spinal cord MNs tend to show steady membrane potentials of around -70 mV (Eccles 1957). The major component of the MN action potential is a rapid positive-going voltage transient, often referred to as a **spike** (Fig. 6.1A). The term 'action potential' is sometimes used as a synonym for 'spike' (as is done in this book), and sometimes it is thought to comprise the spike as well as the after-potentials (see below). Under optimal recording conditions the MN spike may have an amplitude of about 80–90 mV, and it typically shows an **overshoot**, i.e. it briefly reaches positive values of membrane potential. Its duration is about 1–2 ms and it shows a more or less evident break on its rising phase (Fig. 6.1A, IS–SD). If the resting membrane potential is made more negative (hyperpolarized), this break may become accentuated and the upper (later) portion of the spike may become blocked, leaving a smaller spike of only about 30–40 mV (Fig. 6.1A, IS). Experimental evidence has indicated that this remaining spike portion, the **initial-segment spike** (**IS spike**) is generated close to the beginning of the axon. The later portion of the full spike, the **soma-dendrite spike** (**SD spike**) represents the subsequent activation of the soma-dendrite membrane. This spike sequence is seen not only for **antidromic** MN activation (stimulating a ventral root or motor nerve) (Fig. 6.1A), but also when activating the MN synaptically (**orthodromic** activation) (Coombs *et al.* 1955). Because of topographical differences in membrane properties, mainly differences in density of Na^+ ion channels (Dodge and Cooley 1973; Safronov *et al.* 2000), the electrical excitability is higher in the IS region than elsewhere. Because of this arrangement, synaptic effects from both remote dendritic synapses and the soma itself will all be summed at one 'comparison point' near the beginning of the axon (axon hillock or initial unmyelinated segment).

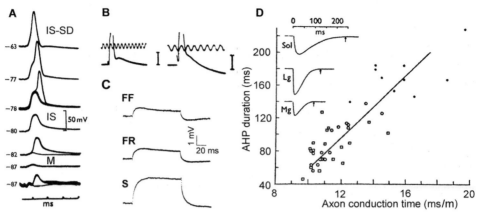

Figure 6.1 Basic electrophysiological MN properties. (**A**) Intracellular responses evoked from a cat lumbar MN by antidromic stimulation while resting membrane potential was held at different levels with injected current (see lefthand labels mV). Block of different spike components at progressively greater hyperpolarization. The lowest record was taken after the amplification had been increased by a factor of 4.5 and the stimulus had been decreased until it was just at threshold for exciting the axon of the motoneurone, showing the M spike. (Reproduced with permission, from Coombs *et al.* 1955.) (**B**) Intracellular recording of the depolarizing after-potential (delayed depolarization) following an antidromic spike in two different MNs of cat spinal cord. Spikes truncated. Calibration 10 mV; time mark 1000 Hz. (Reproduced with permission, from Kernell 1964). (**C**) Membrane potential transients produced by 1 nA step of injected current in cat MNs with different types of muscle units (gastrocnemius medialis) (Reproduced with permission, from Zengel *et al.* 1985.) (**D**) Plot of duration of AHP (ms) versus the time required for conduction along 1 m of the corresponding motor axon (ms/m) in MNs of cat triceps surae. The duration of AHP is longer for cat MNs of slow hindlimb muscles (soleus: Sol, filled circles) than for those with faster contractions (lateral and medial gastrocnemius: Lg and Mg, open symbols). Furthermore, AHPs tend to be longer in MNs with slowly conducting axons than in those with faster axons. In the inset curves of AHPs the arrows indicate the points at which measurements were made. (Reproduced with permission, from Eccles *et al.* 1958a.)

In neonatal MNs, the measured density of Na^+ channels in the soma is often so low that it has even been doubted whether cell bodies of spinal neurones are capable of generating action potentials (Safronov *et al.* 2000). Model calculations have shown that the second spike component, the SD spike, might be an 'axon hillock spike', emerging in cells lacking active spike generation in soma and dendrites (Safronov *et al.* 2000); for calculations on these matters, see also Dodge and Cooley (1973) and Moore *et al.* (1983). A similar topographical differentiation of voltage thresholds appears to be common among neurones of various other kinds, and TTX-labelled Na^+ channels have then indeed been shown to occur in higher densities around the initial portion of the axon than elsewhere (for references, see Safronov *et al.* 2000). Although the established term 'SD spike' will continue to be used in this text for the second spike component of MNs, it should be realized that the membrane supporting it might be that of the axon hillock only, perhaps in combination with spike responses in the dendrites (see below).

Because of the high input resistance of thin dendritic branches, it is likely that local EPSPs might become very large within remote portions of dendritic trees. However, there is no evidence for spikes evoked locally within the dendrites in normal MNs studied *in situ* (cf. different observations in axotomized MNs (Chapter 10, section 10.2.5)). Thus, for distant dendrites of MNs the voltage threshold for the generation of action potentials is probably very high compared with that of the cell body or the initial segment. However, it is still uncertain how far into the dendrites the SD spike is normally conducted and how the electrical excitability is distributed within the dendrites. This is a matter of some importance for understanding how MNs process synaptic information (e. g. Kernell 1971). In organotypic tissue culture, this question has been studied for rat ventral horn cells (presumed MNs) using voltage-sensitive dyes and local patch-electrode recordings (Larkum *et al.* 1996). These experiments demonstrated an active back-propagation of Na^+-dependent spikes along initial portions of the dendrites, sometimes with little or no decrement over distances >100 μm. Furthermore, these dendritic spikes were associated with a substantial amount of Ca^{2+} entry.

When analysed using voltage clamp electrodes in the soma, the MN membrane shows a time and voltage dependence of currents that is qualitatively similar to those of the axon; there is a transient inward Na^+ current and a non-inactivating outward K^+ current with a higher threshold and slower onset (Barrett and Crill 1980). Furthermore, at membrane potentials just below the voltage threshold for evoking a spike in these cells from adult cats, there was little inactivation of the transient Na^+ current. However, in experiments on MNs from neonatal rats, a substantial degree of $I_{Na,t}$ inactivation was seen at threshold membrane potentials (Safronov and Vogel 1995). Details of the various voltage-dependent ion channels of the soma-dendrite MN membrane will be discussed further below (section 6.8).

6.3. **Depolarizing and hyperpolarizing after-potentials**

For a MN in good condition, the SD spike is followed by a depolarizing after-potential (Fig. 6.1B), an 'after-depolarization' or 'delayed depolarization' (DD), which may be smoothly declining or display a more or less distinct hump (Brock *et al.* 1952; Granit *et al.* 1963c; Kernell 1964; Nelson and Burke 1967). After antidromic spikes evoked at resting potential, the DD of a mammalian spinal MN is almost never preceded by a truly hyperpolarizing dip, i.e. under these conditions there is typically no 'fast' after-hyperpolarization (fAHP) of the type evident in, for example, turtle MNs (Hounsgaard *et al.* 1988b). In MNs which show signs of deterioration (run-down or technically bad penetration) the DD may be absent. Following an antidromic spike, the DD may last up to about 5–10 ms before it merges into the after-hyperpolarization, and its amplitude may come close to about 10 mV, i.e. it may approach the voltage threshold for eliciting a spike. The DD depends strongly on Ca^{2+} currents which enter the cell via low-voltage activated (LVA) Ca^{2+} channels (Harada and Takahashi 1983; Umemiya and Berger 1994); it is blocked by replacing external Ca^{2+} with Mn^{2+} (Harada and Takahashi 1983). In addition, capacitive currents from the dendrites appear to make an important contribution to the shape and time course of the DD (Barrett *et al.* 1980). Dendritic recordings in tissue culture have shown large post-spike after-depolarizations associated with Ca^{2+} entry (Larkum *et al.* 1996). A dendritic origin of part of the DD was also suggested by the finding that its amplitude could be influenced by synaptic inputs without any clear relation to shifts of membrane potential (Kernell 1964).

The DD is followed by a more prolonged hyperpolarizing potential, the after-hyperpolarization (AHP) (Fig. 6.1D) (Brock *et al.* 1952; Eccles 1957). In recent neurophysiological literature, this type of after-potential is often referred to as a medium duration after-hyperpolarization (mAHP) to differentiate it from the brief AHP that is sometimes associated with the repolarization of the spike (fAHP; see above) and the much longer hyperpolarizations that may follow trains of repetitive spikes in many types of neurone (slow AHP (sAHP), post-tetanic AHP) (McLarnon 1995; Sah 1996; Sah and Faber 2002). sAHPs have not been well studied in mammalian spinal MNs (cf. suggested absence of sAHP after bursts of SD spikes in hypoglossal MNs (Powers *et al.* 1999)). In this book, the simple term AHP will continue to be used to signify the prolonged after-hyperpolarization following single MN spikes.

As measured from the onset of the spike, the AHP of cat spinal MNs reaches its peak at about 10–20 ms and has a total duration of about 50–200 ms (Figs. 5.5B and 6.1D, and Table 6.1) (Eccles *et al.* 1958a; Kernell 1965c). The amplitude of the AHP becomes larger when a cell is depolarized and smaller when it is hyperpolarized, and the apparent equilibrium potential for the current at the AHP peak is close to -90 mV, i.e. close to the equilibrium potential for K^+ ions (Coombs *et al.* 1955). There are other indications that this current is carried by K^+ ions; for instance, AHP becomes smaller if the external K^+ concentration is increased (Viana *et al.* 1993). This K^+ conductance is not itself voltage

Table 6.1 Basic motoneurone properties

Type	I_{rh} (nA)	R_{in} (MΩ)	τ_m (ms)	AHP_d (ms)	AHP_h (ms)	AHP_a (mV)	TwCT (ms)	CV (m/s)
Cat GM								
FF	21.3	0.6	5.9	65	18	3.0	27	101
Fint	16.8	0.7	5.3	63	17	2.8	26	104
FR	12.0	0.9	8.0	78	22	4.3	26	103
S	5.0	1.6	10.4	161	44	4.9	62	89
Rat GM								
F	5.7	1.8		54	11	2.1	16	62
S	1.8	3.3		75	18	3.7	23	54

Mean values for various electrophysiological parameters of different types of cat and rat hindlimb MNs.

Abbreviations: GM, gastrocnemius medialis muscle; I_{rh}, rheobase, i.e. threshold current for single spike; R_{in}, input resistance; τ_m, membrane time constant; AHP, after-hyperpolarization; AHP_d, total duration; AHP_h, half decay time (from peak to half-peak amplitude); AHP_a, peak amplitude; TwCT, twitch contraction time; CV, axonal conduction velocity.

Cat data from Zengel *et al.* (1985) and, for TwCT and CV, from Fleshman *et al.* (1981). Rat data from Bakels and Kernell (1993b).

dependent, but is activated by Ca^{2+} ions which enter the cell via voltage-dependent channels (Krnjevic *et al.* 1978; Harada and Takahashi 1983; Viana *et al.* 1993). The calcium-dependent K^+ conductance channels ($g_{K,Ca}$) of the AHP are blocked with apamin and belong to the category of SK channels (Sah 1996; Sah and Faber 2002), which are typically activated by Ca^{2+} ions entering via high-voltage activated (HVA) channels of the N and P type (Viana *et al.* 1993; Umemiya and Berger 1994; Sah 1996). These Ca^{2+} channels are pharmacologically distinct from the LVA g_{Ca} channels that are reponsible for the appearance of the DD (Umemiya and Berger 1994). The duration of the AHP is believed to depend mainly on the speed of sequestration of Ca^{2+} ions (Sah 1996); the possible influence of slow kinetics of this $g_{K,Ca}$ channel itself is unclear. In addition, the duration of AHP may be influenced by membrane non-linearities caused by other voltage-dependent permeabilities ('voltage sag') (Gustafsson and Pinter 1985a).

The after-potentials described above (DD, AHP) are associated with the SD spike; no such after-potentials are seen after IS or axon spikes (Coombs *et al.* 1955). These after-potentials, and in particular the AHP, are very important for the repetitive discharge properties of a MN (see below). Thus when a MN is activated synaptically and IS spikes are triggered from the initial axon segment, it is functionally important that these spikes are conducted towards the soma and dendrites as well as towards the muscle fibres in the periphery. Without the 'back-projection' of the IS spikes, triggering SD spikes and after-potentials, MNs would not maintain their normal integrative properties.

6.4. Voltage responses to subthreshold steps of injected current

6.4.1. Input resistance and voltage 'sag'

Figure 6.1C shows examples of the voltage responses to a small intensity of steady injected depolarizing current (1 nA in all three cases). Particularly for the upper record (FF MN), there is a slow 'sag' of voltage following the peak depolarization at around 10–20 ms (Ito and Oshima 1965). A weak hyperpolarizing current delivers a mirror image of these voltage changes. Furthermore, the off-transients look similar to mirror images of the on-transients. Such **voltage sag** behaviour is due to a complex combination of voltage- and time-dependent conductances (cf. Table 6.2); similar behaviour is seen in neocortical cells in which the underlying currents have been analysed in detail (Stafstrom *et al.* 1984).

If voltage is plotted against current for transients like those of Fig. 6.1C, one typically obtains a linear relationship over a wide range of subthreshold membrane potentials. The slope of this relationship gives the apparent input resistance of the MN, by analogy with Ohm's law. For cells with a voltage sag, the value for the apparent input resistance is higher for measurements at the peak of the transient than in the steady state (i.e. at about 10–20 ms compared with 60–80 ms for the upper record in Fig. 6.1C). The input resistance is an important measure of MN excitability: the higher the resistance, the less current is needed for depolarizing the cell to the threshold for spike discharge. In cat spinal MNs, the input resistance varies mainly over the range 0.5–5 MΩ i.e. an input conductance range of 2–0.2 μS (cf. Fig. 6.6A and Table 6.1)

(Coombs *et al.* 1955; Kernell 1966a; Burke and ten Bruggencate 1971; Fleshman *et al.* 1981; Kernell and Zwaagstra 1981; Gustafsson and Pinter 1984c).

6.4.2. Passive on- and off-transients in cells provided with dendrites

A current step causes an initially faster voltage transient when applied to the end of a cable than when uniformly applied to a membrane (Fig. 2.2 C, thin versus thick line). MNs have very extensive dendrites (Fig. 5.3A), and, under conditions extensively explored by Rall (1960, 1977), voltage transients of such cells can be analysed as if all the dendrites were combined into a single **equivalent cable** with a constant diameter (cf. Fig. 7.3A). This can be done if all dendrites branch such that, at each branch point, $D^{3/2} = \Sigma d^{3/2}$, where D is the diameter of the parent branch and d represents the diameters of the daughter branches. Furthermore, the total electrotonic length, as expressed in space constants (see Chapter 2, section 2.4.1), should be the same for terminal branches of all dendrites. Although real MNs do not correspond exactly to such model cells (Rall *et al.* 1992), Rall's equivalent cable simplification has been of great value as an approach to the analysis of MN voltage transients.

The voltage transients that are evoked by steps of current in uniform cables can be regarded as the sum of several exponential transients with different time constants. The component time constants can be determined using simple graphical procedures of analysis such as 'peeling' procedures, often done using plots of dV/dt (for further comments see Rall 1977; Rall *et al.* 1992). The longest time constant corresponds to the conventional membrane time constant τ_m, i.e. the product $R \times C$ (Chapter 2, section 2.4.1). The membrane time constant and the second-longest time constant can be used to calculate the apparent electrotonic length of the equivalent cable (Rall 1969). When performed for cat spinal MNs, such measurements have typically given values of 2–14 ms for the membrane time constant and, on average, about 1.5λ (where λ is the space constant) for the electrotonic length of the equivalent cable (Lux *et al.* 1970; Burke and ten Bruggencate 1971; Gustafsson and Pinter 1984c; Zengel *et al.* 1985). However, with regard to the parameters needed for estimating the electrotonic length, the precision of the peeling method seems satisfactory only for cells with electrotonically relatively short dendrites. Simulations done under realistically noisy conditions suggested that this kind of analysis is unsuitable for discriminating between neurones with different dendritic lengths in excess of about 1.5–2.0λ (de Jongh and Kernell 1982). It should be realized that the extent of dendrites in terms of space constants is an electrical parameter which does not provide information about how many millimetres the dendrites actually reach from the soma.

6.4.3. Membrane resistivity: average value; soma versus dendrites

Theoretically, a value for the average **membrane resistivity** (Ω cm^2) of a MN with uniform membrane properties could be obtained in at least three different ways.

1. By measuring the **membrane time constant** of the MN and dividing that value by its specific membrane capacity, which is usually assumed to be about 1 $\mu F/cm^2$; its precise value can only be determined via other independent measurements of, for example, membrane time constant and membrane resistivity (see below). In a recent study, measurements in spinal MNs of young rats resulted in a high estimated value for membrane capacity of 2.4 ± 0.5 $\mu F/cm^2$ (Thurbon *et al.* 1998). The total input capacitance of a neurone can also be calculated from the analysis of voltage transients, and such data have been used for estimating total neuronal size (Gustafsson and Pinter 1984c; Ziskind-Conhaim 1988).

2. By measuring the **input resistance** of a MN as well as the anatomical dimensions of its soma and stem dendrites (intracellular labelling and subsequent anatomical reconstruction of the MN required). The average membrane resistivity can then be estimated using Rall's equivalent cylinder model and reasonable assumptions (Rall *et al.* 1992).

3. By measuring the **input resistance** of an intracellularly labelled MN and performing a complete anatomical reconstruction of its soma and all its dendrites. Such complete reconstructions and the associated calculations are very time consuming, but this approach gives the least ambiguous results.

The (2) and (3) kinds of measurements have frequently given values of about 1–5 $K\Omega$ cm^2 for specific membrane resistance, assuming uniform membrane properties (Lux *et al.* 1970; Barrett and Crill 1974; Ulfhake and Kellerth 1984; Thurbon *et al.* 1998), and occasionally values up to about 16 $K\Omega$ cm^2 (Kernell and Zwaagstra 1989a). However, an increasing amount of evidence suggests that, at least under normal experimental circumstances (microelectrode in cell body), the membrane resistivity might be higher for the dendrites than for the soma (Iansek and Redman 1973b; Ulfhake and Kellerth 1984; Glenn *et al.* 1987; Clements and Redman 1989; Thurbon *et al.* 1998). At least part of this difference is likely to have been caused by a shunt around the sharp electrode penetrating the soma (Thurbon *et al.* 1998; detailed discussion in review by Powers and Binder 2001). The average membrane resistivity is systematically different for MNs of different size and type (see section 6.9.1).

In extensions of the equivalent cylinder models, Rall and his colleagues (reviewed by Rall *et al,* 1992) have also explored other model versions, including various compartmental models, which are very flexible (each compartment may be given different properties (cf. Fig. 7.3A)). Furthermore, inspired by this work, further calculations have been done (Jack and Redman 1971), and other MN models have been constructed and used as tools for the interpretation of experimental MN measurements (e. g. Durand 1984; Clements and Redman 1989; Burke 2000).

6.4.4. **The voltage and current threshold for spike generation; accommodation to slowly rising currents**

In anaesthetized animals, the voltage threshold for action potential generation in response to a current step or rapid EPSP is often at a depolarization around 10 mV from the resting potential (Eccles 1957).Thus with a resting potential of about -70 mV, the threshold would be at about -60 mV. The stimulating current needed to reaching the threshold (**rheobase** I_{rh}) depends strongly on the cell's input resistance R_{in}. If the 'apparent' voltage threshold V_{th} is calculated as the product $I_{rh} \times R_{in}$, the resulting value tends to be at a less depolarized level than the V_{th} measured as the take-off level for action potentials after stimulation with injected current or by synaptic activation (Gustafsson and Pinter 1984b). Thus, as might be expected, the MN does not behave as a purely passive resistive circuit for all membrane potentials below threshold; close to the threshold potential inward currents are generated which add to the external stimulating current (see section 6.8).

Classical studies of the excitability of axons have shown that, if the intensity of a stimulating current increases too slowly, no spikes will be elicited; motor axons typically have a 'minimal current gradient' for successful activation (Bradley and Somjen 1961). This behaviour may be explained by the presence of a voltage-dependent inactivation of the spike-generating Na^+ conductance. In intracellularly recorded MNs, a minimal current gradient is typically only seen in cells which are abnormally depolarized or show other signs of damage caused by the microelectrode (Bradley and Somjen 1961; Schlue *et al.* 1974). In many other, apparently undamaged, MNs there is also a gradual increase in threshold level for slowly rising currents; however, this increase ultimately reaches a 'plateau' and an action potential may be elicited once the cell becomes sufficiently depolarized ('high-ceiling' versus 'low-ceiling' MNs) (Sasaki and Otani 1961). It seems likely that this rise of threshold current is caused by the mechanism also underlying the voltage 'sag' in response to a depolarizing step of steady current (Fig. 6.1C, FF) (Ito and Oshima 1965; cf. Stafstrom *et al.* 1984). In accordance with this view, both the 'sag' and the threshold increase tend to be more pronounced for fast MNs with brief AHPs than for slower ones with longer AHPs (Sasaki and Otani 1961; Gustafsson and Pinter 1985a; however, see Burke and Nelson 1971).

6.4.5. How 'passive' are the passive membrane properties of MNs?

In electrophysiology, the term 'passive' properties is generally used to indicate the baseline properties of a cell at rest. These measurements include those discussed above concerning the resting membrane potential and data derived from assessments of voltage transients elicted by weak current pulses (e.g. input resistance, membrane capacitance, apparent electrotonic length of the dendrites). However, it should be remembered that the characteristics measured in an inactive, seemingly 'passive', cell may still have been influenced to some extent by various 'active' processes (e.g. ongoing synaptic activity, activated voltage-gated ion channels, electrogenic pumps).

Several kinds of ion channels are known which are differentially gated by voltage over a broad range of subthreshold membrane potentials (Table 6.2). This includes the channels responsible for the voltage 'sag' in response to small intensities of polarizing current (Fig. 6.1C). Moreover, a large MN is covered by tens of thousands of synapses (Chapter 7, section 7.2.5). Even at rest, asleep, or under general anaesthesia, many neurones within the CNS are more or less continuously active, including cells with direct or indirect links to MNs. Furthermore, the great majority of central synapses are of the chemical kind, which are likely to show some degree of spontaneous release of transmitter quanta in the absence of presynaptic action potentials. Much of the membrane 'noise' that is observed during a whole-cell MN recording (often oscillations of 0.5–1 mV) reflects ongoing synaptic activity (Hubbard *et al.* 1967), which might conceivably have had an effect on the average level of membrane potential as well as on the membrane resistivity and time constant. However, in animals investigated under deep general anaesthesia these effects are apparently rather slight. In the spinal cord of cats anaesthetized with pentobarbital, a block of intraspinal action potentials with locally applied TTX produced a 20 per cent decrease in spontaneous miniature PSPs recorded from MNs, but there was no change in either their mean membrane potential or input resistance (Blankenship 1968; see also Hubbard *et al.* 1967).

6.5. **Current-to-frequency transduction: baseline properties**

6.5.1. **Steady currents evoking repetitive spike firing: early insights and experiments**

Long before the mechanisms of neuronal rhythmic firing were investigated, it was well known that repetitive impulse discharges in mechanoreceptors (e.g. muscle spindles) were evoked by maintained 'generator currents' or 'generator potentials' (Katz 1950; Eyzaguirre and Kuffler 1955). These generator currents were, in turn, elicited by mechanical stimuli such as muscle stretch, causing deformation of mechanosensitive membranes in the sensory nerve endings. Early studies of reflex activity suggested that prolonged MN discharges might be produced by similar mechanisms, being caused by maintained postsynaptic 'generator currents' rather than by a pulsating excitatory input (Granit and Renkin 1961; see also Eccles and Hoff 1932). This hypothesis was tested by stimulating MNs directly with steady currents injected through the intracellular tip of a microelectrode and studying the relationship between current intensity and the characteristics of the evoked repetitive discharge (if any) (Fig. 6.2) (Granit *et al.* 1963a,b).

6.5.2. **'Tonic' versus 'phasic' behaviour of intracellularly stimulated MNs**

In most movements, MNs discharge repetitively and it is known from EMG studies that such discharges may continue for very long times (e.g. up to several hours in postural functions). Long-lasting repetitive discharges ('tonic' firing) may also be obtained in many MNs when they are penetrated with sharp electrodes and stimulated with long-lasting depolarizing currents injected via the microelectrode. However, in such experiments, a surprisingly high percentage of the MNs may fail to discharge more than a single spike or a brief phasic burst, whatever the stimulation strength. Initially, this led to the question of whether some MNs might indeed have intrinsic 'phasic' properties, somewhat analogous to phasic mechanoreceptors. In the 1950s it was noted, in reflex studies, that MNs with large axons often fired in phasic bursts and that those engaged in long-lasting tonic discharges tended to have thinner axons; these respective cells were even termed 'phasic' and 'tonic' MNs (Granit *et al.* 1956; 1957), although it was uncertain to what extent the differences in discharge behaviour were caused by differences in how they were synaptically activated or by differences in intrinsic membrane properties (Henatsch *et al.* 1959). We now know that the first of these possibilities was nearest to the truth.

During an intracellular penetration (by a sharp electrode), most cells will eventually show signs of a progressively worsening deterioration of their response properties. One of the first signs of this 'run-down' is that the cell loses its tonic discharge properties and becomes increasingly phasic (Kernell 1965a). More or less in parallel with this change of repetitive properties, the spike amplitude and resting membrane potential decrease. Ultimately, this 'run-down' state will make the cell incapable of discharging any action potential at all (in an intermediate stage, it may fire only the smaller IS spikes after block of the SD spike). It is not yet known whether there are systematic differences between various classes of MNs with regard to their sensitivity to penetration-generated 'run-down', although the existence of such differences has been suggested in some experimental materials (Mishelevich 1969). However, no spinal MN type seems to be immune against this kind of electrode-inflicted deterioration. Furthermore, for MNs in good condition, discharges lasting several minutes may also be evoked in cells known to innervate fast and fatigue-sensitive muscle units (Kernell and Monster 1982a). In muscles with a mixture of fibre types, small enough to follow all individual units simultaneously with EMG recordings, all the units present were capable of long-lasting tonic discharges in response to synaptic activation (Kernell and Sjoholm 1975). Thus the ability to produce prolonged tonic discharges, lasting for many seconds at least, normally seems to be present for all MNs whatever the type of muscle fibre (and thus of the motor tasks).

The nature of the damage that often causes penetrated cells (ultimately) to become phasic is still uncertain. Why such large cells as MNs seem to be so sensitive to the kind of mechanical damage inflicted by a sharp microelectrode remains a physiologically and pathophysiologically interesting question. MNs have a relatively low buffering capacity for Ca^{2+} ions (Lips and Keller 1998, 1999), and inward leakage of Ca^{2+} ions at the penetration site might cause certain ion channels to change their properties. Under these conditions, the loss of tonic properties might be caused by the loss of persistent inward currents that are normally activated at subthreshold membrane potentials and whose presence is required for tonic repetitive firing (see section 6.7.1) (Schwindt and Crill 1977, 1980b; Lee and Heckman 2001).

6.5.3. Current threshold for single spikes versus that for repetitive firing

In healthy MNs, the threshold current I_{rep} for eliciting repetitive firing is typically higher than that needed to evoke a single action potential (rheobase I_{rhe}). On average, the ratio I_{rep}/I_{rhe} is about 1.5 for cat MNs and 1.4 for rat MNs (Granit *et al.* 1963b; Kernell 1965a). The difference between I_{rep} and I_{rhe} seems to be well explained by the voltage 'sag' that often appears on injection of a steady depolarizing current (Fig. 6.1C, FF) (Ito and Oshima 1965), and it implies that, when excited by maintained (synaptic) current steps just above the threshold for single spikes, many MNs will only respond with one or a few action potentials. For stronger stimuli, the same cell will discharge in a 'tonic' maintained fashion (cf. reflex behaviour of Granit's 'tonic' and 'phasic' MNs (Granit *et al.* 1957; Henatsch *et al.* 1959)).

6.5.4. **Frequency versus current relation (*f–I* relation)**

Once a MN is stimulated by a steady current exceeding the threshold for rhythmic firing, a further increase in current will cause an increase in the steady firing rate (Fig. 6.2A). This continues until a current strength is reached which is strong enough to cause a considerable decrease in spike size and, ultimately, to silence the cell (Granit *et al.* 1963b; Kernell 1965a).

The frequency versus current relation (*f–I* relation) of MNs was first determined for a small number of spinal MNs of the rat (Granit *et al.* 1963b). Following a brief initial period of decreasing firing rate (spike-frequency adaptation, see below), the 'steady-state' *f–I* relation could be approximated by a single straight line for all currents up to those causing inactivation. A more extensive analysis of MNs from the cat spinal cord showed

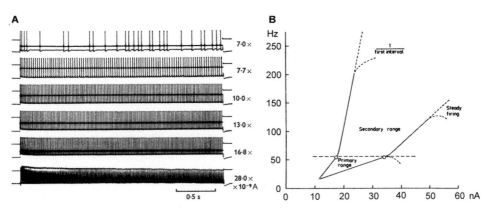

Figure 6.2 Current-to-frequency transduction. (**A**) Intracellular recording from spinal MN of rat (antidromic spike amplitude 81 mV) stimulated with steady currents injected via the intracellular microelectrode. Current intensities (nA) are given beside each record. Change of sensitivity of current-recording beam between 7.0 and 7.7 nA. (Reproduced with permission, from Granit *et al.* 1963b.) (**B**) From spinal MNs of cat. Mean relationship between spike frequency (Hz) and intensity of stimulating current (nA) for the first impulse interval, just after the abrupt onset of stimulation, and for firing following the initial phase of adaptation ('steady firing'). Primary and secondary ranges of spike-frequency as indicated. (Reproduced with permission, from Kernell 1965b.)

that, at least for this species and under these experimental circumstances, the steady-state *f–I* relation could instead often be approximated by two straight lines (Figs 6.2B and 6.4C). Purely descriptively, this behaviour was composed of a lower-frequency 'primary range' and a higher-frequency 'secondary range' (Kernell 1965b), where the slope of the *f–I* relation (*f–I slope*) was higher in the secondary range than in the primary range.

At the very highest rates, the *f–I* curves again tend to become less steep before a final stage of inactivation is reached. This high-rate 'flattening' of the *f–I* curve is regularly seen for the first few intervals and may also be obtained at later periods of the discharge. In maintained firing these higher rates have sometimes been referred to as a 'tertiary range', with an *f–I* slope often flatter but sometimes steeper than in the secondary range (Schwindt 1973).

6.5.5. Initial and late adaptation

When a spinal MN is brought to repetitive activity by a long-lasting step of steady suprathreshold current, its discharge rate shows a gradual decrease (**spike-frequency adaptation**). In cat spinal MNs this decrease takes place in two major phases, an 'initial' phase lasting from a few intervals up to about 0.5–1 s and a 'late' phase lasting about 1 min or more (Figs 6.2B and 6.3A) (Kernell 1965a; Kernell and Monster 1982b); see also data for extracellular stimulation (Spielmann *et al.* 1993) and for turtle MNs (Gorman *et al.* 2005). Both the major phases of adaptation were also seen in hypoglossal MNs of the rat (Sawczuk *et al.* 1995), but in many of the cells investigated the first phase could be further subdivided into an 'initial' and an 'early' phase with a different relation between spike-frequency drop and time (linear for the initial phase and exponential for the early phase). Time constants (mean ± SD) were about 0.2 ± 0.4 s for the early phase (if present) and 22.6 ± 18.5 s for the late phase.

The first phase of adaptation is associated with a pronouced decrease in the slope for the relation between spike frequency and current (Fig. 6.2B), i.e. a drop in '*f–I* gain' (Granit *et al.* 1963b; Kernell 1965a). Only relatively minor drops in *f–I* gain seem to be associated with the late phase of spike-frequency adaptation (Granit *et al.* 1963a; Kernell 1965a; Kernell and Monster 1982b; Sawczuk *et al.* 1995). This difference is important because it indicates that different main mechanisms underlie these various phases of adaptation. During the initial phase of adaptation, the decrease in *f–I* slope occurs in both the primary and secondary range of firing; an upward bend in the *f–I* curve is maintained throughout this phase of adaptation (Fig. 6.2B). Furthermore, the shift of *f–I* slope from the primary to the secondary range occurred at much the same spike frequency early in the discharge as it did later on (Kernell 1965b). This was true even though both the primary and the secondary *f–I* slopes were much higher initially (Fig. 6.2B).

Both the main phases of adaptation are more pronounced for high than for lower intensities of suprathreshold stimulation current, i.e. for high than for lower levels of spike frequency (Figs 6.2B and 6.3B). In spinal MNs, the late adaptation is particularly marked during the initial 30 s of the discharge. However, sometimes a very slow rate of

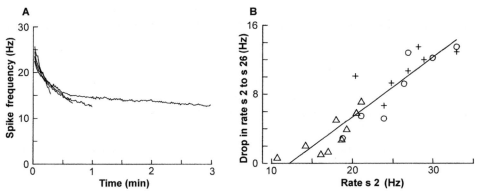

Figure 6.3 Late phase of spike-frequency adaptation. Experiments on cat MNs innervating a hindlimb muscle (medial gastrocnemius). (**A**) Mean relation between impulse rate (Hz) and time (min) for four groups of motoneurones with different durations of firing (Df). All the cells were stimulated with a current of 5 nA above threshold for rhythmic firing. For one group the values were plotted to 18s (40 s > Df > 18 s, $n = 5$), for one group to 40 s (60 s > Df > 40 s, $n = 5$), for one group to 60 s (180 s > Df > 60 s, $n = 6$), and for one group to 180 s (Df > 180 s, $n = 6$). All plots start at second number 2 of the discharge. For consecutive seconds of discharge, mean firing rates are connected by straight lines. For all these cells, firing was regular during the periods for which the illustrated averages were calculated, i.e. for all seconds of firing the standard deviation of the impulse intervals was less than 20 per cent of the mean interval duration (usually much less). (Reproduced with permission, from Kernell and Monster 1982b) (**B**) Drop in discharge rate from second 2 to second 26 of regular firing (Hz) plotted versus the rate of second 2 (Hz) for cells stimulated at 5 nA above threshold for rhythmic firing. The regression line was calculated by the method of least squares ($r = 0.92$, $n = 23$, $P < 0.001$). The contractile properties of the muscle units for all these cells had been measured and categorized as slow fatigue-resistant (S, triangles), fast fatigue-resistant (FR, circles) or fast fatiguable (FF, crosses). Note the low rates and correspondingly low levels of late spike-frequency adaptation in S-MNs. Note also the complete overlap between values for FR- and FF-MNs. (Reproduced with permission, from Kernell and Monster 1982a.)

adaptation seems to take place during at least 4 min of continuous discharge (Kernell and Monster 1982b).

During its initial portion, the first phase of adaptation is associated with a deepening of the AHPs following the spikes (Granit *et al.* 1963b; Kernell 1965a). A radically different behaviour is seen in some young hypoglossal MNs; these cells may show an initial increase in rate during steady current stimulation ('type I cells') (Viana *et al.* 1995). This increase in rate is then associated with a decreasing amplitude of the AHPs seen between consecutive spikes.

6.5.6. **Maximum rate of maintained firing**

For reasons which are still uncertain, many of the cells investigated in the cat spinal cord were not capable of long-lasting repetitive discharges in the secondary range, although they all showed both the main phases of firing initially, i.e. an upward bend of the *f–I* curve above a certain spike frequency (Fig. 6.2B). It should be noted that this is not simply a question of whether the *f–I* curve is straight or bent, but rather it truly concerns differences in spike-frequency range. Cells that lacked a steady secondary range did so because they were incapable of firing steadily at the high spike frequencies belonging to the secondary range, i.e. at steady rates higher than the initial primary–secondary break in their *f–I* curve. For MNs with the same duration of AHP (indicative of MN 'speed'), the maximum steady spike frequency in the primary range is similar irrespective of whether the MN is capable of steady secondary range firing or not (Kernell 1965b,c). The maximum sustainable discharge rate (e.g. maintained for 0.5 s) is much higher for cells capable of firing steadily in the secondary range than for other MNs.

Increases in stimulating current above that producing the maximum rate of sustained firing typically causes a marked decrease in spike size and, ultimately, no firing at all. These reactions are typically reversible; as the intensity of a steady stimulation is decreased, repetitive firing reappears (Granit *et al.* 1963b; Kernell 1965a).

As seen for individual initial spike intervals, the maximum rates of firing of cat spinal MNs may be very high, exceeding 500 Hz. However, such very high rates are only seen for limited periods and only very early in a discharge. During longer periods (0.5 s), the maximum rates within the secondary range are typically around 80–200 Hz (mean 131 ± 45 (SD) Hz). In contrast, maximum rates within the primary range are only 30–100 Hz (53 ± 19 Hz) (Kernell 1965c).

6.5.7. **Minimum rate of steady firing**

In experiments on anaesthetized animals, the minimum steady spike frequency that is obtained with a maintained stimulating current is typically well defined; if there is a small decrease of current below the I_{rep} threshold intensity either firing becomes extremely irregular or the cell becomes completely silent (Fig. 6.2A, topmost trace). In cat spinal MNs, the minimum rate of maintained steady firing, as seen under such conditions, tends to lie between 5 and 25 Hz. In anaesthetized animals, the intervals of this minimum rate of steady firing are close to the duration of AHP as seen after a single spike (Fig. 6.8A) (Kernell 1965c). In non-anaesthetized animals, the maximum intervals of steady firing may be longer than the duration of AHP after a single spike (Carp *et al.* 1991); in such cases slow regenerative phenomena affecting the membrane potential ('local potentials') may be present close to threshold.

Minimum steady rates of firing have also been studied in maintained voluntary contractions in human subjects. If voluntary force is gradually decreased while the discharges of a motor unit are followed, a level will ultimately be reached below which the discharges become increasingly irregular. This was first systematically studied by Tokizane and Shimazu (1964) who measured the relationship between the standard deviation (SD) of interval duration versus the mean interval; below a certain mean rate, the SD–mean curve deviated sharply upwards. The authors made a distinction between 'tonic' T units and 'kinetic' K units; within a given muscle, the upward bend of the

SD–mean curve occurred at lower discharge rates for T units than for K units. Intracellular cat experiments have shown that this upward bend indeed takes place at intervals related to the AHP trajectory (Powers and Binder 2000a). Furthermore, the rates at which the human SD–mean curve deviates upwards (e.g. 8–15 Hz) correspond, roughly, to rates at which human MNs tend to be recruited (Milner-Brown *et al.* 1973a; Grimby *et al.* 1979).

The minimum rate of steady firing is most clearly distinguishable for MNs which are studied under conditions with little synaptic activity, i.e. under general anaesthesia. If the ongoing 'synaptic noise' (i.e. subthreshold synaptic activity) is greater, the spike threshold will occasionally be reached also with steady excitation intensities just below threshold (i.e. below I_{rep}). Random synaptic activity will then be expected to produce highly irregular discharge intervals with a mean rate depending mainly on the amplitude distribution within the synaptic noise and the extent to which stimulation intensity is below I_{rep}(Matthews 1996, 1999); firing at such low 'juxta-threshold' levels has been referred to as firing within a 'subprimary range' (Kudina 1999; see also Kudina and Alexeeva 1992a). Also within this range, the mean firing rate might increase with current intensity because the closer the steady stimulation comes to I_{rep}, the greater is the chance that the threshold for spike initiation will be reached by randomly occurring noise peaks of different sizes. It is still uncertain to what extent such 'subprimary range' firing is actually used in normal motor behaviour; in most accounts and illustrated records of motor unit firing during graded voluntary contractions, motor unit spike intervals seem more regular than those expected for 'subprimary' discharges. It has also been noted that it is 'easier to keep a motor unit firing at higher rates than at the lowest possible rates. This is reflected by a decrease in the regularity at low rates . . . until continuous discharges cannot be maintained at all (about 6/s)' (Freund 1983).

6.5.8. **Doublets**

In MNs that are stimulated with a strong step of injected current, the initial spike intervals are typically much shorter than those seen later on (Fig. 6.2A,B). These initial 'doublets' or 'triplets' arise as a consequence of the steep *f–I* slope prior to initial adaptation, and similar brief intervals are also seen at the onset of ballistic contractions (Bawa and Calancie 1983; Van Cutsem *et al.* 1998). However, 'doublets' of an apparently different type have also been seen in human voluntary contractions, during slow recruitment phases, and/or during later periods of continued firing (Bawa and Calancie 1983; Kudina and Alexeeva 1992b; reviewed by Garland and Griffin 1999). In human contractions, typical doublets have spike intervals of about 2.5–20 ms, appearing during discharges with mean intervals of about 45 ms or more. In patients with spinal cord injury, repeated and interspersed doublets were seen in about 20 per cent of the MNs discharging during spasms (Thomas and Ross 1997). In normal subjects, the appearance of doublets increased after several weeks of training of rapid movements (Van Cutsem *et al.* 1998). Measurements of post-spike excitability in discharging MNs have led to the conclusion that the doublets are likely to emerge on top of the delayed depolarization (cf. section 6.3)

(Kudina and Churikova 1990). Hence their chance of appearance would be increased if this Ca^{2+}-dependent depolarizing after-potential became enlarged. The amplitude of the delayed depolarization in MNs may be influenced by stimulation of brainstem structures and peripheral nerves without any clear relation to the effects on somatic membrane potential (Kernell 1964); perhaps such influence occurs at remote dendritic locations and/or by synaptic effects on voltage-gated membrane channels.

In intracellular recordings from MNs in acute animal experiments, interspersed doublets are not commonly encountered; only very occasionally have cells been recorded in which antidromic spikes were automatically suceeded by a second spike on top of the delayed depolarization (D. Kernell, unpublished observation); similar doublets normally appear in certain other types of neurone in the CNS (e.g. olivary neurones (Crill and Kennedy 1967)). In recordings from cat MNs that were stimulated using extracellular microelectrodes, interspersed doublets were seen in more than 60 per cent of the cells, more commonly in slow-type MNs (Spielmann *et al.* 1993). On the other hand, in walking rats initial doublets (associated with spike-frequency adaptation?) are often seen in units of fast hindlimb muscles but not in those of the slow soleus muscle (Gorassini *et al.* 2000; see also Hennig and Lomo 1985).

6.6. Current-to-frequency transduction: discussion of mechanisms

6.6.1. Early considerations

In classical writings on neurophysiology, two principal mechanisms which might be responsible for the 'rhythmicity' of sensory discharges that were evoked by steady generator currents were discussed. Adrian (1932) suggested that the rhythmicity might depend primarily on spike-dependent transient decreases of excitability, i.e. on phenomena akin to those underlying the period of relative refractoriness following an action potential ('post-spike mechanism'). In this case, a steady current would evoke a discharge in which the latency for the first spike was much briefer than subsequent spike intervals. As an alternative, Hodgkin (1948) suggested that the rhythmicity might be primarily dependent on the rate of change of membrane potential due to slow regenerative phenomena, similar to that actually seen during current-evoked rhythmic firing in crab nerves ('pre-spike mechanism'). In this case, a steady current would evoke a discharge in which the latency for the first spike was approximately equal to subsequent spike intervals.

6.6.2. Role of the AHP: *f–I* slope, minimum rate, and initial adaptation

On the whole, the rhythmic behaviour of spinal MNs shows more similarity to the model proposed by Adrian than to that suggested by Hodgkin, although elements of both kinds of mechanisms are represented. In discharges evoked by steps of steady current, the initial MN impulse interval is typically much longer than the latency of the first spike. Furthermore, at least in spinal MNs of anaesthetized cats, the minimum rate of steady firing takes place at impulse intervals with a duration very similar to that of the AHP following a single spike (Fig. 6.8A), i.e. this firing rate appears to depend strongly on the time course of relative post-spike refractoriness as set by the AHP.

The more the intensity of the stimulating current is increased above threshold, the more the stimulating current would be capable of balancing the hyperpolarizing K^+ current of the AHP and the sooner would the threshold be reached for evoking the next impulse. Hence the time course of the gradually declining conductance changes underlying the AHP would be expected to be of importance for the slope of the f–I relation. In a very simple 'threshold-crossing' MN model, with a fixed voltage threshold for spike initiation and an exponentially declining AHP K^+ conductance following each spike, an approximately linear f–I relation is obtained over a spike-freuency range corresponding to the experimentally observed primary range (Kernell 1968). In this very simple model, the f–I slope would be increased by any of the following changes:

- decreased amplitude of the AHP conductance change
- decreased slowness of AHP conductance decline (i.e. a shorter AHP)
- decreased (i.e. more negative) voltage threshold for spike initiation (cf. effects of monoamines (Fedirchuk and Dai 2004))
- less negative equilibrium potential for K^+.

Experiments in which the AHP amplitude was decreased by serotonin or other synaptic modifiers or blockers have shown that, as expected, this is indeed associated with an increased f–I slope (Zhang and Krnjevic 1987; Hounsgaard et al. 1988a; Hounsgaard and Kiehn 1989; Wallen et al. 1989; Viana et al. 1993; Fig. 7.7, Hultborn et al. 2004; cf. Hornby et al. 2002a). An increased amplitude of the AHP conductance change can probably also explain much of the initial phase of spike-frequency adaptation, which is associated with a decrease in f–I slope. When several spikes are evoked in rapid succession, the AHP following the second spike is larger than that following the first spike; this is true for initial portions of repetitive discharges evoked by steady current as well as for sequences of spikes that are individually evoked by brief pulses of stimulation (Ito and Oshima 1962; Baldissera and Gustafsson 1974). A similar 'summation' of AHPs is also seen in simulations based on voltage clamp equations (Kernell and Sjoholm 1973), where it is due to an incomplete activation of the K^+ conductance mechanism following a single spike; for the second spike, activation of the AHP current would start at a higher level and reach a higher peak. This phase of adaptation can take place without any associated rise in voltage threshold, at least for the first few impulse intervals (Kernell 1972). Furthermore, for a given initial impulse interval, the second interval becomes equally prolonged irrespective of whether the initial spike was evoked by the steady current or inserted prior to the onset of the prolonged current pulse (Kernell 1972).

The 'AHP summation' seems to be able to explain much of the marked adaptation from the first to the second interval of a repetitive discharge (Kernell and Sjoholm 1973; Baldissera and Gustafsson 1974; Baldissera et al. 1978). However, in simulations with voltage clamp equations these mechanisms do not add much to adaptation beyond the second interval, whereas in actual MNs the first phase of adaptation, associated with a decrease in *f–I* slope, may often continue for up to 0.5–1 s (Kernell 1965a), and even longer in some rat hypoglossal MNs (Sawczuk *et al.* 1995). These later periods of initial (and 'early') adaptation might be caused by a progressive increase in voltage threshold caused by Na^+ conductance inactivation (Miles *et al.* 2005). Corresponding increases in the take-off potential for successive spikes have been observed (Schwindt and Crill 1982) and, in model calculations, their occurrrence can be influenced by changing the voltage dependence of the Na^+ conductance inactivation (Powers *et al.* 1999).

Summarizing the role of the AHP current, its duration is important for helping to set the minimum rate of steady firing, its amplitude and rate of post-spike decline are important for the slope of the *f–I* relation, and its 'summation' following consecutive spikes is (partly) responsible for spike-frequency adaptation during the first few impulse intervals. These statements do not, of course, imply that no other mechanisms are involved; almost all voltage-dependent conductances might play an additional role. However, the importance of the AHP is that it serves as a relatively predictable timing device for the neuronal processor.

6.6.3. The secondary range

It is still a matter of discussion as to which mechanisms are responsible for the sharp upward bend in the steady-state *f–I* curve as the firing rate increases from the primary to the secondary range (Fig. 6.2B). In simple threshold-crossing neurone models with an exponentially declining AHP conductance (Kernell 1968), the *f–I* curve indeed deviates upwards at approximately the correct rate of discharge, but the upward turn is less marked and less sharp than that of actual MNs and there is little sign of secondary range firing after the initial phase of spike-frequency adaptation. The Ca^{2+} currents underlying the delayed depolarization might help to produce a more marked upward bend of the *f–I* curve, but in model calculations this did not produce a secondary range behaviour like that of real MNs (Kernell and Sjoholm 1973). A good fit between MN and model behaviour, including secondary range firing, was obtained using measurements of how the AHPs actually summed in MNs ('saturating summation') (Baldissera *et al.* 1978). Thus AHP properties and behaviours appear to be important for the shape of the *f–I* curve and secondary range firing. However, other essential mechanisms may contribute as well.

In the experiments of Schwindt and Crill (1982), membrane potential was measured during repetitive firing in MNs that were also analysed using voltage clamp techniques (Fig. 6.4). The threshold for spike take-off became higher for faster spike frequencies. During secondary-range firing, the interspike membrane potential remained entirely within the range of voltages over which a persistent inward current I_i (probably due to Ca^{2+}) was strongly activated during the voltage clamp. Thus, at these higher rates (and at still more depolarized membrane potentials), I_i was tonically and strongly activated and counteracted the repolarizing outward potassium currents of the AHPs. At slower firing rates (e.g. primary-range firing), the interspike membrane potential oscillated at less depolarized levels and the tonic activation of I_i would then be smaller (Fig. 6.4C,D). Thus,

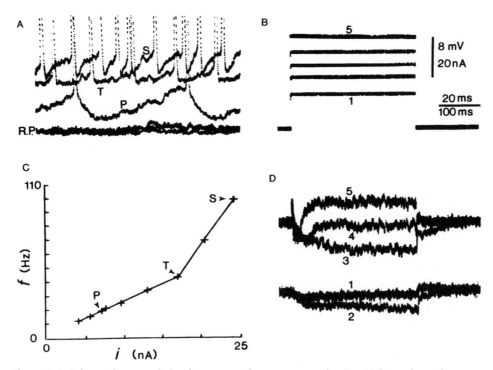

Figure 6.4 Voltage clamp analysis of current-to-frequency transduction. Voltage-dependent persistent inward currents may be required for steady firing in the secondary range. (**A**) Sample voltage records from intracellular recording of cat lumbar MN during repetitive discharge in the primary range (P), in the transition between the primary and secondary ranges (T), and at the upper end of the secondary range (S). (**B**) Somatic voltage clamp steps applied to the same MN. (**C**) Steady-state relation between injected current and firing rate for the same MN. (**D**) Membrane currents (after subtraction of the leak and longest capacitative components) corresponding to the voltage clamp steps in (**B**). Inward currents: downward recording. Note the net persistent inward currents in traces 1, 2, and 3. Traces 1 and 2 have been offset for clarity. Time calibration: 20 ms for (**A**); 100 ms for (**B**) and (**D**). Cat anaesthetized with pentobarbital. (Reproduced with permission, from Schwindt and Crill 1982.)

according to these important results, the high f–I slope within the secondary range is mainly caused by booster functions of I_i, i.e. it is a consequence of slowly inactivating voltage-dependent ion channels (cf also Hultborn *et al.* 2004; Li *et al.* 2004a).

As will be discussed further in section 6.7, the depolarization-induced appearance of persistent inward currents from dendritic ion channels is facilitated by metabotropic receptors for various transmitters, including monoamines (e.g. norepinephrine, serotonin). The monoaminergic innervation of spinal MNs derives from descending tracts originating in the brainstem. Hence, it is interesting that steady firing in the secondary range was found less often in spinalized animals than in cats with the spinal cord intact (Baldissera and Gustafsson 1971). Furthermore, it is of interest in this context that synaptic activation (much of which is likely to arrive at dendritic synapses) causes $f–I$ slopes to change more readily in the secondary than in the primary range (Granit *et al.* 1966b). However, even though I_i booster currents may be important for the effective use and high gain of the secondary range, it does not seem likely that firing within this range is completely a product of dendritic persistent inward currents. As was mentioned above (section 6.5.6), the transition from primary to secondary range firing appears to be frequency rather than depolarization dependent (Kernell 1965b). This is not easily explained as being entirely due to dendritic booster currents. Furthermore, booster currents that are (partly) responsible for the increased $f–I$ slope of the secondary range should have a faster type of kinetics than that typically seen in experiments concerning 'plateau behaviour' (see section 6.7.2). In the latter type of recording, plateau currents often increase slowly over a period of several seconds (see 'counter-clockwise hysteresis' in Fig. 6.5D). However, in experiments without any signs of plateau currents, switching up and down between rates within the secondary-range firing may occur almost instantaneously (cf. switching between 55.9, 64.6, and 54.6 nA in Figs 1 and 2 of Kernell (1965b)). Furthermore, it was noted that 'with weak currents, the same cells always had a primary $f–I$ slope both immediately before and after the application of the stronger current by which the firing rates within the secondary range were determined' (Kernell 1965b).

Very little is known about how far the action potentials of a spinal MN are normally actively conducted into the dendrites (Larkum *et al.* 1996). A major difference between cells with a phasic and those with a tonic secondary range might perhaps be that the latter cells have spikes that actively conduct much further into the dendrites, and thus are less seriously 'loaded' by passive dendritic membranes. Such dendritic conduction might be facilitated (and might even need to be facilitated) by excitatory synaptic inputs from various descending tracts (including those facilitating 'plateau behaviour'), making firing in the secondary range less likely to occur in spinalized animals (Baldissera and Gustafsson 1971).

6.6.4. **The maximum possible rate of discharge**

The AHP is unlikely to be of any particular importance for setting the maximum steady rate of discharge; an increased size or duration of the AHP would make it necessary to use stronger activating currents for reaching a given rate, but it would not change the maximum attainable rate. For cat spinal MNs studied under general anaesthesia, the maximum evocable rate seen in the secondary range in semi-steady firing (i.e. discharge maintained for at least 0.5 s) was about 80–200 Hz, much slower than that maximally attained for initial impulse intervals (Fig. 6.2B). Thus, for relatively maintained firing, the maximum rate was apparently not limited by the absolute refractory period (which tends to be close to spike duration), but probably by the kinetics and voltage sensitivity of the Na^+ conductance inactivation (Barrett and Crill 1980; Safronov and Vogel 1995, 1996). In the voltage clamp experiments of Schwindt and Crill (1982), a g_{Na} inactivation of about 50 per cent was present during maximum rate firing.

6.6.5. **Late adaptation**

With regard to underlying mechanisms, a crucial difference between the first and the late phases of spike-frequency adaptation concerns the behaviour of the *f–I* slope, which decreases markedly during the first phase and changes relatively little later on (Granit *et al.* 1963a; Kernell 1965a; Kernell and Monster 1982b; Sawczuk *et al.* 1995). Thus processes with an influence on the *f–I* slope would seem less likely to be major causes for the late phase of adaptation. These include changes in the size and/or time course of AHP conductances and changes in the voltage threshold for spike initiation. If such mechanisms were mainly responsible for late adaptation, effects on the *f–I* slope must have been largely neutralized by a proper balance of negative and positive influences (e.g. rising voltage threshold combined with a progressively decreasing peak conductance of the AHP, or with a progressive positive-going shift of E_K).

Experiments on late adaptation in adult spinal motoneurones (pentobarbital anaesthesia) showed that the rate drop became more prominent for higher starting frequencies (Fig. 6.3B). This is consistent with a mechanism whereby the repetitive spikes caused some hyperpolarizing current to occur which became stronger for greater numbers of spikes, and that this discharge-evoked outward current counteracted the steady stimulation. Such a mechanism is apparently responsible for a kind of slow spike-frequency adaptation in an invertebrate sensory neurone, the stretch receptor cell of the crayfish (Sokolove and Cooke 1971). In this *in vitro* preparation, current-evoked maintained spike discharges activated an electrogenic Na–K pump, and the discharges were succeeded by a very long-lasting post-discharge hyperpolarization (PDH). The addition of ouabain, which blocked the Na–K pump, also abolished the PDH and most of the late adaptation (Sokolove and Cooke 1971). However, in hypoglossal MNs the PDH was only partly decreased by ouabain and this blocker had no effect on late adaptation (Sawczuk *et al.* 1997). Furthermore, in their *in vitro* experiments, Sawczuk *et al.* (1997) and Powers *et al.* (1999) also found no effect on late adaptation when blocking all Ca^{2+} currents (and hence Ca^{2+}-dependent K^+ currrents) by the extracellular addition of Mn^{2+}. The main mechanisms underlying late spike-frequency adaptation in mammalian MNs are still uncertain (Powers and Binder 2001; Zeng *et al.* 2005).

6.7. **Persistent inward currents (PICs)**

6.7.1. **Subthreshold PICs and the capability for repetitive firing in response to maintained current**

Schwindt and Crill (1977, 1980a,b) found that, in MNs in good condition, a persistent voltage-gated inward current (PIC) was activated already at subthreshold potentials in anaesthetized animals. Even in anaesthetized animals, this PIC was sometimes strong enough to generate self-sustained firing (Schwindt and Crill 1980a, Fig. 9c). This persistent current (I_i) was very sensitive to presumed microelectrode damage. Two of the earliest signs of such damage were the disappearance of the persistent inward current and the loss of 'tonic' repetitive discharge properties. These observations were recently extended by Lee and Heckman (2001), who also noted that steady injected currents cause no repetitive firing in a MN unless there was activation of a persistent inward current (probably carried by Na$^+$ ions) at subthreshold potentials. Thus the disappearance of this current might be a major cause of the loss of 'tonic' discharge properties on rundown. These subthreshold-activated PICs are probably necessary for creating 'local potentials' that bring the membrane potential to V_{th} sufficiently rapidly to avoid a dangerous degree of Na$^+$ conductance inactivation. In MN models provided with axonal membrane properties and long-lasting MN-like AHPs, no 'tonic' repetitive firing was possible unless a decrease was introduced in the Na$^+$ conductance inactivation seen at V_{th} (Kernell and Sjoholm 1973).

6.7.2. PICs as booster currents; plateau behaviour

Voltage-gated PICs become much more powerful in the absence of anaesthesia, particularly when facilitated by modifying neurotransmitters such as the monoamines norepinephrine and serotonin (5HT) (for synaptic aspects of PICs and plateau behaviour, see Chapter 7, section 7.5.1). In such situations, an excitatory depolarization (e.g. injected stimulating current) will affect the MN membrane such that it supplies a functionally significant part of its own activating current. Thus this PIC represents a kind of 'autostimulation' which will be added to any synaptic or injected currents that activate or inhibit the cell. In this book, this kind of phenomenon will sometimes be referred to as **booster PICs** (elsewhere also often referred to as 'plateau currents' or signs of 'bistability'). Behaviours resulting from such booster PICs are illustrated in Fig. 6.5 showing results from the experiments of Hounsgaard, Hultborn, Kiehn, and their colleagues on MNs in decerebrate cats (Hounsgaard *et al.* 1986, 1988a; Hultborn *et al.* 2004). According to the initial descriptions, plateau currents were predominantly carried by Ca^{2+} ions, which entered the cell through L-type voltage-gated Ca^{2+} channels (Hounsgaard and Kiehn 1989; Delgado-Lezama *et al.* 1997). Later, however, other kinds of powerful 'self-stimulating' PICs were also described, including currents carried by Na$^+$ ions (Powers and Binder 2003; Li *et al.* 2004a).

In Fig. 6.5A, a brief depolarizing pulse evokes a repetitive discharge which continues after the end of the stimulation. This 'plateau' discharge is stopped by a brief injected hyperpolarization. In this case, the PIC was strong enough to keep the cell depolarized above its threshold for PIC generation, i.e. the 'auto-generated' discharge continued in the absence of external driving current. Because of the voltage dependence of the PIC, the discharge could be stopped by a brief hyperpolarizing pulse. In Fig. 6.5B, the stimulating pulse is longer and it is evident that there is a gradual acceleration of discharge during the steady injected current, i.e. the booster PIC did not start instantaneously but had a slow onset phase (arrow). Thus, under these conditions, MNs behave as if there were a 'negative' spike-frequency adaptation. In Fig. 6.5C,D, slowly activated plateau currents produce a 'counter-clockwise hysteresis' of the frequency–current relation. In the absence of plateau behaviour, this kind of saw tooth stimulation would give a 'clockwise hysteresis', with spike-frequency adaptation causing lower rates to occur for the

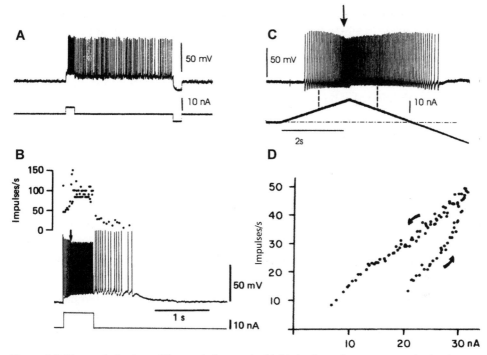

Figure 6.5 Plateau behaviour. All records from spinal MNs in decerebrate unanaesthetized cats. (A),(B) Sustained shifts in MN discharge behaviour triggered by depolarizing and hyperpolarizing currents injected intracellularly. Upper traces are intracellular voltage recordings. Lower traces indicate the amount and timing of the injected current. (A) Sustained repetitive firing in a MN initiated by a short depolarizing current pulse and terminated by a short hyperpolarizing pulse. (Reproduced with permission, from Hounsgaard *et al.* 1984.) (B) Record from another MN during rectangular stimulus current pulse. Note the gradual spike-frequency acceleration during steady stimulation (arrow), signalling the onset of a plateau current. This cell was from a decerebrate cat with a spinal cord transection and i.v. administration of 5-hydroxy-DL-tryptophan (5-HTP), a precursor of 5HT. (Reproduced with permission, from Hounsgaard *et al.* 1988a.) (c), (D) Firing pattern during injection of triangular current pulse. (c) Spike activity in a MN (upper trace) and triangular profile of the injected current (second trace). The broken vertical lines indicate the difference in firing frequency at similar current intensities during the ascending and descending phase. The broken horizontal line shows the zero level for injected current. (D) Plot of instantaneous spike frequency versus intensity of injected current for the data of (c). Note the counter-clockwise hysteresis. (Reproduced with permission, from Hounsgaard *et al.* 1984.)

descending intensities of stimulating current than for the earlier ascending intensities (Hounsgaard *et al.* 1988a; Hounsgaard and Kiehn 1989). During steady or intermittent stimulation, booster PICs are typically activated with a time constant of the order of seconds. A sequence of depolarizing pulses, repeated during the course of tens of seconds, will give a progressively increasing PIC intensity ('warming up', 'wind up' (Svirskis and Hounsgaard 1997; Bennett *et al.* 1998a); compare increasing effects of repeated 'reflex' stimulation in humans (Collins *et al.* 2002). A plateau discharge may have a self-limiting duration (e.g. after the end of the stimulation pulse in Fig. 6.5B), i.e. there then appears to be a slow inactivation (or deactivation) of the PIC process.

There are strong indications that many of the PIC-generating channels are located far out on the dendrites; they can be activated more easily by synaptic inputs than by depolarizing currents injected at the soma (Bennett *et al.* 1998b; Lee *et al.* 2003; Heckman *et al.* 2005). However, as most of the membrane in a MN is dendritic, a dendritic dominance might be expected even if the PIC channels were rather evenly distributed over the MN. Rather surprisingly (but fortunate for computational simplicity), the strengths of different synaptic inputs seem to add linearly even in the presence of facilitated PIC-generating channels (Prather *et al.* 2001). This may be related to the intriguing 'all-or-none' behaviour of plateau potentials and currents (Hounsgaard *et al.* 1988a); the phenomenon seems continuously graded with time but often less readily so with stimulation intensity.

6.8. Ion channels of the soma-dendrite membrane

The Na^+ and K^+ channels of the axon also seem to be represented in the soma region. In addition, there are several other types of K^+ channels, some other kinds of Na^+ channels, and, most importantly, several kinds of Ca^{2+} channels. Brief descriptions of the best understood ion channels of those so far identified in MNs, including some of their probable functions, are given below and in Table 6.2. The ligand-gated channels, which are important for synaptic functions, are not included here (see Table 7.1). However, it is of great importance that many of the voltage- or ion-gated channels may become influenced by synaptic transmitter substances ('modifying' synaptic effects) (Table 6.2). The synaptic modification of ion channels will be discussed further in Chapter 7, section 7.5. For more details concerning ion channels of (moto)neuronal membranes, see reviews by McLarnon (1995), Rekling *et al.* (2000), Hille (2001), Powers and Binder (2001), and Sah and Faber (2002).

6.8.1. Na^+ channels

The opening of Na^+ channels causes an inward (depolarizing) current. The fast transient $I_{Na,t}$ channel is reponsible for the rising phase of the action potential, and the non-inactivating $I_{Na,p}$ is essential for repetitive impulse firing (see section 6.7.1).

6.8.2. Ca^{2+} channels

The opening of Ca^{2+} channels may have several, partly competing, electrophysiological effects:

- an inward (depolarizing) current I_{Ca} directly resulting from the increased Ca^{2+} conductance

Table 6.2. MN ion channels

Current (conductance)	Ions	Activation	Inact	Modified by transm	Function	Blocker
$I_{Na,t}$	Na^+	$\sim V_{th}\uparrow$	fast		spike rise & fall	TTX
$I_{Na,p}$	Na^+	$<V_{th}\uparrow$	slow		rep firing	riluzole
I_i	(Ca^{++})	$<V_{th}\uparrow$	slow		rep firing, (sec-range)	
$I_{Ca,T}$ (LVA)	Ca^{++}	$\sim V_{th}\uparrow$	fast	$\uparrow$5HT	DD	
$I_{Ca,L}$ (HVA)	Ca^{++}	$\sim/>/>>V_{th}\uparrow$	slow	$\uparrow$5HT, NE,Glu-m, ACh-m	plateau-current	nifedipine
$I_{Ca,N}$ (HVA)	Ca^{++}	$>>V_{th}\uparrow$	fast		(AHP)	ω-Conotoxin-GVIA
$I_{Ca,P/Q}$ (HVA)	Ca^{++}	$>>V_{th}\uparrow$	slow		(AHP)	ω-agatoxin-IVA
I_K or $I_{K,\,dr}$	K^+	$<V_{th}\uparrow$	slow		spike fall, fAHP, V_{sag}	TEA, Cs^+
I_A or $I_{K,A}$	K^+	$\sim/>V_{th}\uparrow$	fast	$\uparrow$NE	spike fall	4-aminopyridine
$I_{K,Ca(BK)}$	$(I_{Ca} \rightarrow) K^+$	$Ca^{++}, >V_{th}\uparrow$			spike fall	TEA
$I_{K,Ca(SK)}$	$(I_{Ca} \rightarrow) K^+$	Ca^{++}		$\downarrow$5HT, NE	AHP	apamin
I_{Kir}	K^+	$<V_{th}\downarrow$				
I_h	Na^+, K^+	$<V_{th}\downarrow$		$\uparrow$5HT, NE	V_{sag}	Cs^+
I_{leak}, I_L	K^+ (& Other)			$\downarrow$5HT, NE, TRH,etc.	$\uparrow R_{in} \rightarrow \downarrow I_{rh}$	
Na/K pump	$3Na^+$ out & $2K^+$ in	Na_i^+			MP_r	ouabain

Examples of functionally important ion channels in MN membranes. *Abbreviations for currents (I_{xx}; corresponding conductances would be denoted g_{xx})*: $I_{Na,t}$, transient sodium current; $I_{Na,p}$, persistent sodium current; I_i, persistent inward current (probably Ca^{++}); $I_{Ca,T}$, $I_{Ca,L}$, $I_{Ca,N}$, $I_{Ca,P/Q}$, calcium currents of types T, L, N, P or Q, respectively; *HVA*, high-voltage activated; *LVA*, low-voltage activated; I_K, $I_{K,\,dr}$, delayed rectifier current; I_A, $I_{K,A}$, transient outward current; $I_{K,Ca(SK)}$, $I_{K,Ca(BK)}$, calcium-activated potassium channels with small (SK) and big unitary conductances (BK, also voltage-gated); I_{Kir}, inward rectifier channel; I_h, hyperpolarization-activated cation channel; I_{leak}, I_L, leak current (complex and heterogeneous group of channels, see text); *Na/K pump*, also referred to as Na/K-ATPase. *Indications concerning manner of normal activation*: for voltage-activated currents and conductances it is indicated whether they are modified by membrane potential at levels negative to ($<$), about equal to ($\sim$) or positive to ($>$, $>>$) the voltage threshold for spike initiation (V_{th}). Furthermore, it is indicated whether a conductance would increase ($\uparrow$) or decrease ($\downarrow$) for a positive-going shift of membrane potential. *Other abbreviations*: *Inact*, relative speed of channel-inactivation during constant membrane potential (valid for voltage-gated channels; 'slow' includes cases with (almost) no inactivation); transm, transmitter; *5HT*, serotonin; *NE*, noradrenalin; *Glu-m*, *ACh-m*, glutamine (Glu) or acetylcholine (ACh) acting via metabotropic receptors; *TRH*, thyrotropin releasing hormone (acting as transmitter); *rep firing*, repetitive spike firing in response to maintained activating currents; V_{sag}, voltage sag during subthreshold current injection (cf. Fig. 6.1C); R_{in}, input resistance; I_{rh}, threshold current (rheobase); MP_r, resting membrane potential. For further information and references on these and other ion channels, see text and reviews (Binder *et al.* 1996; McLarnon 1995; Rekling *et al.* 2000; Hille 2001; Sah and Faber 2002).

- for some Ca^{2+} channels, a superimposed outward (hyperpolarizing) current resulting from Ca^{2+} activated K^+ channels
- incoming Ca^{2+} ions may, in addition, have many and complex effects on various intracellular (biochemical) mechanisms, some of which might also affect ion channels in the surface membrane.

A distinction is often made between LVA and HVA Ca^{2+} channels (Table 6.2). The intracellular functional effects of Ca^{2+} ions that are entering a neurone via a particular set of channels may be effectively compartmentalized to only a minor portion of the total cell. This spatial limitation is partly due to the rapid and distributed mechanisms for Ca^{2+} sequestration. For instance, only some of the various Ca^{2+} channels are localized such that they activate neighbouring Ca^{2+}-gated K^+ channels (Umemiya and Berger 1994).

The kinetics of the Ca^{2+} channels and their effects is very complex. The time course of the effects depends on the kinetics of the membrane channel itself (e.g. speed of voltage-dependent activation and, possibly, inactivation and deactivation), the kinetics of secondary effects (if any) triggered by Ca^{2+}, and the speed of Ca^{2+} sequestration by various mechanisms working in parallel (binding to Ca^{2+} buffers, transport into Ca^{2+}-accumulating organelles such as mitochondria, outward transport across the surface membrane). One of the electrophysiologically important functions of inward Ca^{2+} currents is their contribution to the generation of after-potentials (Table 6.2).

6.8.3. K^+ channels

The opening of K^+ channels has a hyperpolarizing effect, counteracting excitation. In biological membranes, there are many different species of K^+ channels (Hille 2001), and only some of the varieties that are well known in MNs are included in Table 6.2. Some of the K^+ channels are directly voltage gated (I_K, I_A) and other important ones are Ca^{2+} gated ($I_{K,Ca(SK)}$) or Ca^{2+} and voltage gated ($I_{K,Ca(BK)}$). The SK channels ($I_{K,Ca(SK)}$) are responsible for the K^+ current underlying the AHP (Sah and Faber 2002); these channels and the AHP are blocked by apamin. Other K^+ channels are of importance for the time course of the action potential (I_K, I_A, $I_{K,Ca(BK)}$) and aspects of subthreshold rectification (I_K).

6.8.4. 'Paradoxical' channels

There are two classes of ion channel that increase their permability on hyperpolarization and close when depolarized. In one class the current is carried by K^+ ions, which means that its direction will normally be outward. Such channels are often referred to as inward rectifiers (I_{Kir}); they exist in several varieties (Hille 2001), and evidence for a function in MNs is mainly derived from studies of brainstem MNs (for further information, see Rekling *et al.* 2000). The other class of hyperpolarization-activated channel will normally pass an inward current (reversal potential at around -20 mV) which is mainly carried K^+ and Na^+ ions. This current is often referred to as I_h (Table 6.2), and it has slow activation kinetics.

6.8.5. 'Leak' channels

The resting conductance of the membrane depends partly on voltage-sensitive channels that are gated at subthreshold membrane potentials (Table 6.2), and to an important extent on channels that are not very effectively voltage gated, which are often referred to as 'leak' channels (I_L). These latter channels are often selective for K^+ ions, and their membrane density is probably one of the main factors responsible for the resting membrane resistivity. Hence these channels are important for the input resistance and electrical excitability of the neurone. There are many types of such channels, including varieties with a so-called 4TM architecture and a two-pore-domain; at least 14 mammalian genes code for such channels (reviewed by Hille 2001; Bayliss *et al.* 2003). The 4TM channels may be gated by various mechanisms other than voltage, including second messengers, changes in pH, and inhalation anaesthetics (e.g. halothane). Some leak channels are also gated by neurotransmitters, which will affect the electrical excitability of the cell (Table 6.2).

6.9. Differentiation of motoneurone characteristics in relation to muscle fibre properties

There are two main ways in which intrinsic MN properties are adapted to the contractile properties of their muscle units.

1 MNs with weak, slow, and fatigue-resistant muscle units and slow axons have *higher input resistances* and are therefore activated with *smaller excitatory currents* than those generally needed for MNs with stronger, faster, and more fatigue sensitive units and faster axons (Figs. 6.6, 6.7). Such differences in intrinsic excitability will promote a recruitment hierarchy favouring the weak, slow, and fatigue-resistant units in weak muscle contractions, which is functionally advantageous (e.g. for postural contractions) ('recruitment gradation match', see Chapter 8, section 8.2).

2 MNs with slow-twitch units and slow axons have *longer AHPs* and slower *minimum steady spike frequencies* than those innervating faster units (Fig. 6.8A,B). These differences are such that the range of steady discharge rates of a MN is matched to the tension–frequency characteristics of its muscle unit ('rate gradation match', Fig. 6.8C,D).

In addition there are also other differences in membrane properties between F- and S-unit MNs (e.g. non-linear membrane properties). Details concerning these various types of MN–muscle unit matching are commented on further below.

6.9.1. Intrinsic excitability (current threshold)

Within a given MN pool, the average current threshold I_{rep} is higher for MNs with fast axons than for those with slower ones (Fig. 6.7A) (Kernell 1966a; Kernell and Monster 1981). Units with fast axons also tend to have stronger muscle units (Chapter 3, section 3.7.3). In terms of unit types, consistent threshold differences are found such that

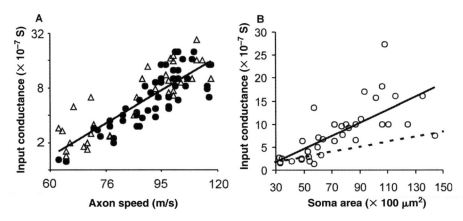

Figure 6.6 Distribution of input conductance versus measures of MN size. The input conductance (inverse of input resistance) for cat hindlimb MNs is positively correlated with both (**A**) axonal conduction velocity (logarithmic coordinates) and (**B**) soma area (correlation coefficients (**A**) 0.84 and (**B**) 0.72; $P < 0.001$). The broken line in (**B**) shows the expected values if input conductance varied in direct proportion to soma membrane area (which it does not). This lack of a direct proportionality between soma area and input conductance could not be explained by differences in the number and size of dendritic stems emerging from the various MNs (Kernell and Zwaagstra 1981). Filled symbols in panel (**A**), data from Kernell (1966a). Open symbols in panels (**A**) and (**B**), cells labelled by intracellular injection of HRP and afterwards reconstructed and measured from serial sections of the spinal cord (data from Kernell and Zwaagstra 1981). Panel (**A**) is replotted from Kernell and Zwaagstra (1981).

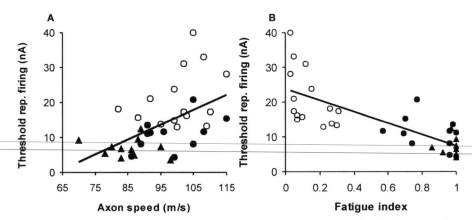

Figure 6.7 Distribution of electrical excitability within a MN population. Threshold current for repetitive firing plotted versus (**A**) axonal conduction velocity and (**B**) muscle unit fatigue index for MNs of cat gastrocnemius medialis muscle. MNs with muscle units clasified as FF (open circles), FR (filled circles), and S (filled triangles). Correlation coefficients were (**A**) +0.53 and (**B**) −0.77; both were statistically significant ($P < 0.001$). Panel (**A**) is replotted from Kernell and Monster (1981); panel (**B**) is plotted from unpublished data from the same study.

S < FR < FF (Table 6.1), and there is also a correspondingly prominent difference between MNs with fatiguable and fatigue-resistant muscle units (Fig. 6.7B). It is notable here that FR and FF units differ systematically in electrical excitability even though they may have the same axonal conduction speed (Table 6.1 and Fig. 6.7A; (I_{rh}, Fleshman *et al.* 1981; I_{rep}, Kernell and Monster 1981). Differences in current threshold may be due to two main mechanisms:

- differences in the amount of current needed per millivolt of depolarization (i.e. differences in neuronal input resistance R_{in})
- differences in the amount of depolarization needed for discharging action potentials (i.e. differences in voltage threshold V_{th}).

Cells with a high current threshold tend to have a smaller input resistance than that found for cells with a lower current threshold (Kernell 1966a; Fleshman *et al.* 1981; Gustafsson and Pinter 1984b); the input resistance is the most important parameter determining intrinsic differences in electrical excitability. However, within a given MN pool, the range of variation in current threshold is often wider than the range for input resistances. For instance, for types of cat gastrocnemius medialis MNs, mean current threshold varied by a factor of 4.3 and input resistance by only a factor of 2.7 (I_{rh}, Table 6.1) (Zengel *et al.* 1985). Thus, in addition to the differences in input resistance, there were also covarying differences in non-linear membrane properties (e.g. for producing depolarizing 'local potentials' below V_{th}) and/or in voltage threshold. Some indications exist that the voltage threshold may indeed be systematically lower for S than for F MNs (Pinter *et al.* 1983; Gustafsson and Pinter 1984b), but these differences are smaller and less consistently present than those found for input resistance.

The input resistance of a neurone depends on the combined effects of two main parameters:

- the size and shape of the neurone, determining the effective membrane area across which (injected) currents will flow
- the (mean) resistance of a unit membrane area at subthreshold membrane potentials (membrane resistivity R_m (Ω cm^2)).

Differences in MN size are certainly of importance for differences in MN input resistance. The input conductance (reciprocal of resistance) is systematically lower for MNs with slow axons than for those with faster axons (Fig. 6.6A) (Kernell 1966a; Burke 1968b; Fleshman *et al.* 1981; Ulfhake and Kellerth 1984; however, cf. Dum and Kennedy 1980a), and the average soma size is larger for MNs with fast and large axons than for those with slower and smaller ones (Fig. 5.5A) (Cullheim 1978; Kernell and Zwaagstra 1981). It has also been shown directly that MNs with small cell bodies indeed have a smaller G_{in} than those with larger cell bodies (Fig. 6.6B) (Kernell and Zwaagstra 1981; Burke *et al.* 1982; Ulfhake and Kellerth 1984). Smaller somas carry a smaller total load of dendritic stems than larger cell bodies (sum of dendritic holes is positively correlated with soma size) (Kernell 1966a; Kernell and Zwaagstra 1981; Ulfhake and Kellerth 1981), i.e. their total membrane area is smaller. However, the apparent differences in total soma-dendrite size are too small to be solely responsible for the differences in input conductance (compare data points with broken line in Fig. 6.6B; see caption for details). These and other measurements (e.g. of membrane time constant (Gustafsson and Pinter 1984c)) indicate that the average membrane resistivity is greater for small than for larger MNs (Kernell and Zwaagstra 1981; Burke *et al.* 1982; Gustafsson and Pinter 1984c; Ulfhake and Kellerth 1984). This has important consequences for the synaptic recruitment thresholds of the various MNs (see Chapter 8, section 8.2.1.3). In terms of unit type, MN membrane resistivity is ranked as S > FR > FF (Burke *et al.* 1982; Ulfhake and Kellerth 1984).

6.9.2. Voltage 'sag'

Within much of the range of subthreshold membrane potentials, several types of ion channels are differentially gated by changes in membrane potential (Table 6.2 and section 6.8). One result of these subthreshold non-linearities is the 'voltage sag' seen in response to a rectangular current step (Fig. 6.1C and section 6.4.1) (Ito and Oshima 1965), which tends to be less prominent in S than in F MNs (Gustafsson and Pinter 1985a). Such differences are probably reponsible for the fact that the threshold for rhythmic firing (I_{rep}) seems to be further from the rheobase (I_{rh}) in fast than in slow cells; weak suprathreshold currents will tend to produce phasic bursts in fast low-resistance MNs but not in slower MNs with a high input resistance (Schwindt 1973). Thus such differences in membrane properties favour the appearance of 'phasic' reflex bursts in MNs with large axons and fast muscle units, as was also noted in early MN studies (cf. 'phasic' versus 'tonic' units in Granit *et al.* (1956; 1957).

6.9.3. Rhythmic properties

6.9.3.1. Early observations

In one of the earliest EMG studies of single motor unit activity, Denny-Brown (1929) observed that the units of slow muscles (mainly soleus) tended to discharge at comparatively slow rates, which seemed to be in general accordance with the slow isometric speed of their contraction (Cooper and Eccles 1930). Several later observations have confirmed that, in voluntary or reflex contractions, MNs of slow muscle units have a range of regular spike frequencies extending down to slower rates than those seen for faster units (e. g. Kernell and Sjoholm 1975; Grimby *et al.* 1979).

After the introduction of intracellular MN recording, Eccles *et al.* (1958a) found that MNs of slow muscles had longer postspike after-hyperpolarizations (AHPs) than MNs innervating fast muscles. They also found a significant negative correlation between axonal conduction speed and AHP duration (Fig. 6.1D), and they suggested that the prolonged AHPs of slow-muscle MNs might be of importance for limiting their discharges to slow rates.

6.9.3.2. Minimum steady firing rate versus duration of AHP

As mentioned in section 6.5.7, F_{min} is strongly correlated with the duration of the single-spike AHP; the intervals at F_{min} are similar to the duration of AHP when studied in hindlimb MNs of anaesthetized cats (Fig. 6.8A) (Kernell 1965c). In addition to the AHP, subthreshold changes in voltage-gated permeabilities will also have an influence on low-frequency firing behaviour. Therefore it is not surprising that, in some preparations, the correlation between minimum rate of steady firing and AHP duration after a single spike might be lower than that seen for the anaesthetized hindlimb MNs in Fig. 6.8A (Jodkowski et al. 1988; Carp et al. 1991; Viana et al. 1995). However, also under such more complex circumstances, the AHP will be one of the major factors setting the minimum rate.

6.9.3.3. Duration of AHP versus twitch speed

At the time of the study of Eccles et al. (1958a), whole muscles were compared and the mixed-unit composition of single muscles had not yet been explored. Further investigations of the relationship between twitch speed and AHP duration revealed that at the level of single units there was also often a positive correlation between AHP duration (or half-decay time) and a measure of twitch time course (time to peak, half-relaxation time) (Hammarberg and Kellerth 1975b; Dum and Kennedy 1980a; Zengel et al. 1985; Cope et al. 1986; Gardiner 1993). Using indirect methods, Gossen et al. (2003) obtained similar results from humans. Direct comparisons showed that, on average, isometric twitch duration was very similar to AHP duration (Fig. 6.8B) (Kernell 1983; Bakels and Kernell 1993 a, b), which means that F_{min} would be set to a rate close to the lowest value producing a partial 'summation' of twitches in repetitive activation, i.e. at the lower end of the steep portion of the T–f curve (Fig. 6.8 C,D). The correlation between isometric twitch speed and the minimum and maximum rates within the primary range has also been demonstrated experimentally (Kernell 1979, 1983). On average, 'speed-matching' between AHP and twitch duration generally seems to be present in MN pools of single muscles. However, in some muscles with a rather narrow range of variation of muscle unit isometric speed, the mean twitch duration is similar to the mean AHP duration without a continuous correlation between the two measures (true for tibialis anterior of the rat (Bakels and Kernell 1993a); weak correlation in pretibial flexors of cat (Dum and Kennedy 1980a)). Thus, for the relationship between AHP versus twitch duration, the mean and the continuous matching might be independently controlled.

6.9.3.4. Maximum rates of steady firing in fast versus slow MNs

In cat hindlimb MNs studied under general anaesthesia, the maximum steady rates of firing showed a positive correlation with the inverse of AHP duration (1/AHP) (Kernell 1965c). As there is no evident causal link between AHP and maximum firing rate (section 6.6.4), this correlation suggests that, for cat hindlimb MNs, there is a systematic covariation between AHP duration and, perhaps, the voltage dependence of g_{Na} inactivation.

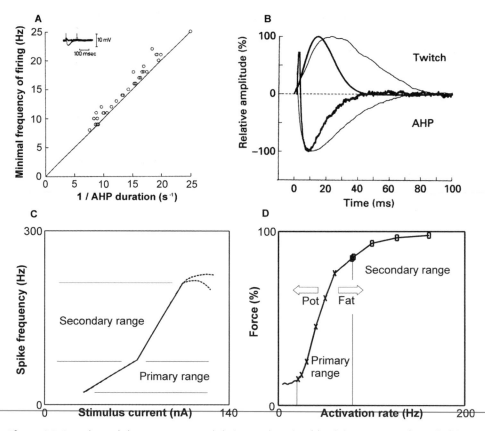

Figure 6.8 Speed match between MNs and their muscle units. (**A**) Minimum rates of steady firing in discharges evoked by maintained injected current plotted versus 1/AHP duration. The diagonal line is plotted for $y = x$. Inset: AHP of MN, threshold antidromic stimulation, 15–20 superimposed sweeps. Hindlimb MNs, anaesthetized cat. (Reproduced with permission, from Kernell 1965c.)
(**B**) Averaged recordings of AHP and twitch for a slow (thin lines) and a fast (thick lines) MN muscle unit combination (rat, gastrocnemius medialis). Twitches and AHPs are all drawn with normalized amplitudes and a common timescale. Action potentials preceding the AHPs are not shown (elicited at time zero). Note the similarity of duration for the AHP and the twitch of the same motor unit. (Reproduced with permission, from Bakels and Kernell 1993b.) (**c**),(**D**) Schematic illustration of how the repetitive properties of MNs and the contractile properties of their muscle units are functionally matched to each other. (**c**) Motoneuronal relation between steady discharge rate and the intensity of a constant activating current (*f–I* curve). (**D**) Muscle unit relation between isometric force and activation rate (*T–f* curve). The lower and upper limits of spike frequency for the primary and secondary range are indicated by (**c**) horizontal and (**D**) vertical lines. The plotted firing rates are those obtained after the initial phase of spike-frequency adaptation. Note that firing rates of the primary range correspond to the most effective activation rates for changing muscle force. The numerical dimensions on the *x*- and *y*-axes of (**c**) and (**D**) are those characteristic for relatively fast units of cat hindlimb muscles (for (**D**) as studied at the muscle length giving a maximum twitch force). A rightward shift of the *T–f* curve will cause less force to be generated for a given intermediate spike frequency (Fat, fatigue) and a leftward shift gives the opposite effect (Pot, potentiation). For stimulus currents exceeding those of the linear secondary range, the *f–I* relationship generally flattens off or declines (see dotted curves in (**c**)) and, finally, firing stops ('spike inactivation'). (Reproduced with permission, from Kernell 1995.)

In the absence of a causal link, the relationship between AHP and maximum spike frequency might conceivably be quite different for different neuronal populations. For instance, in turtle MNs, low-threshold MNs (MN-1) and high-threshold MNs (MN-4) differed in maximum rate, while there were no significant differences in AHP duration or minimum rate (Hornby *et al.* 2002b). Also in the turtle, the minimum rate was, on average, rather close to 1/AHP (mean for all: F_{min} = 6.4 Hz versus 1/AHP = 5.1 s^{-1}).

For an optimal use of muscle, the maximum rates of a MN should be high enough to elicit a fused maximum tetanic contraction. For cat hindlimb MNs, this requirement seems fulfilled with regard to the properties of hindlimb muscle fibres (Fig. 6.8D). Higher rates would be needed for the twitch fibres of extraocular muscles (Cooper and Eccles 1930; Shall and Goldberg 1992) and, correspondingly, extraocular MNs may have adapted *f–I* relations extending up to rates of several hundred hertz (Grantyn and Grantyn 1978).

6.9.3.5. The *f–I* slope and the range of required driving currents

Reports have been inconsistent with regard to the presence of systematic variations of 'gain' (i.e. the slope of the relation between spike frequency and stimulating current (*f–I* slope)) between different kinds of cat hindlimb MNs. In an early study of mixed hindlimb MNs, in which the contractile properties of muscle units were not investigated, cells with a high input resistance and a low current threshold (i.e. MNs of presumed S units) were found to have a less steep *f–I* slope than those with a lower input resistance and a higher current threshold (Kernell 1966a). In a later study, the average steady-state *f–I* slope was 1.4 Hz/nA, and no significant correlation was found between *f–I* slope and muscle unit characteristics (MNs of cat gastrocnemius medialis) (Kernell 1979). Thus, within the hindlimb as a whole, some highly excitable (slow?) units may have MNs with rather low *f–I* slopes, but this tendency may not be significantly present within each MN pool. It should be noted that these comparisons concern absolute measures of *f–I* slope (Hz/nA). If large and small cells have the same absolute *f–I* slope, the slope with regard to current density (*f–I$_d$* slope) would be greater in the larger cell (less current density for the same absolute intensity of stimulation). Conversely, if the *f–I$_d$* slopes were equal for large and smaller MNs, the absolute *f–I* slope would be expected to be steeper for the MNs with slower axons; this is opposite to the experimental findings (Kernell 1966a, 1979). Thus both these series of investigations actually indicate that the *f–I$_d$* slope is lower in small MNs than in larger and faster ones. As a consequence, smaller changes of firing rate would be expected in slow than in faster MNs if both types were influenced by similar shifts in synaptic current density.

Based on the combined knowledge concerning the excitability of cat triceps surae MNs (Kernell 1979; Kernell and Monster 1981) and the relationship between AHP duration and the range of firing rates (Kernell 1965c), it can be calculated that a slow MN with an AHP of 200 ms might reach a maximal firing rate in the secondary range of about 55 Hz when activated with a current intensity of about 27 nA (threshold current 3 nA). At the other extreme, an FF MN with an AHP of 50 ms might need 105 nA to reach about 210 Hz (threshold current 30 nA). These numbers are very approximate and intended only for roughly indicating which range of postsynaptic excitatory currents would be needed to drive MN repetitive discharges (cf. Chapter 7, section 7.4.2).

6.9.3.6. Spike-frequency adaptation

As was discussed earlier, there are two main phases of spike-frequency adaptation in MNs which depend on different main mechanisms. The first phase is typically very brief and is partly caused by a 'summation' of the AHP currents of the first few spikes. This phase of spike-frequency adaptation is well matched to the muscle-controlling task of MNs. A maximum rate of rise of muscle force requires much higher rates than those needed for the maintenance of maximum tension (Buller and Lewis 1965c). Thus the high initial firing rate produced at the onset of a rectangular current pulse helps to produce a fast rise of force in response to a fast rise of stimulation, i.e. in this sense the initial phase of adaptation helps to 'linearize' the relation between synaptic input and force output for the MN–muscle unit complex. These aspects of the initial spike-frequency adaptation have been extensively explored by Baldissera and his colleagues (Baldissera and Parmiggiani 1975; for further references, see Baldissera *et al.* 1987).

In their analysis of the late phase of spike-frequency adaptation, Kernell and Monster (1982a) found less adaptation in S-type MNs than in those of F units when all cells were activated with a stimulating test current of 5 nA above the rhythmic threshold. However, the amount of late adaptation in each individual neurone, as well as across the tested population of cells, was markedly dependent on the starting rate of a discharge: the higher the starting rate, the more adaptation (i.e. more decline in spike-frequency). Presumably because of their long AHPs, the S units fired at lower initial rates for the standardized test current, and this might have been responsible for much of their low degree of late adaptation (Fig. 6.3B, triangles). Thus the small amount of late adaptation in S units might be a secondary (and useful) consequence of their low rates of discharge. Of course, there might also be frequency-independent differences in late adaptation between slow and fast MNs. Such differences might be investigated by comparing the currents needed for clamping a steady firing rate at the same spike frequency in long-lasting discharges of slow versus fast MNs.

6.9.3.7. Match between f–I and T–f curve

Direct comparisons between the f–I curve of a MN and the T–f curve of its muscle unit (or of units of corresponding speed) show that the steep portion of the T–f curve corresponds to rates within the primary range of firing for the MN (Fig. 6.8C,D) (Kernell 1965c, 1966b, 1979). The secondary range, with a steep f–I slope, corresponds to the upper portion of the T–f curve with a less steep T–f slope. Thus, in this upper range of spike-frequencies, the steep f–I slope partly compensates for the declining slope of the

T–f relation, helping to linearize the relation between motoneuronal excitation and muscle unit force. At least for isometric contractions at the optimum muscle length, firing within the secondary range would be needed to produce the final 15–30 per cent of the maximum attainable force of a muscle unit.

6.9.3.8. Plateau behaviour

As described in section 6.7.2, MNs in good condition may start to generate 'self-stimulating' PICs above a certain level of depolarization. This capacity for self-stimulation is facilitated by various kinds of metabotropic transmitter-receptor interactions, including those of

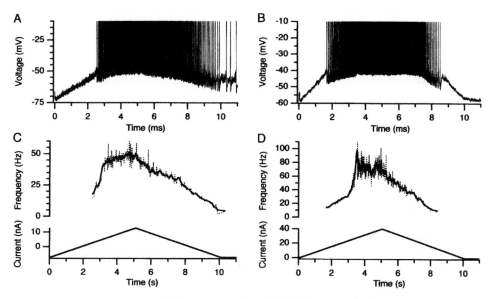

Figure 6.9 Plateau currents in different categories of hindlimb MNs. Plateau currents are more easily evoked in (presumed) slow MNs than in fast MNs. Intracellular stimulation of a 'fully bistable cell' (left) and of a 'partially bistable cell' (right). (**A**),(**B**) Changes in membrane potential in response to a triangular injected current (10 s total duration, spikes truncated for clarity). (**C**),(**D**) Firing frequency versus time for data from (**A**) and (**B**). Dotted curve, instantaneous firing rate; bold curve, smoothed firing rate (moving average of five interspike intervals); solid line (below), injected current intensity. In the fully bistable cell, the threshold for repetitive firing coincided with that for the plateau current (i.e. initial firing rate acceleration). In the partially bistable cell, firing rate acceleration occurred at a stimulating current ~8 nA higher than that required for initiation of firing. Decerebrate cat; noradrenergic α_1 agonist (methoxamine) applied to ventral surface of the spinal cord. Compared with fully bistable cells, the partially bistable MNs had a higher rheobase and more rapidly conducting axons. (Reproduced with permission, from Lee and Heckman 1998b.)

monoaminergic synapses. The generation of booster PICs in spinal MNs of different functional categories was investigated by Lee and Heckman (1998a,b) who found that the phenomenon had a lower threshold in presumed 'slow' MNs (Fig. 6.9A,C) than in presumed 'fast' MNs (Fig. 6.9B,D (cell categories were assessed by measurements of axonal conduction velocity and current threshold). As a result, under their experimental conditions a maintained plateau discharge could more easily be generated in the presumed 'slow' MNs ('fully bistable cells') than in the 'fast' MNs ('partially bistable cells'); in the fully bistable cells, PICs were generated even below the threshold level for action potentials. Furthermore, compared with the partially bistable neurones, deactivation of the PICs was less rapid and occurred at less depolarized levels in fully bistable cells. Prolonged plateau discharges in slow MNs might be useful for the maintenance of postural contractions. In 'fast' MNs the PICs would appear above a certain frequency of repetitive firing, shifting the firing rate to a higher level (Fig. 6.9B,D; cf. Fig. 6.5C,D) ('bistable' firing), which might be useful for the performance of fast movements. These differences between presumed fast and slow MNs might reflect genuine differences in membrane properties (e.g. different thresholds and kinetics of voltage-gated Ca^{2+} channels), differences in Ca^{2+} sequestration parameters, and/or differences in the localization of PIC-generating membranes within the dendritic trees.

6.10. **Pathophysiological issue: motoneurone disease**

Amyotrophic lateral sclerosis (ALS), also known as Lou Gehrig's disease in the USA, is the most common adult MN disease (reviewed by Bruijn *et al.* 2004). The disease causes a selective dysfunction and death of neurones in the motor pathways, including both the MNs with peripheral axons and large cells in the corticospinal pathways ('lower motoneurones' and 'upper motoneurones' respectively in neurological terminology). Patients usually die within 1–5 years of onset, mostly from respiratory failure. Only about 5–10 per cent of all cases are inherited. The lifetime risk is about 1:2000, and the typical age of onset is around 50–60 years.

The causes of ALS are still largely unknown. Among the familial cases (i.e. 5–10 per cent of all cases), approximately 20 per cent are apparently caused by particular kinds of mutations (dominantly inherited) in the protein Cu/Zn superoxide dismutase (SOD1). The best-known function of this enzyme is to convert superoxide, a toxic byproduct of mitochondrial oxidative phosphorylation, to water or hydrogen peroxide. However, SOD1-mutation-mediated toxicity in ALS is not due to a loss of SOD1 function but instead to the emergence of toxic properties of the changed SOD1-protein, independently of the levels of SOD1 enzyme activity. Thus, for instance, SOD1 knock-out mice do not develop any disease resembling ALS. However, certain types of SOD1-mutant mice do indeed develop a MN disease, and three types of SOD1-transgenic mice (SOD1-G85R, SOD1-G37R, and SOD1-G93A) have been extensively characterized and explored as models of ALS. In such mice, weakness typically starts in the hindlimbs at between 3 and 12 months of age. This hindlimb weakness coincides with a loss of spinal cord MNs, and the pathology mimics many aspects of the human ALS disease.

Electrophysiological MN properties of presymptomatic SOD1-G93A-mutant transgenic mice (SOD1-mice) have been extensively investigated using tissue culture techniques (Kuo *et al.* 2005). The MNs from SOD1-mice had repetitive spike-discharge properties that differed from those of normal mice; the *f–I* slope was steeper and the maximum firing rate was higher. These changes were more evident in cells with a low input resistance, i.e. presumably in larger MNs. The increased excitability was due to an increased PIC for Na^+ ions (PIC_{Na}), which could be selectively blocked with riluzole. In high-input-resistance MNs, the depolarizing effects of this increased PIC_{Na} were counteracted by other mechanisms. Interestingly, ALS preferentially kills the larger MNs (Sobue *et al.* 1983), and riluzole is known as a drug that slows down the progress of ALS symptoms and prolongs life in both humans and mice (Bensimon *et al.* 1994; Gurney *et al.* 1996). However, riluzole also has a variety of other actions, such as inhibition of glutamate release and enhancement of glutamate uptake (Doble 1996; Dunlop *et al.* 2003). In a vulnerable MN, an increased rate of spike firing due to the increased PIC_{Na} might possibly cause a dangerous increase of Ca^{2+} entry; high intracellular levels of Ca^{2+} are toxic. There is also other evidence indicating that Ca^{2+} ions play an important role in ALS; MNs that are well provided with Ca^{2+} buffering systems are relatively resistant to ALS and survive longer than other MNs (e.g. extraocular MNs, containing high levels of parvalbumin and/or calbindin 28K (Alexianu *et al.* 1994)). Normal MNs of the types that are sensitive to ALS often have a dangerously low calcium-binding capacity (low concentrations of calcium buffer) (Ladewig *et al.* 2003).

Among the several mechanisms that might play a role in ALS, one must not forget the possible importance of MN–muscle interactions; MNs may become more vulnerable and die because of a decreased of provision of crucial substances from the muscle (see Chapter 10, section 10.2.6, and Chapter 12, section 12.6). However, such a lack apparently does not concern the classical neurotrophic substances because they have even been found to be *increased* in muscles of deceased ALS patients (Kust *et al.* 2002).

Chapter 7

Motoneurones: synaptic control

7.1. General issues

A central problem in neuroscience concerns the question of how the hundreds to thousands of synapses on a neurone are used to control its activity. These processes have been extensively studied for MNs. During the last 10–20 years, an increasing amount of evidence has been accumulated concerning the important dichotomy between synapses with primarily a 'driving' function (the conventional excitation and inhibition) and those with primarily a 'MN-modifying' function (changing the manner in which MNs respond to changes in synaptic drive). Furthermore, several types of synaptic input to MNs have been studied in unusual detail at cellular level; the best known instance is the monosynaptic MN projection of type Ia afferents from muscle spindles.

7.2. Individual synapses: cytology and physiology

7.2.1. Electrical versus chemical synapses

During early embryonic development, direct connections called 'gap junctions' are commonly seen between (future) nerve cells in the CNS. In electron microscopy (EM) such structures are characterized by a very small distance of 3.5 nm between pre- and postsynaptic membranes; this small gap is bridged by a varying number of very thin tubular channels (**connexons**) which allow the passage of molecules up to a diameter of about 1.5 nm (Kandel and Siegelbaum 2000a; Alberts *et al.* 2002). Small molecules (e.g. amino acids) and inorganic ions, but not proteins and other macromolecules, can pass through these connexons. In electrophysiology, gap junctions are often referred to as 'electrical' or 'electrotonic' synapses. Most of the early connections ultimately disappear. By far the majority of the synapses in the adult mammalian CNS (and onto the MNs) show the EM characteristics of chemical synapses (Fig. 7.1):

♦ pre- and postsynaptic membranes are separated by a synaptic cleft of width about 20–40 nm

♦ small synaptic vesicles are accumulated in the presynaptic terminal

♦ electron-dense specializations are commonly seen in apposing pre- and postsynaptic membranes.

These general EM characteristics are similar to those of the neuromuscular junction (Fig. 4.1), an extremely large chemical synapse. In the CNS, most axon terminals end in

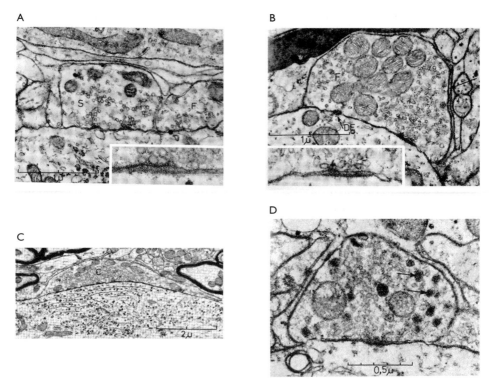

Figure 7.1 Types of synapses on spinal MNs. Electron micrographs of characteristic types of presynaptic boutons on cat spinal MNs. (**A**) S type (spherical synaptic vesicles, see inset). Abouton of the F type (flattened synaptic vesicles) can be seen on the right of this panel. (**B**) F type (flattened vesicles, see inset). Scales for (**A**) and (**B**): main panel, bar = 1 μm; inset, bar = 0.42 μm. (**C**) C-type bouton on the proximal part of a motoneuron dendrite. Note the abundance of granular endoplasmic reticulum below the bouton. Scale bar = 2 μm. (**D**) Bouton with several dense-core vesicles. Scale bar = 0.5 μm. Electron-dense membrane specializations along the synaptic cleft ('active regions') are most clearly seen in the high-magnification panels (insets to (**A**) and (**B**); (**D**)). (Reproduced with permission, from Conradi and Skoglund 1969.)

a slightly thickened 'terminal bouton', which typically has an average diameter of about 1–2 μm (Fig. 7.1), i.e. such boutons can, if suitably stained, be counted even under light microscopy. It should be remembered that only part of the area of close apposition between pre- and postsynaptic membranes appears to contribute to the synaptic function. These 'active regions' appear as thickenings in suitably prepared EM sections (Fig. 7.1). The space between the boutons is occupied by processes of astroglia.

7.2.2. Different morphological types of chemical synapse

In EM studies of synapses, several attempts have been made to distinguish between different types based on their morphology. One of the most common distinctions concerns the shape of the synaptic vesicles, sometimes as seen after pretreatment with certain EM fixatives (Kandel and Siegelbaum 2000c). Based on such criteria, synapses on MNs are often classified as follows (Conradi and Skoglund 1969):

- S-type synapses with spherical vesicles, assumed to be excitatory (Fig. 7.1A); sometimes an L-type subcategory of synapses is used for those with spherical vesicles and long appositions (>4 μm) (Brannstrom 1993)
- F-type synapses with flat or pleomorphic vesicles, assumed to be inhibitory (Fig. 7–1 B)
- synapses with large dense-core vesicles, assumed to be monoaminergic or peptidergic (Fig. 7.1D)
- synapses with small irregular vesicles, typically seen in synapses onto other boutons and likely to be responsible for **presynaptic inhibition**, i.e. a synaptically evoked decrease of the effect of excitatory synapses.

In addition to these characteristics, there is one type of morphological arrangement which has attracted particular attention—the so-called 'C synapses' which show, on the postsynaptic side, cisternae (membrane bags) with ribosomes, indicating that they as sites for protein synthesis (Fig. 7.1C). Such synapses might be of particular interest in relation to MN plasticity and 'trophic' influences. Interestingly, these synapses are apparently cholinergic and associated with muscarinic postsynaptic membrane receptors (Nagy *et al.* 1993; Hellstrom *et al.* 2003). C synapses constitute about 10 per cent or less of all synaptic boutons (11 per cent on soma, 6 per cent on proximal dendrites of monkey MNs , Starr and Wolpaw 1994), and they are not present on presumed gamma MNs (cat, Destombes *et al.* 1992). Apparently, the cholinergic terminals which end in C synapses do not include those of the MN collaterals onto MNs (cf. Chapter 8, section 8.5.2) (Lagerback *et al.* 1981b).

On primate triceps surae MNs, 56–58 per cent of all boutons are type F and 33–36 per cent are type S (soma and dendrites, Starr and Wolpaw 1994). Also, for the soma and proximal dendrites of cat MNs, type F boutons tend to be more common than those of type S (Conradi *et al.* 1979; Kellerth *et al.* 1979; Brannstrom 1993).

7.2.3. Different cytochemical types of presynaptic terminals and their distribution

In order to identify a transmitter substance clearly it is not sufficient to demonstrate its presynaptic localization. Its activity-dependent neuronal release and appropriate postsynaptic effects also need to be shown. Such complete proofs are difficult to deliver, and most of the evidence concerning the transmitter identity of synapses converging onto MNs is limited to observations of the following:

- high presynaptic intravesicular concentrations of the transmitter candidate
- adequate postsynaptic reactions of MNs when the compound is artificially applied (**micro-iontophoresis**; may be done via microelectrodes, also inside the CNS)
- transmitter-specific postsynaptic receptor molecules, identified using pharmacological tools (receptor-specific antagonists and agonists).

In EM studies, most synapses on MNs contain clear vesicles which are either round (S type) or flat (F type) (Fig. 7.1A,B) (Conradi *et al.* 1979; Kellerth *et al.* 1979; Brannstrom 1993; Starr and Wolpaw 1994). Correspondingly, the vast majority of synapses on MNs contain either the excitatory transmitter glutamate or one or both of the inhibitory transmitters glycine and GABA (Table 7.1) (Ornung *et al.* 1996, 1998). These excitatory and inhibitory synapses are probably mainly responsible for producing the driving currents needed for eliciting and controlling MN discharges.

MNs receive roughly 1.4–3.7 times as many inhibitory as excitatory synapses; this is indicated by both the distribution of different ultrastructural bouton types (type F

Table 7.1 Major transmitter-containing presynaptic terminals on MNs

Transmitter	% Prox	% Dist	Rec-i	Funct-i	Rec-m
GABA[a]	72	55	GABA$_{A,C}$	I: $\uparrow g_{Cl}$	GABA$_B$
Glycine[a]			Gly		
Glutamate	21	40	AMPA	E: $\uparrow(g_K$ and $g_{Na})$	mGluR
			Kainate	E: $\uparrow(g_K$ and $g_{Na})$	
			NMDA	E: $\uparrow(g_K, g_{Na},$ and $g_{Ca})$	
Others	7	6			
Probably including:					
Serotonin (5HT)[b]			5HT$_3$		5HT$_{1,2,7}$
Norepinephrine (NE)					$\alpha_1, \alpha_2,$
Dopamine					D$_1$, D$_2$
Acetylcholine (ACh)					Muscarinic
Furthermore:					
ATP, adenosine, TRH[b],					
neurokinins (e.g.					
substance P)[b], other					
neuropeptides[b]					

MNs from cat spinal cord. %prox and %dist are the percentages of synaptic terminals on MN dendrites that were immunoreactive to glutamate or to GABA and/or glycine (Ornung *et al.* 1998, Tables 2–3). %prox gives percentages calculated for stem dendrites, and %dist for the rest of the dendritic trees investigated. Measurements from the soma have indicated a coverage of about 69 per cent for GABA/glycine and 19 per cent for glutamate, i.e. a factor of 3.7 times less (Ornung *et al.* 1996; Linda *et al.* 2000). The category 'Others' are those boutons that were not labelled for GABA, glycine, or glutamate (excluding the C boutons), i.e. in these cases the transmitters were not identified.

Abbreviations: Rec-i, ionotropic receptor(s); Funct-i, function of ionotropic receptor; Rec-m, metabotropic receptor(s); I, inhibition; E, excitation.

[a]Co-localization very common.

[b]Co-localization common.

Metabotropic receptors may mediate slow PSPs and often have MN-modifying functions (see text and Table 6.2). For further information concerning transmitters and their receptors see Rekling *et al.* (2000).

versus S, section 7.2.2) and the distribution of boutons containing different transmitters (GABA, glycine, or glutamate) (Table 7.1). However, this does not necessarily mean that the total of all inhibitory synaptic effects would be stronger than that of the excitatory ones. Consider a membrane like that in Fig. 2.2A with a resting potential of E_m, and a resting input conductance of g_m (= $1/R_m$). The cell is kept at threshold membrane potential V_{th} with a combination of postsynaptic excitation and inhibition. The excitatory current is generated by the ionic conductance g_e with equilibrium potential E_e, and the inhibitory current is generated by conductance g_i with equilibrium potential E_i. In the steady state there are no capacitive currents, and the following equations apply:

$$i_m + i_e + i_i = 0 \qquad (7.1)$$
$$i_m = g_m(V_{th}-E_m) \qquad (7.2)$$
$$i_e = g_e(V_{th}-E_e) \qquad (7.3)$$
$$I_i = g_i(V_{th}-E_i). \qquad (7.4)$$

In MN physiology (Eccles 1964), E_m is usually considered to be about -70 mV, V_{th} is around -60 mV, E_e is close to 0 mV (e.g. for glutamate excitation), and E_i is close to -80 mV (e.g. for GABA or glycine inhibition). Inserting these values and combining the equations gives the following expression for the amount of excitatory postsynaptic conductance change needed for keeping membrane potential at threshold:

$$g_e = (g_m/6) + (g_i/3). \qquad \text{Eq.7–5}$$

Thus, for synapses close to the soma (or close to each other, with the same V_{th}), one unit of excitatory conductance change balances three units of inhibitory change because of the pronounced differences in driving potential (60 mV for excitation, 20 mV for inhibition). Thus, when taking such biophysical characteristics into account, MNs appear to be provided with functionally roughly equivalent total amounts of synaptic inhibition and excitation; there is apparently (almost) enough total inhibition available to balance all the excitation. Furthermore, this simple example illustrates that, when considering the effects at a given membrane potential (e.g. the threshold potential), 'shunting' effects of inhibition are unimportant and excitatory and inhibitory currents simply add (cf. absence of shunting effects in repetitive impulse firing (Fig. 7.5A–C)).

In a minority of synapses (probably roughly 6–7 per cent, Table 7–1), a multitude of other types of (potential) transmitter substances are accumulated, including monoamines and several kinds of neuropeptides. In many cases, different combinations of such transmitters are co-localized in different boutons. Such synapses are probably largely engaged in MN-modifying functions, changing the manner in which the MN responds to excitatory and inhibitory driving currents, e.g. by facilitating the appearance of booster-PICs and/or by changing the excitability or frequency-current relation of the MN.

Some of the synaptic supply to MNs might be of a dynamic nature, changing with the hormonal state of the animal (e.g., effects of oestrogen, cat, Vanderhorst and Holstege 1997a; monkey, Vanderhorst et al. 2002).

7.2.4. **Different kinds of postsynaptic receptors**

The postsynaptic effect of a neurotransmitter (or transmitter combination) depends on the type and the amount of expression of postsynaptic membrane receptors. Pharmacological and immuno-histochemical studies have demonstrated that synapses using the same transmitter can be separated into many different functional types with regard to their postsynaptic receptor molecules. This variability has long been known for the peripheral nervous system, starting with the distinction between ACh receptors of two main types: nicotinic (agonist nicotine; blocker curare) and muscarinic (agonist muscarine; blocker atropine). The list of different postsynaptic receptor molecules is continuously growing for each type of small-molecule transmitter (for examples, see Table 7.1).

A major dichotomy with regard to postsynaptic characteristics is that between 'ionotropic' and 'metabotropic' receptors (Siegelbaum *et al.* 2000). In synapses expressing ionotropic receptors, the transmitter molecule will directly cause an ion receptor channel to open, thus directly giving rise to a rapid change of postsynaptic current and potential. The vast majority of all the synapses on MNs seem to be of the ionotropic kind (Table 7.1). In synapses with metabotropic receptors, the transmitter molecule will trigger off a cascade of biochemical events in the cytoplasm, typically mediated by G proteins which are linked to the receptor. Various intracellular 'second messengers' are involved (e.g. cyclic AMP (cAMP) and cyclic GMP (cGMP)) and, ultimately, the biochemical events may result in the opening of ion channels through the membrane, causing a postsynaptic potential. Thus metabotropic synapses may also generate excitatory or inhibitory currents. Such postsynaptic effects may last for seconds to minutes, i.e. much longer than those mediated by ionotropic receptors. In metabotropic-receptor-mediated synaptic transmission, the ionic conductance is ultimately modulated via the phosphorylation of an ion-gating protein separate from that of the receptor itself. In addition, the intracellular 'signalling cascade' may lead to other changes inside the cell and/or in its membrane properties. For instance, metabotropic synapses of various kinds are known to influence the properties of voltage-gated ion channels (MN-modifying synapses) (see Tables 6.2 and 7.1, and section 7.5).

In activated excitatory ionotropic glutamate synapses with kainate or AMPA receptors (Table 7.1), the postsynaptic ion channels typically allow the passage of K^+ and Na^+ ions, producing a net depolarizing current with an equilibrium potential close to 0 mV, i.e. postsynaptic effects similar to those generating the EPP at the neuromuscular junction (Chapter 4, section 4.3.5). In a resting cell, single-spike activation of such a synapse generates an excitatory postsynaptic potential (EPSP), a phenomenon similar to the EPP but very much smaller. Like the EPP, the EPSP of 'fast' (ionotropic) synapses has a rapid rising phase and a subsequent more gradual falling phase which largely reflects the passive MN membrane properties (cf. Figs 7.2A and 7.4B,C). In the endplate, the EPP generated by a single axon may be about 30 mV (Fig. 4.2B), much larger than the value needed for discharging a postsynaptic action potential. In the MN, a single presynaptic axon often evokes an EPSP of 0.1–0.2 mV or less (**unitary EPSP**) (Fig. 7.2A–C), i.e.

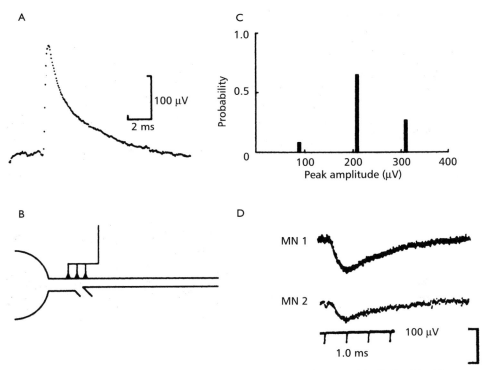

Figure 7.2 Unitary postsynaptic potentials in MNs. All records from cat hindlimb MNs. (**A**) Average time course of unitary EPSP generated by a single Ia afferent axon. This axon and the MN were anatomically reconstructed after being labelled with intracellular injection of HRP. (**B**) Three boutons were found on a proximal dendrite. (**c**) When activated repeatedly, the EPSP amplitude fluctuated between three quantal levels. (Reproduced with permission, from Redman and Walmsley 1983a.) (**D**) Unitary IPSPs generated in MNs by an inhibitory interneurone. In each case, spikes recorded from a single Ia inhibitory interneurone were used for spike-triggered averaging of the membrane potential responses in a target MN. Averaged potentials shown for the effects of the same interneurone on two different MNs. (Reproduced with permission, from Jankowska and Roberts 1972.)

1–2 per cent or less of the depolarization typically needed to evoke a MN action potential. Thus MNs can only be made to discharge by the summed effects of nearly simultaneous activations of many synapses.

A special and relatively complex example of an ionotropic excitatory mechanism is that of the NMDA receptor (Table 7.1) (reviewed by Rekling *et al.* 2000), in which glutamic acid may cause the opening of channels that allow the passage of Ca^{2+} ions in addition to Na^+ and K^+; the Ca^{2+} current will add to the excitatory (depolarizing) effect. However, in these receptors, the ion channels are normally blocked by Mg^{2+} ions, which will be removed only if the postsynaptic membrane is sufficiently depolarized (e.g. by activation of other synapses, including those with AMPA receptors). Thus in this case the synapse is only fully functional if other synaptic inputs have provided the necessary background depolarization for the cell, i.e. the NMDA synapse can be said to be voltage gated. In addition to the direct excitatory actions of such synapses, caused by the net inward current, the Ca^{2+} influx may also have numerous effects on intracellular biochemical processes. Therefore NMDA receptors and the synaptic regulation of Ca^{2+} entry have attracted much attention as a possible mechanism for long-term effects of synaptic activity on cell properties (cf. similar possible effects of metabotropic receptors). Monosynaptic EPSPs generated in MNs by Ia afferents from muscle spindles are largely produced via AMPA receptors and may include a slower component evoked via NMDA receptors (Rekling *et al.* 2000).

In activated ionotropic inhibitory synapses (transmitter glycine and/or GABA), the postsynaptic current is usually carried by Cl^- ions and its equilibrium potential is about -80 mV. In a resting cell with a membrane potential close to V_{th}, single-spike activation of such inhibitory synapses generates an inhibitory postsynaptic potential (IPSP) which looks like a mirror image of the rapid EPSP and is about equally small for single-axon activation (**unitary IPSP**) (Fig. 7.2D). Activation of inhibitory synapses produces currents that tend to drive the membrane potential in a direction negative to V_{th}, thus directly counteracting synaptic excitatory currents (see equations (7.4) and (7.5)). Examples of ionotropic 'fast' IPSPs are those generated by Renshaw cells and by Ia inhibitory interneurones (reciprocal inhibition) (Fig. 7.2D).

7.2.5. **Numbers of presynaptic inputs per motoneurone**

Bouton counts have been done in several studies during the past four decades. Often, synaptic packing densities for spinal MNs have been reported to be around 10–25 boutons per 100 μm^2 membrane area (e.g. Ornung *et al.* 1998). Synaptic densities on dendrites have been found to be rather similar to those for the soma, but the distal dendritic boutons are smaller in size. In primate MNs, synaptic terminals covered 39 per cent of the cell body membrane, 60 per cent of the proximal dendritic membrane, and 40 per cent of the distal dendritic membrane (Starr and Wolpaw 1994). Measurements of total MN soma-dendritic size are given in Chapter 5 (see Table 5.1). Combining this evidence with the data for bouton densities has provided an estimated total number of synapses of about 50 000–140 000 for a cat spinal MN (Ornung *et al.* 1998).

Very commonly, several of the branches of presynaptic central axons terminate on each postsynaptic cell (e.g. a MN). Thus the total number of synapses on a MN is considerably larger than the number of presynaptic neurones delivering these synapses. The only carefully measured system from this point of view concerns the monosynaptic connections from Ia axons onto MNs. In this case each axon has, on average, about 10 boutons on a homonymous MN and six boutons on a heteronymous MN (Burke and Glenn 1996). If this is taken as a representative case, a MN with 100 000 synaptic boutons on its membrane would be commanded by a total of roughly 10 000–20 000 presynaptic neurones.

The number of presynaptic neurones does not tell us directly how many presynaptic functional entities are concerned in driving a MN because, almost certainly, each presynaptic neurone is just one individual in a functional population of pre-motoneuronal cells. At this level, the uncertainty becomes very great. Again, Ia axons provide an interesting example. A functional population of Ia axons might be considered to consist of the Ia afferents coming from the same muscle (cf. Table 2.1, number of spindles). This would result in a characteristic population size of roughly 50 per functional set. As applied to the total synaptic input of single MNs, this might mean that the number of presynaptic functional entities (i.e. command populations) which together 'manage' a MN (or a MN population) might be roughly 200–400, which is still a large number but more 'manageable' than 100 000 synapses. In this context, it is interesting to note that there are roughly 30 times as many neurones as MNs in a spinal cord segment (Gelfan and Tarlov 1963). There are large numbers of descending fibres from other parts of the spinal cord (propriospinal paths) and from the brain, and most of these do not contact MNs directly but are connected to various kinds of other intraspinal neurones ('interneurones'). The Ia monosynaptic connections from various hindlimb muscles to a hindlimb MN account for only about 500–1000 synapses (Burke and Glenn 1996), i.e. 1–2 per cent or less of all its synaptic boutons.

The spinal command unit for the control of a skeletal muscle is a MN population, and individual intraspinal axons distribute their synapses to many MNs within the same pool, i.e. to large portions of the total muscle command unit. This has been most directly investigated for individual Ia afferents from muscle spindles, which distribute monosynaptic connections to the great majority of MNs innervating the same homonymous muscle (Mendell and Henneman 1971). Similarly broad distribution patterns are also likely to exist for other synaptic inputs, which explains why different MNs within a MN pool often tend to vary their discharge rates more or less in parallel (see Fig. 8.4) (Adrian and Bronk 1929; Milner-Brown *et al.* 1973a; Kernell and Sjoholm 1975; Monster 1979; De Luca and Erim 1994; however, cf. Tansey and Botterman 1996). However, for individual presynaptic axons the amount of innervation to different MNs may show systematic quantitative variations along the rostro-caudal extent of the MN pool: e. g. excitatory effects of Ia synapses (Clamann *et al.* 1985; Luscher *et al.* 1989); inhibitory effects from Renshaw cells (Van Keulen 1981); inhibitory effects via MN axon collaterals and Renshaw cells (Hamm *et al.* 1987).

The presence of, possibly, 200–400 command systems (excitatory, inhibitory, or modifying) converging onto a single MN pool raises the interesting question of how many of the excitatory input systems would have to be activated together in order to produce a maximum voluntary contraction. An answer to this question is closely linked to the intricate problem of how strongly a MN might become activated by all its excitatory synapses; this will be discussed further in section 7.4.

7.2.6. Soma-dendritic location of synapses and postsynaptic effects

The time to peak of fast EPSPs and the time course of their more prolonged declining phase are mainly dependent on passive neuronal properties like the membrane time

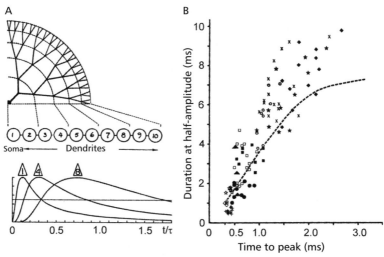

Figure 7.3 Influence of dendritic location on unitary EPSP shape. (**A**) Model calculations of expected EPSP shapes for different locations. Upper panel: correspondence between a model dendritic tree (with soma) and a chain of 10 compartments. Lower panel: calculated shape of EPSPs from each of three different numbered compartments. (**B**) 'Shape index' plot of EPSPs: half-width (i.e. duration at half-maximum amplitude) plotted against time to peak. Comparison between experimental measurements for unitary Ia EPSPs (different symbols for different Ia afferent fibres) (cf. Burke 1967a) and theoretical shape index values for different dendritic localizations of synaptic input (broken line), calculated with a standardized set of general assumptions using the model in (**A**). (After Rall *et al.* 1967.)

constant and, for dendritic locations, the electrotonic distance to the soma and the architecture and membrane properties of the dendrites (Fig. 7.3).

Ia EPSPs belong to the very few postsynaptic events that have been directly analysed in relation to MN architecture. Even for the same MN, the time course of individual unitary EPSPs may be very different, with some being much slower than others. Using MN reconstructions and corresponding models, much of this variability in time course could be explained as being due to variations in the electrotonic distance along the dendrites from the activated Ia synapses to the point of recording, i.e. presumably the soma (Fig. 7.3) (Burke 1967a; Jack *et al.* 1971; Mendell and Henneman 1971). These conclusions were validated by a few recordings of EPSPs from synapses whose location within the dendritic tree was directly determined by the combined intracellular labelling of the target MN and the stimulated Ia axon (Fig. 7.2A–C) (Redman and Walmsley 1983b; Burke and Glenn 1996). Such experiments demonstrated that the synapses of a single Ia axon were often distributed over a wide spatial and electrotonic range of dendritic locations (Burke and Glenn 1996), although a limited spatial distribution was seen by Brown and Fyffe (1981). Thus the differences in shape may indicate average differences in location between groups of synapses rather than unique synaptic locations (Burke and Glenn

1996). Unexpectedly, recordings failed to show that the slow EPSPs of remote synapses were systematically smaller than the faster ones generated closer to the soma (Iansek and Redman 1973a; Jack *et al.* 1981a,b). The explanation for this paradox is still uncertain.

Rapid IPSPs in MNs, including those evoked by Ia afferent stimulation, are caused by increased Cl⁻ conductance. This was demonstrated in the classical experiments of Eccles and colleagues (reviewed by Eccles 1964) by studying the effects on the IPSPs of injecting Cl⁻ ions into the cell via a penetrating microelectrode. Such an injection would shift E_{Cl} in a positive direction and, consequently, cause a decrease in IPSP hyperpolarization or even cause this PSP to become a depolarizing potential. The equilibrium potential for IPSP currents is normally about −80 mV. Cl⁻ injection may even shift this potential to a level more positive than the threshold for initiating action potentials; IPSPs will then, paradoxically, become capable of activating the MN. Ia IPSPs are generally relatively easy to change by Cl⁻ injection, and this suggests that they are generated quite near the soma.

7.2.7. Effects of stimulation pattern on PSPs

It is well known from other synaptic systems that a period of intense repetitive activation may have prolonged after-effects: post-tetanic depression and/or potentiation. Furthermore, similar effects may also be seen during the repetitive synaptic activation; they are then often referred to as frequency-dependent synaptic depression or facilitation. As synapses will almost always be activated by repetitive spike discharges, these effects are important for the synaptic input–output relations. There are only two synaptic input systems to MNs for which effects of stimulation patterns have been reasonably well tested: the monosynaptic effects onto MNs from Ia afferents and, in primates, the monosynaptic effects evoked by corticospinal fibres.

7.2.7.1. Ia synapses

Monosynaptic EPSPs evoked in MNs by Ia afferents from muscle spindles may show frequency-dependent facilitation as well as depression. With regard to these reactions, there are characteristic differences between synapses on MNs with different kinds of muscle fibres. In MNs with fast fatiguable muscle units (FF MNs), the Ia EPSPs tend to become facilitated during and after a stimulation train, whereas in those with slow fibres (S MNs) they tend to become depressed (Fig. 7.4B,C) (Koerber and Mendell 1991). Normally, S MNs have larger Ia EPSPs than the FF MNs of the same muscle. Thus, the changes during repetitive activation are such that the Ia EPSPs will become more equal to each other for the two categories of MNs. Interestingly, the same Ia afferent shows these different reactions for its synapses with different types of MN (Koerber and Mendell 1991), i.e. these characteristics seem to be controlled by the MN itself (see also Chapter 10, section 10.2.5, and Chapter 11, section 11.4.3.2).

The average steady-state size of compound Ia EPSPs varies in a complex manner with stimulation frequency (Fig. 7.4A) (Curtis and Eccles 1960). Following a high-frequency tetanic stimulation, single Ia EPSPs show post-tetanic potentiation (Curtis and Eccles

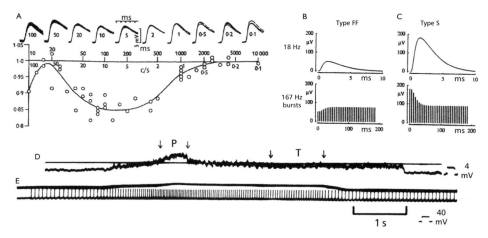

Fig. 7.4. Repetitive activation of synapses. (**A**) Compound Ia EPSPs elicited in a biceps-semitendi-
nosus MN by electrical stimulation of its muscle nerve (cat). Stimulation was given at different
steady rates. Upper curves: superimposed traces of EPSPs recorded at different stimulation frequencies, as indicated (Hz). Lower curve: relative EPSP amplitude versus pulse interval of stimulation (log scale). Lower scale on x-axis: frequencies of stimulation. (Reproduced with permission,
from Curtis and Eccles 1960) (**B**), (**C**) Examples of differences in high-frequency modulation of
unitary Ia-EPSPs for MNs with (**B**) fast fatiguable (FF) and (**C**) slow (S) muscle units (cat). Upper
panel: unitary Ia-EPSP. Lower panel: peak amplitude of unitary Ia-EPSP versus time during
167 Hz stimulation. (Reproduced with permission, from Mendell *et al*. 1994) (**D**), (**E**) Effects of
normal asynchronous repetitive activation of synapses on MN (**D**) membrane potential and (**E**)
spike discharge. Triceps surae MN from anaemically decerebrated cat, light additional anaesthesia. (**D**) Maintained depolarization ('steady EPSP') produced by a 10 mm ramp-and-hold stretch
of the triceps surae muscle. 'Phasic' (dynamic) and 'tonic' components of the response labelled
P and T respectively. (**E**) Repetitive spike discharge initiated in the MN by maintained depolarizing
injected current of 14 nA. About 1.5 s after the onset of this discharge, the triceps surae muscle
was again stretched, as signalled by the upper trace of this record. This caused an increase in
spike frequency in the MN. (Reproduced with permission, from Granit *et al*. 1966a.)

1960), which tends to be greater for initially small EPSPs than for the larger ones
(Lev-Tov *et al*. 1983; Luscher *et al*. 1983). Very little is known about the endurance of
monosynaptic Ia EPSPs in MNs (or of any other type of MN monosynaptic input), i.e.
how much the postsynaptic effect might decline after several minutes of continuous
activation.

7.2.7.2. Synapses onto MNs from decending fibres

The monosynaptic connections from corticospinal fibres to primate MNs produce a
pronounced initial facilitation of EPSP amplitude during brief bursts of stimulation (Muir
and Porter 1973). This facilitation is apparently more marked than that seen for other
descending systems with motoneuronal synapses (reviewed by Burke and Rudomin 1977).

7.3. **Postsynaptic currents driving repetitive spike discharges**

7.3.1. **Steady-current effects of maintained synaptic activity**

In Chapter 6, section 6.6 a description was given of the relation between activating currents and spike frequency, as investigated with stimulating currents injected via a microelectrode. A crucial question in this context is whether the effects of such artificially applied currents on the firing frequency correspond to those generated by synaptic activity. When testing this idea, one must first consider the nature of the natural drive to MNs.

In a state of maintained increase of synaptic drive to a MN, many of the activated synapses are firing asynchronously, with each of them producing only a very small shift in membrane potential (Fig. 7.2). Synchronicity between different unitary inputs does exist but can usually only be detected using advanced statistical techniques (e.g. for detecting shared innervation input to different MNs) (reviewed by Farmer *et al.* 1997). A state of essentially asynchronous synaptic drive may be produced experimentally by means of natural stimulation, such as muscle stretch which produces an asynchronous repetitive discharge of muscle spindle afferents and, correspondingly, a maintained depolarization in the MN (Fig. 7.4D) (Granit *et al.* 1966a; Burke 1968a). Alternatively, high-frequency electrical stimulation might be applied to a peripheral nerve or to appropriate sites within the CNS (Fig. 7.5A–C). The activation should then be given at a rate which is too high for simple one-to-one following of all the activated elements and chains of synapses (e.g. at 200 Hz or more) (Granit *et al.* 1966a). In a silent MN, such types of synaptic activation will indeed produce a maintained shift of membrane potential in a depolarizing or hyperpolarizing direction. The same stimulation given during current-evoked repetitive firing will change the discharge rate (Figs 7.4E and 7.5B).

7.3.2. **Simple effects of synaptic 'driving-currents' on spike frequency**

The graphs in Figure 7.5C,D illustrate that, over the whole of the primary range of firing, a constant amount of additional synaptic current will usually cause a constant shift of firing rate, i.e. the *f–I* relation is shifted in parallel (Granit *et al.* 1966a; Kernell 1969). Thus in such cases injected currents appear to have effects very similar to those of synaptic currents (in Fig. 7.5 they are generated by electrical activation of a peripheral nerve or by muscle stretch). Within the secondary range, the synaptic effects are generally larger and more variable (Granit *et al.* 1966b). Effects such as those shown in Fig. 7.5 are characteristic of the actions of many synaptic inputs, as tested in anaesthetized or lightly anaesthetized decerebrate animals.

A particularly thorough series of investigations of this kind has been published by Binder, Heckman, Powers, and their colleagues (reviewed by Powers and Binder 2001). These investigators used many different sources of maintained synaptic activation, including muscle vibration (i.e. activating Ia spindle afferents) and electrical repetitive stimulation of various sites within the CNS (see caption to Fig. 7.6). Postsynaptic current intensity was measured using voltage clamp techniques, and the current intensity at

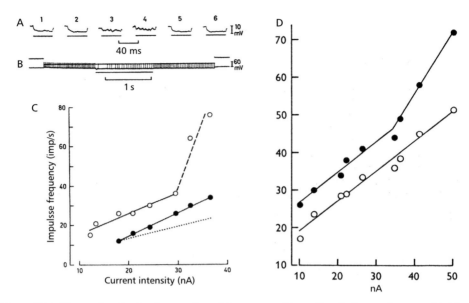

Figure 7.5 Effects of maintained synaptic activity on repetitive spike discharges in MNs. (**A**)–(**c**) Effects of net postsynaptic inhibition on membrane conductance and discharge rate in a lumbosacral MN (cell receiving monosynaptic excitation from the popliteal nerve) (decerebrate cat). (**A**) Change in membrane potential caused by a 7.8 nA pulse of hyperpolarizing current before (1–2), during (3–4), and after (5–6) a maintained tetanic stimulation at 439 s^{-1} to the common peroneal nerve. Duration of test current pulses is given by horizontal bars. On average, the amplitude of the voltage transients decreased by 41 per cent, i.e. there was a substantial increase in membrane conductance. (**B**) Repetitive impulse discharge elicited by a maintained depolarizing current of 29.6 nA. During the time indicated by the horizontal bar, a maintained tetanic stimulation was given to the common peroneal nerve (same stimulation parameters as in panels A3–A4). (**c**) Impulse frequency versus intensity of injected current for discharges similar to that in panel (**B**). Open circles: average firing rate during 0.5 s just before onset of peroneal stimulation. Filled circles: average firing rate at 0.55–1.05 s after onset of peroneal stimulation (with weak injected currents the firing rate was zero, or extremely irregular and slow, at times earlier than about 0.55 s after the onset of peroneal stimulation). The regression lines for values within the primary range calculated by method of least squares. The two highest firing rates of the control discharges are well up in the secondary range. The dotted line was drawn with a slope which is 59 per cent of that referring to control values (open circles) for the primary range; this line shows the expected change of *f–I* slope if the current-to-frequency transduction process had been shunted by the synaptically increased membrane conductance (which it apparently was not). (Reproduced with permission, from Kernell 1969.) (**D**) Impulse frequency (Hz) versus intensity of injected current (nA) for discharges in ankle extensor MN (anaemic decerebrate cat, slight additional anaesthesia). Maintained postsynaptic excitation caused by 10 mm stretch of the gastrocnemius-soleus muscle, rising in 1.4 s (cf. Figure 7.4D-E). The control curve (open circles) is the mean of values measured before and after stretch (1.0 s before onset of stretch and from 0.5 to 1.0 sec after cessation of stretch). The facilitated curve (filled circles) was measured from 0.5 to 2.5 s after the onset of stretch. (Reproduced with permission, from Granit *et al.* 1966b.)

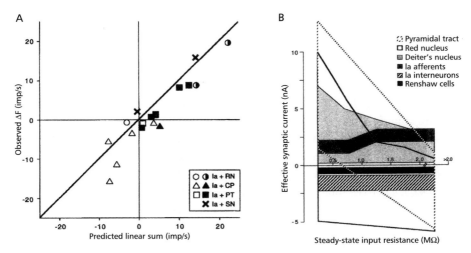

Figure 7.6 Summation of synaptic 'driving currents' and their intrapool distribution. Experiments on lumbar MNs of anaesthetized cats. (**A**) Effects of maintained synaptic activity on the spike frequency of repetitive discharges elicited with steady injected currents in MNs of triceps surae muscle (cf. Fig. 7.5). Synaptically evoked changes in firing rate during the concurrent activation of two synaptic inputs plotted versus the linear sum of the rate changes produced by each input alone. Open symbols represent cases in which the combined input produced a >20 per cent decrease in the steady-state input resistance of the cell, whereas filled symbols represent cases in which a <20 per cent decrease in resistance occurred. Half-filled circles are two cases in which effective synaptic currents and synaptically evoked changes in input resistance were not measured. Sources of synaptic effects: Ia, Ia muscle afferents; RN, red nucleus; CP, common peroneal nerve; PT, pyramidal tract; SN, sural nerve. (Reproduced with permission, from Powers and Binder 2000b). (**B**) Graphical representation of the effective synaptic currents seen in MNs of different input resistance for six different input systems. Measurements in lumbar MNs at rest. Synaptic currents shown for activation of the contralateral pyramidal tract (excitation and inhibition,dotted lines) (Binder *et al.* 1998), contralateral rubrospinal neurones (excitation and inhibition, thick lines) (Powers *et al.* 1993), ipsilateral Deiter's nucleus (excitation, grey band) (Westcott *et al.* 1995), homonymous Ia afferent fibres (excitation, upper dark band) (Heckman and Binder 1988), Renshaw interneurones (inhibition, lower dark band) (Lindsay and Binder 1991), and Ia inhibitory interneurones (inhibition, lower hatched band) (Heckman and Binder 1991a). (Reproduced with permission, from Binder *et al.* 1998).

threshold membrane potential ('effective synaptic current', I_{syn}) was calculated. The results of these studies essentially confirmed that, in anaesthetized animals, injected and synaptic currents have similar effects on firing within the primary range (Powers *et al.* 1992). Some minor differences were noticed: for excitatory or inhibitory Ia inputs, the effects on firing rate were, on average, somewhat greater than predicted from the combination of measured I_{syn} and *f–I* slope (Powers and Binder 1995), and the effects of two coactivated synaptic inputs were often a little less than that predicted from the linear sum of their effective synaptic currents (Fig. 7.6A) (Powers and Binder 2000b). However, under these circumstances the synaptic currents largely acted on MNs according to their intrinsic *f–I* relation. Such synaptic effects, whether excitatory (Fig. 7.5D) or inhibitory (Fig. 7.5C), will be referred to below as the effects of postsynaptic **driving currents**.

In anaesthetized animals, simple driving current effects of synaptic activity are commonly encountered (Figs 7.5 and 7.6), but even under these conditions more complex effects have also been described. Thus, in response to certain sources of synaptic activation (including brainstem stimulation) the slope of the *f–I* relation increased even within the primary range and alterations were observed in the minimum rate of steady firing (Kernell 1965d, 1966b). Similarly, as noted above, the synaptic effects were often more complex and larger for discharges at the higher rates of the secondary range than in the primary range (Granit *et al.* 1966a, b), perhaps reflecting the combined effects of postsynaptic driving currents and voltage-activated persistent inward currents (PICs) from dendrites. Postsynaptic effects on repetitive firing properties and the actions of voltage-activated and synaptically facilitated PICs will be dealt with further in section 7.5.

7.3.3. **Absence of postsynaptic 'shunting' effects on firing frequency in primary range**

One of several major differences between injected currents and common types of synaptic driving currents is that the latter are generated by, and thus associated with, increases in membrane conductance. It is known that, in accordance with Ohm's law, an increase in postsynaptic conductance will cause a decrease in the size of long-lasting postsynaptic potentials. However, counter-intuitively, such 'shunting' effects are of no importance for the synaptic effects on repetitive firing.

In the experiment illustrated in Figure 7.5A–C (Kernell 1969), stimulation of a peripheral nerve generated a persistent strong postsynaptic inhibition which was associated with a marked decrease in the neuronal input resistance (see decreased size of test pulses in Fig. 7.5A). However, the addition of the same postsynaptic inhibition to different current intensities for generating repetitive firing did not decrease the effects of the injected currents on firing rate; within the primary range, the *f–I* relation was shifted in parallel but there was no decrease in its slope (Fig. 7.5C). These results have been confirmed in other experiments including measurements of input resistance (Schwindt and Calvin 1973) and in 'dynamic clamp' experiments (Brizzi *et al.* 2004), and they are in accordance with many other observations concerning synaptic effects on repetitive firing in anaesthetized animals (Granit *et al.* 1966a; Powers and Binder 2001). Furthermore, the results shown in Figure 7.5C correspond well with the repetitive discharge behaviour of simple MN models in which the rhythmic properties depend mainly on the characteristics of the postspike AHP conductances. In these models, an increased leak conductance causes no decrease in the slope of the *f–I* relation (Kernell 1968; Kernell and Sjoholm 1973); actually, the main effect might be a small increase in slope because of the decreased membrane time constant. In AHP-dependent repetitive firing, the current increase needed to decrease the impulse interval from x to y depends mainly on the difference in

AHP conductance between postspike times x and y. Hence, with such a discharge mechanism, the $f-I$ relation largely reflects the time course and size of the AHP conductance, independently of the leak conductance. Therefore, when discussing repetitive firing, it may be misleading to think of the synaptic drive in the conventional terms of postsynaptic potential. Voltages are essential when considering the threshold currents needed for starting a neuronal discharge; for this aspect of neuronal excitability, the input resistance is very important (see Chapter 6, section 6.9.1). However, when considering the effects on firing of different intensities of maintained suprathreshold activation, the most relevant parameter is clearly the current and not the postsynaptic potential.

7.4. Available amount of postsynaptic driving current in motoneurones

In the consideration of MN discharges, a crucial question concerns the total driving capacity of the synapses on the soma and dendrites of a MN. Measurements of the repetitive response properties of cat MNs have indicated that, for a large hindlimb MN with a fast-twitch muscle unit, the maximum rate (and the maximum evocable unit force) may require a stimulation intensity at the soma of about 105 nA. In a slower and smaller MN, about 27 nA might be sufficient for maximum firing (AHP durations of 50–200 ms are assumed (see Chapter 6, section 6.9.3.5); calculations based on the equations of Kernell (1965c)). As will be discussed later (Chapter 8, section 8.4.3), there is good evidence that forces close to the maximum evocable force may indeed be approached in reflex or voluntary contractions. However, paradoxically, MN physiology has so far met with difficulties in trying to explain how (and whether) such intense activation is achieved.

7.4.1. Experimental assessments of postsynaptic current intensity

The maximum postsynaptic currents measured in response to the electrical activation of various sets of MN synapses have often been surprisingly weak compared with the currents needed for the whole range of MN activation (cf. Figs 7.6B and 6.2B). The weakness of the postsynaptic effects might have been partly caused by the the general anaesthesia used in these experiments. Furthermore, electrical stimulation of the brain is a relatively coarse and indiscriminate method of evoking central neuronal activity, and it might not be capable of generating an optimal selection of strongly activated command neurones, such as that required for a strong voluntary contraction. What range of excitatory currents might be theoretically expected?

7.4.2. Theoretical considerations

7.4.2.1. A (too) simple calculation

About 20–40 per cent of the synapses on a spinal MN are excitatory (Table 7.1). Assume that each of these synapses possesses the properties of the best known example, the Ia monosynaptic synapse. At threshold membrane potential and with a release probability of about 0.5 (the correct value is difficult to estimate, cf. Redman and Walmsley (1983a)), such a Ia terminal would produce a mean postsynaptic current of about 0.075 pA when firing at 1 Hz (for equations and references, see Cushing *et al.* 2005). If we now assume that 20–40 per cent of all the 140 000 terminals on a large MN are excitatory (i.e. 28000–56000) and that each fired at 50 Hz, then together they would generate a summed current of about 105–210 nA, provided that no attenuating mechanisms were operating. Thus, in this case the maximum current generated would approach or exceed the 105 nA needed for a maximum rate of MN discharge (see Chapter 6, section 6.9.3.5). Similar relative results would be obtained for the smallest MNs; the current needed for a maximum discharge would be about 25 per cent of that for the largest MN, and their total membrane area (and, consequently, total number of synapses) would also probably be roughly 25 per cent or less of that for the largest MN. Thus, in both cases, the maximum current generated seems to be roughly 1–2 times as large as that needed for a maximum output. However, the calculations have not taken into account how currents would be summed and transmitted along the dendrites, which drastically attenuates the outcome.

7.4.2.2. Attenuation along passive dendrites

Cushing *et al.* (2005) (see also Rose and Cushing 1999) recently published an intriguing set of calculations based on their detailed reconstructions of cervical MNs. Their MNs had a smaller total number of synapses (estimated number of excitatory synapses, about 16 000 or less) than that provisionally assumed for a large spinal MN (about 28 000–56 000). With all excitatory synapses activated at 100 Hz and the soma membrane potential clamped close to threshold (−55 mV), the total excitatory current at the cell body was only about 24–40 nA, i.e. far too low to drive a large spinal MN to its maximum rate (but probably sufficient for a small spinal MN). Furthermore, the attenuation was markedly non-linear and of a saturating character, i.e. the greater the number of active synapses, the smaller was the effect of an additional synapse. The attenuation was partly due to the cable properties of the dendrites; in addition to the 'normal' cable attenuation (cf. Fig. 2.2D), the increase in postsynaptic conductance would worsen the transmission characteristics of the cable by decreasing its characteristic length. The major portion of the attenuation, as calculated by Cushing *et al.* (2005), was due to a loss of the driving potential for dendritic postsynaptic currents, depending on the large postsynaptic depolarizations caused in small dendrites with a high input conductance (see also Taylor and Enoka 2004). The calculations of Cushing *et al.* (2005) were done for neck MNs, and higher (but not proportionately higher) currents would have been obtained with the greater estimated number of synapses for spinal MNs (see above). When performing this type of calculation it is important to remember that the attenuation of synaptic current takes place independently for each dendritic tree. Thus a large number of dendritic stems would be favourable for achieving a high maximum current intensity at the soma.

With regard to the dendritic attenuation of synaptic current transfer, it is important to consider the possible effects of voltage-dependent ion channels in the dendrites, producing PICs. Such PIC channels, perhaps strategically placed between distal dendrites and soma, might intensify the currents that ultimately reach the action potential trigger zones close to the soma (reviewed by Binder 2002; Heckman *et al.* 2003; Hultborn *et al.* 2004). On the other hand, such channels might also have a saturating effect, pushing the membrane potential close to the equilibrium potential for the driving current and making locally activated synaptic channels of the same dendrite ineffective (cf. conceivable function of PICs in frequency saturation, Chapter 8, section 8.4). For less intense non-saturating intensities of excitation, dendritic voltage-sensitive PICs might help to counteract attenuation of dendritic postsynaptic currents by acting as if the dendritic length constant were prolonged (Crill 1996, 1999). Finally, the dendritic attenuation problems might also be counteracted by the presence of action potential conduction and AHP generation along the dendrites following initiation of action potentials at the initial segment of the axon; local dendritic AHPs would help to restore an effective driving potential for dendritic excitatory currents. Antidromic conduction of action potentials into the dendrites has been recorded for MNs in organotypic spinal cord culture (Larkum *et al.* 1996), and evidence for orthodromic spike-like processes in MN dendrites has often been observed after axotomy (see Table 10.1).

7.5. **Motoneurone-modifying synapses and their effects on motoneurone firing**

Two important inputs for modifying synaptic effects to spinal MNs and interneurones come from cells in the brainstem with descending fibres travelling down the spinal cord: the raphe nuclei containing serotoninergic (5HT) cells and the locus coeruleus with noradrenergic neurones. The 5HT cells are preferentially activated in combination with motor output and are thought to facilitate motor activities and suppress sensory processing (Jacobs and Fornal 1993). Cells of the locus coeruleus are particularly activated in threatening or challenging situations, and are thought to play a role in defence reactions (Levine *et al.* 1990).

7.5.1. **Facilitation of plateau firing and persistent inward currents**

In the 1980s Hultborn, Hounsgaard, Kiehn, and their colleagues were searching for the explanation of certain strikingly long-lasting after-effects of stretch reflex activation, as seen in MNs of decerebrate cats (Hultborn *et al.* 1975). A few repeated muscle stretches could start a rhythmic MN activity that lasted for minutes. Moreover, this activity could easily be interrupted by a short-lasting activation of inhibitory inputs to the MNs. The original hypothesis was that this prolonged discharge behaviour might be caused by some kind of neuronal reverberating circuit. However, an intracellular analysis quickly showed that there was instead a drastic change in the properties of individual MNs. Thus, even in response to direct intracellular activation of a single MN (i.e. no reverberating circuits), a discharge could sometimes be started that continued even after removal of the injected stimulation current (Fig. 6.5A,B) (Hounsgaard *et al.* 1984; see also Schwindt and Crill 1980a). In the single MN, this 'plateau firing' could be interrupted by a brief pulse of hyperpolarizing current (cf. effect of inhibition in the case of the prolonged reflex discharge). The continued analysis of this phenomenon was performed in spinal MNs of decerebrate cats (Conway *et al.* 1988; Crone *et al.* 1988; Hounsgaard *et al.* 1988a) and on *in vitro* preparations of turtle spinal cord (Hounsgaard *et al.* 1988b; Hounsgaard and Kiehn 1989). In both preparations, the occurrence of plateau behaviour could be facilitated by monoamines, norepinephrine (NE), and 5HT in cats, and by 5HT in the turtle. Later, other metabotropic synaptic receptors were identified which also influenced L-type Ca^{2+} channels and the appearance of plateau behaviour (e.g. facilitation by glutamate and acetylcholine and downregulation by GABA(B) receptors (Alaburda *et al.* 2002)). Thus, various transmitter substances apparently promote the appearance of voltage-sensitive PICs which may also be seen in MNs, to a lesser extent, without the explicit addition of transmitters (Schwindt and Crill 1980b). For further details concerning such 'booster PICs', see Chapter 6, section 6.7 and Figures 6.4, 6.5, and 6.9).

7.5.2. Synaptically evoked changes of AHP and firing properties

There are other MN-modifying effects besides the facilitation of booster PICs. In addition to facilitating plateau behaviour, 5HT causes a decrease in AHP amplitude which elicits an increase in the *f–I* slope of MNs; for example, turtle MNs (Hounsgaard and Kiehn 1989; Hornby *et al.* 2002a), lamprey MNs (Wallen *et al.* 1989), neonatal rat hypoglossal MNs (Berger *et al.* 1992), and guinea pig trigeminal MNs (Hsiao *et al.* 1997). In Fig. 7.7, these effects were evoked by brainstem stimulation in a region containing monoaminergic cells with axons descending into the spinal cord (Hultborn *et al.* 2004). It is still uncertain how closely linked these different effects of monoamines are, and to what extent PIC facilitation and AHP depression are independently controlled.

An interesting illustration of MN-modifying synaptic effects is provided by the MN characteristics during fictive locomotion, a rhythmic locomotion-like motor activity pattern which can be evoked in decerebrate cats using repetitive electrical stimulation of the brainstem. Intracellular MN recordings during such burst discharges show that the AHPs are drastically decreased in size, firing is irregular and takes place at a relatively high rate, the firing rate is insensitive to added depolarizing current, and firing can be stopped altogether by small steps of hyperpolarizing current (Brownstone *et al.* 1992). The results suggest that each fictive locomotion burst is caused by a synaptically facilitated plateau potential combined with a synaptically evoked AHP decrease (almost elimination). The MN might largely fire on noise peaks superimposed on the plateau potential (cf. 'noise-generated' firing mode (Calvin 1975)) and, for this reason, its discharge rate might be irregular but also relatively insensitive to depolarizing current. Plateau potentials are voltage-gated phenomena and therefore may often be stopped by a hyperpolarizing pulse (Fig. 6.5A). It is not known how representative this fictive locomotion firing is for the types of MN discharge seen in normal motor behaviour. One

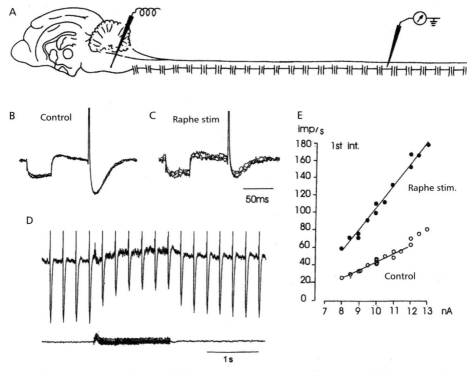

Figure 7.7 Synaptic modulation of AHP and transduction gain (*f–I* slope). (**A**) Experimental set-up. Cat under barbiturate anaesthesia, intact CNS. Intracellular recording from lumbosacral MNs. Stimulation of caudal raphe nuclei, i.e. activation of descending monoaminergic fibre tracts. (**B**) Intracellular recording of MN membrane potential: superimposed voltage transients produced by injected hyperpolarizing test current followed by spike (truncated) with AHP; the spike was elicited by a brief injected current pulse. (**C**) Same as (**B**), but during 20 Hz tetanic stimulation of the caudal raphe nuclei. (**D**) Upper trace: spikes (truncated) with subsequent AHPs elicited by injected current pulses at a frequency of 5 Hz before, during, and after a short train of stimuli to the raphe nuclei (time of raphe stimulation indicated in the lower trace). (**E**) Plot of spike frequency (Hz) versus steady stimulating current (nA) for first interspike interval, as tested with 1 s injected rectangular current pulses. Open circles: control data obtained without raphe stimulation; filled circles: experimental values obtained during raphe stimulation. Note the decreased AHP amplitude and increased slope of frequency–current relation (f−*I* slope) during raphe stimulation. (Reproduced with permission, from Hultborn *et al.* 2004.)

notable property of ficitive locomotion seems to be that such bursts of muscle activation can be increased by recruitment gradation but not by MN rate modulation (see discussion in Brownstone *et al.* 1992). This contrasts with many kinds of voluntary motor behaviour in which MN rate gradation plays a prominent role (e.g. Fig. 8.4) (Adrian and Bronk 1929; Freund 1983), including normal locomotion in the cat (Hoffer *et al.* 1981).

7.5.3. **Synaptically evoked changes of other MN response properties**

As PSPs are typically generated by increases in ionic membrane conductance, a strong synaptic activation will be associated with a marked change (generally decrease) of neuronal input resistance. However, postsynaptic effects also exist that involve an increase in membrane resistivity, typically due to a decrease of leak conductance, which would cause a depolarization and increase MN excitability. Such effects can be elicited by several different substances, including 5HT (Hsiao *et al.* 1997), NE, ACh (muscarinic receptor), substance P, and TRH. In addition, various voltage-gated ion channels of importance for subthreshold rectification processes may also be modified by transmitters, including the channels for the hyperpolarization-activated inward current I_h (increased by 5HT) (Hsiao *et al.* 1997), and a transient outward K^+ current (increased by NE) (for further references and details, see Rekling *et al.* 2000; Powers and Binder 2001).

Under most circumstances, the rhythmicity of repetitive MN discharges seems to depend mainly on spike-linked mechanisms, such as the AHP. However, it has also been noted that, in the subthreshold range of membrane potentials, a slow voltage oscillation may emerge when MNs are under the appropriate pharmacological influence (including *in vitro* stimulation of NMDA receptors). So far, the oscillations seen under such circumstances (which are usually ≤1 Hz) seem too slow to generate regular repetitive spike firing (Guertin and Hounsgaard 1998; Hochman and Schmidt 1998; Kiehn *et al.* 2000). However, if evoked by natural synaptic activity, such oscillations might be of importance for regulating the rhythmicity of bursting activity such as that seen in locomotion or respiration.

7.6. **Innervation of motoneurones controlling different categories of muscle unit**

How the various kinds of MNs and muscle units are actually used by the CNS will be analysed in the next chapter (Chapter 8). This is, of course, dependent on the distribution of excitation and inhibition to the various MNs and on their intrinsic properties. Questions concerning motor control and muscle coordination fall outside the scope of the present monograph; the general principles for the management of individual MNs, MN pools, and muscles are the main concerns here.

By far the best known synaptic input to MNs is the monosynaptic excitation from primary muscle spindle afferents, which has served as a model system for other synaptic MN connections. Because of the technical problems involved, quantitative studies of the distribution of postsynaptic effects (e.g. maximum EPSP sizes) to MNs of different muscle unit type and axon size (i.e. axonal conduction velocity) have been performed for very few synaptic systems. Only in some of these cases was the distribution such as to favour the common type of orderly recruitment according to the 'size principle', i.e. an ascending force order of recruitment (Table 2.2), as is indeed the case for the monosynaptic effects from Ia spindle afferents (cat, Fig. 7.6B) (Eccles *et al.* 1957; Burke and Rymer 1976; Dum and Kennedy 1980b; Heckman and Binder 1988)). On the other hand, monosynaptic EPSPs from type II spindle afferents tend to be about equally large in MNs of different MU types (cat) (Munson *et al.* 1982), and this is also true for mono-synaptic EPSPs of ventral and medial descending spinal fibres or of the medial longitudinal fasciculus (cat) (Burke and Rymer 1976; Dum and Kennedy 1980b). An even more extreme difference from the distribution of monosynaptic Ia excitation has been observed in cat lumbar MNs for the polysynaptic influence from cortico- and rubrospinal fibres (Fig. 7.6B) and from skin nerves (Burke *et al.* 1970; Dum and Kennedy 1980b); these effects are generally mainly inhibitory to the 'slow' MNs (cells with thin axons and weak muscle units) and excitatory to (many of) the 'fast' cells (thicker axons and stronger but fatigue-sensitive units). However, somewhat unexpectedly, the monosy-naptic excitatory effects from the primate motor cortex to MNs are instead distributed like the monosynaptic Ia effects (Clough *et al.* 1968b); monosynaptic corticospinal con-nections are lacking in cats. Thus, in the rather few cases for which quantitative data about the distribution of postsynaptic excitatory effects to different categories of MN are available, these distributions are strikingly different. However, when the CNS is executing motor programs the various distributions of postsynaptic effects do not generally upset the hierarchy of intrinsic MN excitabilities (Fig. 6.7), favouring the ascending force order of recruitment (Table 2.2 and Chapter 8, section 8.2). The variability of synaptic distri-butions within MN pools is of interest not only for questions of recruitment hierarchies but also for problems concerning possible variations in 'recruitment gain' (Chapter 8, section 8.4.4).

In cats, MNs with slow (S) and fast (FR, FF) muscle units have been found to differ in their dendritic synaptic density and organization: S MNs have a larger preponderance of F-type boutons on the soma and, moreover, in the most distal dendritic regions they have more than 50 per cent higher values for the percentage of covering, packing density, and total number of boutons (Brannstrom 1993). This last difference might possibly promote the apppearance of larger synaptic current densities in S than in F MNs, which is of interest with regard to recruitment problems. However, in monkeys, the coverages and frequencies for different EM types of synaptic boutons were not correlated with cell body diameter (Starr and Wolpaw 1994).

For inhibitory MN inputs, there are size-ordered distributions of the amplitudes of reciprocal Ia IPSPs and recurrent Renshaw IPSPs, but not of the underlying currents (Fig. 7.6B) (Burke and Rymer 1976; Friedman *et al.* 1981; Hultborn *et al.* 1988a; Heckman and Binder 1991a; Lindsay and Binder 1991), i.e. in these cases the differences in IPSP amplitude were mainly caused by the differences in neuronal input resistance.

Chapter 8

Motoneurone populations and the gradation of muscle force

8.1. General issues

The fact that muscles are organized into populations of non-overlapping motor units implies that muscle force may be graded by two mechanisms:

- by activating a larger or smaller number of units ('recruitment gradation')
- by grading the degree of activity for already recruited units ('rate gradation').

Elsewhere within the mammalian CNS, many functions are also likely to be controlled, in a similar 'two-dimensional' manner, by neuronal populations rather than by single cells. However, for most neurones within the mammalian CNS, functional populations are difficult to trace, define, and record from; in this respect, the neuromuscular system offers important advantages.

8.2. Recruitment gradation in motoneurone pools

8.2.1. The 'size principle'

8.2.1.1. Initial observations and functional relevance

The rate and recruitment mechanisms for muscle control became evident in the very first series of investigations of voluntary contractions using electromyographic techniques (Adrian and Bronk 1929): in weak maintained contractions only one or a few units were active, firing repetitively at regular rates. In stronger contractions, the spike-frequencies of already activated units might increase and, in addition, new units would become recruited. Furthermore, Denny-Brown (1929) had already noticed that the motor units of slow muscles were generally more easily activated by reflexes than were those of synergistic fast muscles. This kind of recruitment hierarchy was later found to be valid also for the gradation of unit activity within single muscles, as was shown in a series of papers published in the 1960s by Henneman and his colleagues (e.g. Henneman *et al*. 1965; reviewed by Henneman and Mendell 1981; see also Henneman 1957). Their first set of experimental measurements were extracellular recordings of unitary action potentials from ventral root filaments of decerebrated cats, and the MNs were activated by stretching hindlimb muscles (gastrocnemius, soleus), i.e. by stretch reflexes caused by the activation of muscle spindles (Fig. 8.1A). It was then consistently observed that units with small extracellular action potentials were recruited more easily than those with larger action

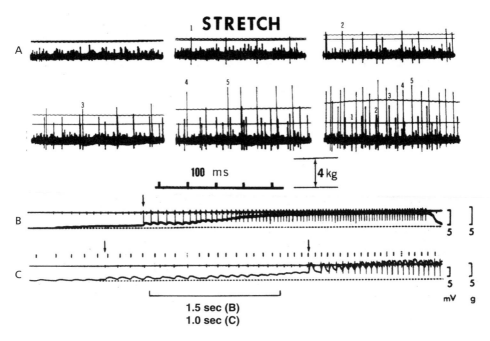

Figure 8.1 Recruitment hierarchy of MNs. (**A**) Orderly recruitment of MNs in response to increasing degrees of stretch of the triceps surae muscle in a decerebrate cat. Degree of stretch signalled by the separation of the two upper traces. Consecutive sections shown from the same continuous discharge. The lower thick trace is the extracellular recording from a multi-fibre ventral root filament: small deflections indicate firing of gamma MNs; large deflections represent rhythmic firing of alpha MNs. Note the recruitment of five MNs (numbered) in order of increasing spike size, i.e. presumably in order of increasing size of the respective motor axons. (Reproduced with permission, from Henneman *et al.* 1965.) (**B**),(**c**) Recruitment of motor units in the first deep lumbrical muscle of cat's foot by (**B**) prolonged electrical stimulation of the contralateral motor cortex and (**c**), reflexly, by pinching the plantar cushion of the foot containing the muscle. Panels (**B**) and (**c**) are from two different cats, anaesthetized with pentobarbital. In each record, the upper trace shows the electromyogram, and the lower trace the isometric muscle tension. Baseline for the myograms (zero active tension) is indicated by dotted lines. In (**B**), two motor units are recruited; the arrow indicates the time of recruitment of the second (larger) motor unit. The smaller unit in (**B**) continued to fire throughout the contraction (checked by simultaneous recording at high gain). In (**c**), both the mechanical stimulation and the resulting impulse activity of a small motor unit had already started before the beginning of the illustrated record. The occurrence of impulses in this small motor unit (checked by simultaneous recording at high gain) is indicated by vertical bars above the record. Times of recruitment of a second and a third motor unit are indicated by arrows. In (**B**) and (**c**), note the recruitment in order of increasing contractile force. (Reproduced with permission, from Kernell *et al.* 1975.)

potentials. There was a continuous hierarchy of such differences in recruitment excitability—the larger the axon spike, the higher the recruitment threshold. Derecruitment occurred correspondingly in the reverse order: the last units to be recruited were the first units to be derecruited.It should be remembered that, in the present context, the term 'recruitment order' should be understood to mean ranking order in a hierarchy (Freund *et al.* 1975; Desmedt and Godaux 1977), i.e. all units with a lower rank can be activated without activity in units of higher rank. For practical purposes, this is often tested by scrutinizing how MNs (or muscle units) are recruited during very slow ramps of increasing or decreasing force (Fig. 8.1).

For biophysical reasons, differences in the sizes of extracellularly recorded spikes are likely to reflect differences in axonal diameter. Furthermore, Henneman *et al.* (1965) argued that MNs with large axons would probably also have large soma-dendrite regions (direct proof of this belief came later (Cullheim 1978; Kernell and Zwaagstra 1981; Burke *et al.* 1982)). Hence, Henneman *et al.* (1965) concluded that recruitment excitability was graded according to the axonal and soma-dendrite size of the MNs. They speculated about the possible mechanisms, for instance that MN excitability was related to size-associated differences in neuronal input resistance (actual measurements added later (Kernell 1966a)).

In their initial papers, Henneman *et al.* stressed the functional advantages of a recruitment hierarchy associated with MN size (see Henneman and Mendell 1981). Because of the general matching between neuronal and muscle unit properties, small alpha MNs with thin axons are likely to be associated with muscle units that are relatively weak, slow, and fatigue resistant (Chapter 3, section 3.7.3). Such units would be optimal for the initial gradation of force; with recruitment according to the 'size principle', weak units producing small force steps would be grading weak muscle forces. In this way an almost constant relationship might even be preserved between the size of recruitment steps and overall muscle force, which would optimize the smoothness of force gradation by recruitment (**force–gradation match** between MN recruitment and unit force). Furthermore, weak long-lasting contractions will often be used for the maintenance of posture. Therefore it is appropriate that the most easily recruited MNs are those with fatigue-resistant slow muscle fibres; slow fibres are metabolically cheap in isometric contractions (cf. Chapter 3, section 3.3.2.1) (posture versus movement match). The shortening contractions that we need for the production of movements may have to be performed rapidly and at great power, i.e. fast (F) units would then be most suitable. In strong contractions, muscle circulation may temporarily become ineffective or blocked because of pressure on blood vessels from contracting muscle fibres. Correspondingly, the F units are good at rapidly extracting energy from intramuscular glycogen stores, even without immediate access to oxygen.

8.2.1.2. Confirmations, modifications and extensions

In several later series of experiments, Henneman and his colleagues confirmed the presence of a recruitment hierarchy according to characteristics associated with axonal size (e.g. extracellular spike amplitude (Fig. 8.1A), conduction velocity), and they stressed the relatively 'noiseless' character of this hierarchy, showing few exceptions (Clamann and Henneman 1976; Bawa *et al.* 1984). Furthermore, the relation between recruitment rank and axonal conduction velocity was also valid within MN populations of the same muscle unit type (e.g. within the uniformly slow soleus of the cat (Binder *et al.* 1983)). Corresponding statistical hierarchies of recruitment have been seen in numerous other laboratories in both human subjects (Milner-Brown *et al.* 1973b; Freund *et al.* 1975) and animal experiments (Kernell and Sjoholm 1975; Zajac and Faden 1985); for further references see Henneman and Mendell (1981), Stuart and Enoka (1983), and Cope and Pinter (1995). In a later extension of the 'size principle' experiments, Sokoloff *et al.* (1999) showed that a size principle hierarchy of recruitment is also valid within a wider functional group of units from a pair of closely synergistic muscles (lateral and medial gastrocnemius).

There is typically a strong correlation between the contractile force of a muscle unit and the conduction velocity of its axon (Emonet-Denand *et al.* 1988). Hence an ascending size order in terms of axon dimensions will largely correspond to a similar size order in terms of muscle unit twitch amplitude or maximum tetanic force, a physiological parameter of more direct and obvious relevance for motor behaviour than the axon or MN soma diameter. The characteristic recruitment behaviour of units with different forces is illustrated in Fig. 8.1B,C, which shows recordings from a very small muscle of the cat's foot (first deep lumbrical muscle, which often contains only two to ten units (Kernell and Sjoholm 1975)). A positive correlation was found between the relative recruitment threshold and unit force for each one of two synaptic inputs: electrical stimulation of the motor cortex, and reflex activation by pinching the cat's footpad. However, some unit pairs showed a 'reversed' recruitment behaviour (activation of stronger prior to weaker unit) with either type of stimulation and, for the same set of individual units, such 'exceptions' concerned different pairs for different synaptic inputs. Such cases emphasize that the 'size principle' should typically be regarded as a statistical pattern of recruitment rather than an absolute hierarchy with no exceptions.

Initially it was wondered whether the 'size principle' might be valid mainly for postural contractions, but perhaps not for fast voluntary movements. However, experiments in humans showed the same recruitment hierarchy for pairs of units irrespective of whether they were used in slow or ballistic voluntary movements (Desmedt and Godaux 1977).

8.2.1.3. Possible causes

For a given synaptic input, the hierarchy of recruitment must depend on the combination of two factors:

- ◆ the distribution of electrical excitability among the MNs
- ◆ the distribution of synaptic input across the MN population.

As described in Chapter 6, section 6.9.1, there is a strong positive correlation between MN input conductance and a measure of axon size (axonal conduction velocity; see Fig. 6.6A) (Kernell 1966a; Burke 1967b, 1968b; Fleshman *et al.* 1981; Kernell and Zwaagstra 1981; Gustafsson and Pinter 1984c). There is also a significant correlation between axon speed (size) and MN electrical excitability, as tested with current injection into the soma-dendrite region via a microelectrode (Fig. 6.7A) (Kernell 1966a; Kernell and Zwaagstra 1981). Thus MNs with small axons and high input resistances need less current for spike activation than those with larger axons and smaller input resistances: single-spike threshold I_{rh} (see Table 6.1) (Fleshman *et al.* 1981; Zengel *et al.* 1985); threshold for repetitive discharge I_{rep} (Kernell and Monster 1981). These differences in input resistance and electrical excitability are caused partly by the differences in size and partly by the high membrane resistivity of the small slow-twitch MNs (note higher τ_m values in Table 6.1 (see Chapter 6, section 6.9.1) (Kernell and Zwaagstra 1981; Burke *et al.* 1982; Gustafsson and Pinter 1984c; Ulfhake and Kellerth 1984). The differences in membrane resistivity are important because they mean that, even if all the MNs of different sizes were randomly innervated with the same synaptic density from a given source, the small MNs would still tend to be those most easily recruited. However, size as such still has no known causal relation with the 'size principle' of recruitment; the term is a useful descriptive label for the integrated property-ranked features of the normal recruitment hierarchy, but it is not (as far as is yet known) related to the mechanisms involved.

The distribution of synaptic inputs across MN pools was described in Chapter 7, section 7.6. It is interesting to note that, with regard to synaptic current intensity, most of those inputs that have been quantitatively investigated are not distributed in such a way as to favour the 'size principle' of recruitment (Fig. 7.6B). The vast majority of inputs have not yet been measured from this point of view. However, the available data (Fig. 7.6B versus Figures 6.6 and 6.7) suggest that the distribution of MN excitabilities is the dominant factor responsible for the appearance of a recruitment hierarchy according to the 'size principle'.

8.2.2. Recruitment behaviours deviating from the 'size principle'

8.2.2.1. Seemingly random recruitment behaviours during relative rest

In long-lasting EMG recordings (tens of minutes or even hours) from single motor units in awake and resting animals, individual units which were initially silent may suddenly start discharges which may continue long after those of other units, recruited later, have stopped (Eken 1998). Thus in such cases a certain degree of 'uncoupling' seems to exist between an individual unit and the rest of the population. It is assumed that this behaviour is due to the emergence of plateau potentials and plateau discharges in individual MNs (see Chapter 6, section 6.7).

8.2.2.2. Cases with preferential recruitment of fast rather than slow muscle units

It was noted as early as the classical studies of Denny-Brown (1929) that while slow extensor muscles were typically more easily activated than synergistic fast muscles (e.g. in postural reflexes, decerebrate cat), these muscles were as readily (sometimes even more easily) activated in transient contractions caused by moving the head. However, there were no detailed follow-up studies of these 'kinetic reflexes'. In a later series of experiments on awake cats, the relative recruitment of slow and fast synergistic muscles (soleus and gastrocnemius) were compared in the so-called 'paw shake' behaviour, in which a cat rapidly moves its hindpaw back and forth to shake something off. In this behaviour the prolonged relaxation phase of a slow muscle would be cumbersome and, indeed, the fast muscle was selectively recruited (Smith *et al.* 1980).

As was described in Chapter 7, section 7.6, the reflex effects from skin afferents tend to be distributed such that fast units are more strongly excited than slower ones (Burke *et al.* 1970). In accordance with these observations, the recruitment order seen in a reflex or voluntary contraction may indeed be modified by skin stimulation, apparently favouring the normally high threshold fast-twitch units (Kanda *et al.* 1977; Garnett and Stephens 1981). Even if no recruitment reversal takes place, inputs with a distribution of MN-targeted synaptic effects like that of skin afferents will influence recruitment in terms of its 'gain' (see section 8.4.4).

Another apparent deviation from an orthodox 'size principle' behaviour was seen in a comparison of active shortening and lengthening contractions in human calf muscles (foot plantar flexors; again recordings concerning the soleus and the gastrocnemius) (Nardone *et al.* 1989). During shortening movements units were preferentially activated in the slow mixed soleus, but under lengthening conditions many units were activated in the fast mixed gastrocnemius. Also in this case, the 'inverted' recruitment pattern might have conferred a functional advantage by avoiding slow relaxation rates that would impede the speed of muscle lengthening. A selective preferential recruitment of different units during shortening and lengthening contractions was also observed for an intrinsic hand muscle (Howell *et al.* 1995), whereas no evidence for such differential behaviour was found for lengthening contractions in wrist flexors (Stotz and Bawa 2001) or knee extensors (Beltman *et al.* 2004).

8.2.3. Task-associated switching of recruitment thresholds; voluntary influence on recruitment

In their analysis of unit activity during cat locomotion on a treadmill, Hoffer *et al.* (1987) noticed that, within the sartorius muscle, different individual units were discharging during different parts of the step cycle. As they all seemed to lie within the same portion of the muscle, and there was no mechanical reason for having a different choice of units in different phases of the walking, Hoffer *et al.* (1987) suggested that this organization indicated that different MNs belonged to different 'task groups', having the same efferent target but different synaptic inputs. In several other cases, a similar appearance of 'task groups' was seen for units with a different localization within the muscle (see section 8.2.4).

At low muscle forces, human subjects may learn to preferentially activate different individual units within the same muscle (Basmajian 1963; Thomas *et al.* 1978). It seems probable that these 'selections' actually represent task-associated differences in relative recruitment threshold, and that subjects try to perform different motor actions with their arms and hands when making the choice between different units. In experiments where such 'task variations' were less likely, using a muscle with a single mechanical function, very little voluntary control of unit recruitment was observed (extensor indicis proprius muscle) (Henneman *et al.* 1976). A 'rank de-ordering' with the direction of a movement, but not with its speed, has also been directly observed in human muscles (Desmedt and Godaux 1981).

8.2.4. Topographically heterogeneous recruitment behaviour in MN pools

8.2.4.1. Regional activation in 'multi-torque' muscles: equivalent to choice of different muscles

When discussing topographic aspects of MN recruitment, it should be remembered that muscles that have been given single names by anatomists may still represent several functional units in terms of force directions. A striking example is the deltoid muscle of the shoulder, which is fan shaped and contributes to elevation of the upper arm in anterior or lateral directions, depending on which muscle portion is activated (Wickham and Brown 1998). Another example is found in the cat hindlimb; the posterior part of the biceps femoris muscle is a knee flexor but its anterior part is a hip extensor. In such cases, the activation of different muscle portions is equivalent to the activation of different muscles as required for appropriate motor coordination.

With regard to muscle choice in coordination, it should be remembered that the same joint torque may often be produced with several different alternative combinations of synergistic muscles or mucle portions; such differences may be one of the reasons for individual variations in recruitment strategy (Loeb 1993; Wolf *et al.* 1998). Furthermore, different individuals may have different motor habits which will also contribute to sometimes striking variations in muscle activation (Hensbergen and Kernell 1998). All the topographic discussion below concerns muscles (or muscle portions) with an apparently single force direction.

8.2.4.2. Topographical differences associated with intramuscular fibre type regionalization

As was described in an earlier chapter (Chapter 3, section 3.6.2), muscles are typically heterogeneous with regard to the intramuscular topographic distribution of different fibre types; the slow and fatigue-resistant type I fibres often tend to be preferentially accumulated towards one side of the muscle, mostly towards the side facing the limb centre (Armstrong 1980; Wang and Kernell 2001a,b). Thus if all the MNs of a given muscle belonged to the same task group, sharing the same input and being recruited according to the size principle, recruitment behaviours would typically be heterogeneous with regard to intramuscular topography. Units lying in 'red' slow portions (or compartments) would consistently be more easily recruited than those lying in 'white' faster portions. Such distinctions have also been repeatedly observed in large and clearly

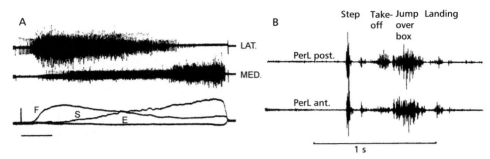

Figure 8.2 Intramuscular distribution of activity during different motor tasks. (**A**) Upper two panels: electromyographic (EMG) recordings from lateral and medial portions of the long head of biceps brachii muscle in a human subject. Lower panel: isometric force (torque) measured at the wrist in three different directions (F, elbow flexion; S, forearm supination; E, humerus exorotation). At the onset of this contraction, the subject exerted an elbow flexion force, which was then slowly released while lower-arm supination force slowly increased (i.e. outward rotation). For both force directions, the torque contributions of active units were about the same for medial and lateral muscle portions. However, EMG activity was predominantly medial during supination and lateral during flexion. Time bar, 2 s; force (torque) bar, 2.7 Nm flexion (F), 0.6 Nm supination (S), and 0.6 Nm exorotation (E).(Reproduced with permission, from ter Haar Romeny *et al.* 1984.) (**B**) EMG recordings from anterior and posterior regions of cat peroneus longus muscle (PerL) during voluntary unrestrained movements. The cat took a step and then jumped over a small box lying on the floor (box height, 20 cm). Note the varying relationships between anterior and posterior EMG during the different phases of motor behaviour; posterior EMG dominates during jump take-off and anterior EMG during the landing from the jump. The EMG recordings were obtained from bipolar thin-wire electrodes with a relatively restricted recording area, and there was no significant cross-talk from adjoining muscles (controlled by simultaneous EMG recordings from neighbouring muscles). Data from experiments of Hensbergen and Kernell (1992). (Reproduced with permission, from Kernell 1992.)

regionalized and/or compartmentalized muscles (Gordon and Phillips 1953; English 1984; Chanaud *et al.* 1991).

8.2.4.3. **Intramuscular unit position and task-associated differences in recruitment threshold**

In the experiments of Hoffer *et al.* (1987), the units belonging to different task groups did not seem to have any preferential or different localizations within the muscle. However, in several other sets of experiments, differences in relative recruitment threshold for different coordination tasks have been observed between units lying in different, but mechanically equivalent, muscle portions. One example concerns the long head of biceps brachii in humans (ter Haar Romeny *et al.* 1984), which contributes to the torques of arm flexion as well as supination (outward hand rotation). A preferential recruitment of medial units was found for supination, and units that were located more laterally were recruited for elbow flexion (Fig. 8.2A). It was ascertained, using local stimulation, that units in both locations exerted similar torques on the hand (ter Haar Romeny *et al.* 1984). Another example of topographical organization in relation to task concerns the peroneus longus muscle of the cat. In this species, the peroneus longus is a foot everter and dorsiflexor, and it acts via a single long slender tendon attached to the foot. As the cat prepares to jump, EMG activity within this muscle concerns predominantly posterior units; when the cat expects to land there is an activation of mainly anterior units (Fig. 8.2B) (Hensbergen and Kernell 1992). For peroneus longus, differences between the recruitment of anterior and posterior units have also been seen under anaesthesia in a comparison of the activation in a flexion reflex (peripheral nerve stimulation) with that caused by electrical activation of the motor cortex (Kandou and Kernell 1989). There is no difference between the density of the slow type I fibres in the anterior and posterior portions of the cat peroneus longus (Kernell *et al.* 1998).

Differences in pool innervation between MNs with topographically different targets within a muscle might be related to the location of the respective MNs within the spinal cord. MN nuclei are very long (Fig. 5.2C,D), and it seems unlikely that all portions of a pool would be homogeneously innervated by all synaptic inputs. It is known that in some single-unit inputs the effects are stronger for MNs lying topographically close to the input than for those located further away, for example Renshaw inhibition (McCurdy and Hamm 1994) and Ia monosynaptic excitation (Clamann *et al.* 1985; Luscher *et al.* 1989). It is also known that anterior portions of the cat peroneus longus are predominantly innervated by MNs lying more cranially within the cord, and vice versa for posterior portions (Fig. 5.6) (Donselaar *et al.* 1985). It should be noted that these topographic recruitment preferences do not have to imply that only part of the pool is reached by each individual task input. All the MN pool of the muscle might possibly be activated for very strong task inputs.

8.2.5. Daily aspects of MN recruitment: for how long are different units and muscles used?

The functional properties of muscle fibres are markedly influenced by training, i.e. by their patterns of daily use (Chapter 11, section 11.3). As a background to the analysis of such aspects of muscle unit plasticity, it is essential to know how much the various muscles are used normally. The simplest kind of measurement in this context is to record during how much time per day muscles are at all active. Such measurements have been done for various muscles in humans for 8 h working days (Monster *et al.* 1978), for sessions of up to 24 h (Fuglevand *et al.* 1995), and for sessions of up to 10 h (Kern *et al.* 2001), and during 24 h sessions for hindlimb muscles in rhesus monkeys (Hodgson *et al.* 2001), cats (Alaimo *et al.* 1984; Pierotti *et al.* 1991; Hensbergen and Kernell 1997; 1998), and rats (single units) (Hennig and Lomo 1985). The differences in daily duty time for single units are enormous; presumed FF units of the extensor digitorum longus muscle were only active in brief bursts covering, on average, about 0.11 per cent of total recording time, whereas presumed S units of soleus had daily duty times of about 30 per cent (Hennig and Lomo 1985). Similarly, in the monkey, EMG amplitudes that approximated the recruitment of all fibres within a muscle occurred for only 5–40 s/day in the various muscles, i.e. the daily duty times for the least excitable units were only about 0.006–0.05 per cent of total time (Hodgson *et al.* 2001).

Of course, measurements of daily activity times for whole muscles will only concern the discharge durations of their most easily recruited units (i.e. the S units). However, there are remarkable differences in daily duty time between various muscles from the same hindlimbs; in cats duty times range from about 2 per cent of total time per day for extensor digitorum longus up to about 14 per cent or more for the soleus (Fig. 8.3A) (Hensbergen and Kernell 1997). One of the longest average duty times published so far concerns human hand and arm muscles (18 per cent of total time) (Kern *et al.* 2001). A positive correlation has been found between the daily duty time and the percentage of slow type I fibres in humans (Monster *et al.* 1978) and in cats (Kernell *et al.* 1998); however, there is a lack of correlation when comparing only selected human hand and leg muscles (Kern *et al.* 2001). Long duty times are presumably related to the time periods that muscles are used for maintained postural contractions. Such contractions would be more important during active parts of the day than in rest periods. Correspondingly, in cats, intermuscular differences in duty time were much less pronounced or even absent at night (when these cats rested) than during the day (Hensbergen and Kernell 1998). When compared within the same species and limb, muscles with prolonged daily duty times apparently have a low 'postural threshold', i.e. a relatively high proportion of their total fibre population might be engaged in postural tasks and develop the appropriate functional characteristics. These relationships might be quantitatively different for muscles from different species and different limbs. The percentage of type I fibres is very much higher in humans than in corresponding muscles of cats, although the daily duty times might be quite similar (Fig. 8.3B).

8.3. **Rate gradation in motoneurone pools**

8.3.1. **Minimum rates of steady firing**

As already discussed in Chapter 6, section 6.5.7, the regular firing rate of a MN cannot be continuously varied down towards zero; there is typically a fairly well-defined minimum rate of steady firing for discharges evoked with artificial stimulating currents as well as for those elicited via the CNS. Thus, as voluntary or reflex muscle force is very slowly increased, newly recruited MNs tend to start discharging at a rather regular rate which is characteristic for that cell (Fig. 8.1). The recruitment rates may be systematically higher at short compared with longer muscle lengths (Vander Linden *et al.* 1991), and in slow concentric compared with isometric contractions (Tax *et al.* 1989). Such adaptations to muscle use are functionally relevant because the tension–frequency relation shifts toward higher rates at short muscle lengths (Fig. 3.2B). The mechanisms underlying the adjustments of minimum steady rate to muscle use are still unknown (synaptic modification of MN membrane properties, possibly leading to changes in AHP time course? (cf. Chapter 7, section 7.5)).

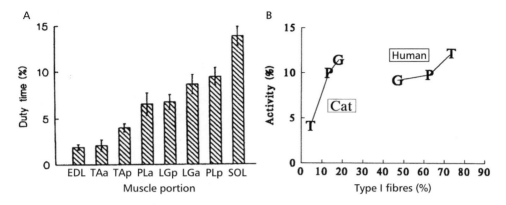

Figure 8.3 Durations of daily muscle use. (**A**) Comparisons between different muscles (and muscle portions) of the cat hindlimb. The daily duration of spontaneous activity (duty time) was determined using 24 h EMG recordings and expressed as a percentage of total time spent in activity. The bar graph shows means ± SE for the following eight recording sites, displayed in order of ascending duty time: EDL, extensor digitorum longus; TAa, anterior side of tibialis anterior; TAp, posterior side of tibialis anterior; PLa, anterior side of peroneus longus, LGp posterior side of gastrocnemius lateralis, LGa anterior side of gastrocnemius lateralis, PLp posterior side of peroneus longus, SOL soleus. (Reproduced with permission, from Hensbergen and Kernell 1997.) (**B**) Comparisons between cat and human with regard to the mean daytime duration of spontaneous activity (given as a percentage of total sampling time) and the mean percentage of type I fibres in tibialis anterior (T), lateral gastrocnemius (G), and peroneus longus (P). The human activity data were taken from measurements by Monster *et al.* (1978), which concerned an 8 h working day. For comparison, the plotted cat data are averages from highly active periods around noon (Hensbergen and Kernell 1998). Histochemical data were taken from Kernell *et al.* (1998) for the cat peroneus longus and tibialis anterior, from Ariano *et al.* (1973) for cat gastrocnemius, and from Johnson *et al.* (1973) for humans. Whenever applicable, mean values were computed for anterior and posterior measurements. (Reproduced with permission, from Kernell *et al.* 1998.)

8.3.2. Maximum rates of steady firing

Information about the upper end of the gradation range is more limited because of the technical problems involved in obtaining reliable electromyographic unit recordings at high force levels. However, there is an intriguing discrepancy between the average rates recorded during human maximum voluntary contractions (often in the range of 20–30 Hz; cf. Fig. 8.4) and those apparently required for a maximum isometric force in human muscles (about 30–100 Hz, often in the range 80–100 Hz; for detailed data and references, see Enoka and Fuglevand (2001)). Either the maximum voluntary force of these contractions was far below the maximum evocable force (however, see section 8.4.3), or some factor other than mean firing rate was of importance for the forces achieved (for further discussion, see Enoka and Fuglevand 2001). Rates in the range 80–100 Hz or above have occasionally been recorded in human voluntary contractions, but

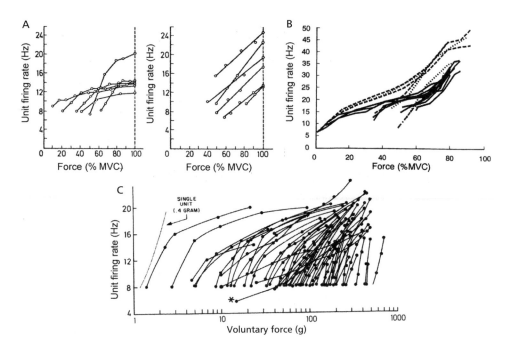

Figure 8.4 Recruitment and rate gradation of motor units in voluntary contractions. Electromyographic unit recordings from isometric voluntary contractions of human muscles. (**A**) Biceps brachii. Impulse rate versus isometric force of elbow flexion. Observations from the same single unit connected by straight lines. Force given as a percentage of maximum voluntary contraction (MVC). Left- and right-hand panels show units with different types of behaviour. (Reproduced with permission, from Gydikov and Kosarov 1974.) (**B**) Tibialis anterior (foot dorsiflexion), display as in (**A**). (Reproduced with permission, from De Luca and Erim 1994). (**c**) Extensor digitorum communis, diplay as in (**A**). Forces of wrist extension in absolute units (note logarithmic X-scale). The MVC force was about 700–800 g. (Reproduced with permission, from Monster and Chan 1977.)

only under special circumstances (e.g. in muscles with very few active units, permitting a selective recording up to high levels of activity (Marsden *et al.* 1971)).

8.4. **Force gradation: recruitment and rate gradation combined**

In weak contractions, recruitment and rate gradation typically take place in parallel; an increase in voluntary or reflex contraction strength is caused by recruiting new units and, simultaneously, increasing the rate of those already recruited (Figs 8.1 and 8.4). Ultimately, in a moderately strong voluntary contraction, all units will have been recruited and only rate gradation will remain as a means of force gradation. However, units discharging at such high levels of force are technically very difficult to investigate and there is a significant amount of uncertainty about muscle unit behaviour at these levels. Such studies have mostly been performed with human subjects who can easily be instructed as to how to vary voluntary force.

In maintained submaximal contractions, the firing rates of active MNs might decrease while other MNs are recruited (Person and Kudina 1972; Garland *et al.* 1994). This behaviour is expected as a result of the late phase of spike-frequency adaptation in the MNs (Fig. 6.3A and Chapter 6, section 6.5.5). In accordance with this interpretation, a constant firing rate in individual MNs can only be maintained by gradually increasing the excitation to the MN pool, as indicated by an increasing level of total EMG (Johnson *et al.* 2004).

In descriptions of experiments with multi-unit recordings and gradually increasing voluntary force levels, it is often stated that the first units recruited also reach the highest final rates (Freund *et al.* 1975; Freund 1983; De Luca and Erim 1994) (cf. Fig. 8.4B). However, in some investigations in which units could be followed up to high relative forces, the opposite sometimes seems to be true; units recruited at relatively high forces tended to increase their rate proportionately faster than units recruited at the lowest rates and, ultimately, some late recruits may reach the highest final rates (Fig. 8.4A) (Gydikov and Kosarov 1974; see also Tokizane and Shimazu 1964; Grimby *et al.* 1979). This would fit expectations from experimental work on MN repetitive properties; presumed fast MNs would be expected to reach higher final rates than presumed slow MNs (Kernell 1965c).

In voluntary contractions the rates of some low-threshold units tend to 'saturate' as muscle force is increased (Fig. 8.4A, left panel) and, as force approaches the MVC, the discharge frequencies of these various units will tend to overlap. Possible mechanisms underlying such pool behaviours have been analysed and discussed using detailed models and experimental data concerning the intra-pool distribution of synapses and cell properties (Heckman and Binder 1993a,b). There is evidence indicating that MNs may be truly insensitive to extra postsynaptic stimuli while firing at saturation rates (e.g. tested with muscle vibration activating Ia afferents (Fuglevand and Johns 2004)). The activation of dendritic voltage-gated permeabilities (Chapter 6, section 6.7) (reviewed by Heckman *et al.* 2005; Hultborn *et al.* 2004) might possibly be strong enough to occlude the transfer of synaptic current along (selected) dendrites (cf. Lee *et al.* 2003).

8.4.1. **Force range for recruitment gradation**

On the basis of a few detailed investigations, a difference seems to exist between different muscles with regard to the force range for voluntary recruitment gradation (i.e. the relative force at which recruitment reaches 100 per cent) (Kukulka and Clamann 1981; De Luca *et al.* 1982). In two intrinsic hand muscles (adductor pollicis, first dorsal interosseus), this force was at about 40–50 per cent MVC. In two larger muscles of the upper arm (biceps brachii, deltoid), some recruitment continued up to 70–90 per cent MVC. These observations may suggest a systematic difference in the distribution of synapses and/or intrinsic excitabilities between these two kinds of MN pools. However, such conclusions should be treated with some caution. For instance, the flexion torque at

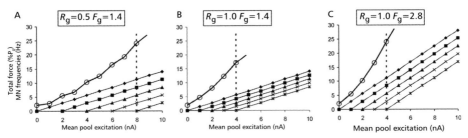

Figure 8.5 Model illustration of changes in rate gain and recruitment gain. Plots of MN firing rates (lower five lines) and total muscle force (%P_0, upper line, open circles) in a simple model of a MN pool, illustrating some general effects of changes in the gains for rate and recruitment gradation. This simple pool model had five MNs which differed only in their intrinsic excitability (current threshold for repetitive firing, I_{rep}). All cells received the same fraction of total pool input, i.e. the mean pool excitation is also the current intensity received by each individual MN. Only intensities that were suprathreshold for pool activation are plotted, and the spike frequencies are those exceeding the rate obtained on recruitment (F_{min}). In the 'control' case of panel (**A**), each MN had an *f–I* slope of 1.4 Hz/nA and the recruitment gain was 0.5 MN per nA. Once recruited, each MN fired at F_{min} and evoked a mean force of 10 %P_0 from its muscle unit. For rates above F_{min} (i.e. those plotted) force increased at a rate of 2.5 %P_0/Hz. Total force (open circles) is the sum of all the unit forces. In (**B**) and (**C**) recruitment gain was twice that in (**A**), and in (**C**) the rate gain was also doubled. Forces at completed recruitment (broken vertical lines) were (**A**) 24 per cent, (**B**) 17 per cent, and (**C**) 24 per cent. Forces for 10 nA mean pool excitation were (**A**) 31 per cent, (**B**) 38 per cent, and (**C**) 66 per cent.

the elbow is produced by three synergic muscles, two of which (brachialis, brachioradialis) were not included in these measurements.

A relatively low-level limit for completed recruitment gradation will be attained if the recruitment thresholds are close together (high recruitment gain) (see section 8.4.4), allowing all the units to be recruited while firing at relatively low rates (compare Figs 8.5A and 8.5B), which might be advantageous for counteracting fatigue. Recruitment thresholds also seem to be more closely clustered for slow low-threshold units than for those with higher thresholds (Bakels and Kernell 1994).

8.4.2. **Tremor**

At low levels of maintained activation, it is advantageous to have many weak units firing out of phase with each other in order to decrease the force oscillations caused by non-fused contractions. Some force oscillations normally remain in human contractions (**physiological tremor**), typically with a peak at around 6–10 Hz and partly due to some still existing synchronization of MN discharges with unfused unit contractions (Dietz *et al.* 1976; Allum *et al.* 1978; Deuschl *et al.* 2001). This low-level synchronization is probably mainly caused by shared synaptic inputs. Other possible sources of tremor in voluntary contractions are oscillations in the stretch reflex loop (Fitzpatrick *et al.* 1996). Furthermore, there is evidence for a pulsatile input to MNs from central neurones during smooth movements (Vallbo and Wessberg 1993; Wessberg and Vallbo 1995, 1996). There

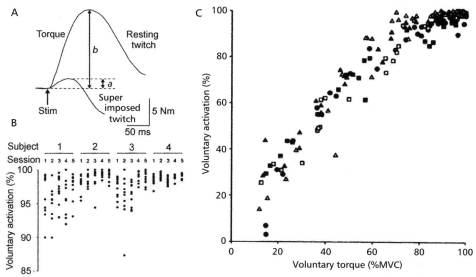

Figure 8.6 Degree of activation in maximum voluntary contractions. Method of twitch interpolation, as applied to voluntary contractions of muscles plantar flexing the ankle joint. (**A**) Plantar
flexion torque following a supra-maximum electrical stimulus over the triceps surae muscle while
at rest (resting twitch, indicated by 'b') and during a maximum voluntary contraction (superimposed twitch, indicated by 'a'). The relative voluntary activation (percentage of maximum) was
quantified as: $(1 - a/b) \times 100$, i.e. when a muscle is truly maximumly activated an interpolated
twitch stimulation should be incapable of evoking any superimposed contraction. (**B**) Degree of
activation in repeated maximum voluntary contractions and testing sessions in four different
subjects. Note the relative scarcity of 100 per cent values and clustering of most contractions in
the range 95–100 per cent. (**c**) Relation between degree of voluntary activation and voluntary
contractile torque during brief submaximum and maximum contractions. Results from each subject are shown with different symbols. Note the smaller slope of the curve in the range 80–100
per cent. (Reproduced with permission, from Todd *et al.* 2004.)

is also an unsteadiness of maintained force with lower frequencies of superimposed
oscillation (e.g. 1–2 Hz), which is probably related to central mechanisms; this kind of
unsteadiness is exacerbated with stress and is more pronounced in ageing individuals
(Laidlaw *et al.* 2000; Christou *et al.* 2004).

8.4.3. **Total extent of attainable (and CNS gradable) force**

A crucial question of importance in many contexts of neuromuscular physiology concerns the upper limit of the normal working range. Does voluntary or reflex gradation of
force cover all tensions up to and including the maximum tetanic force, also referred to
as the 'maximum evocable force' (MEF) (Gandevia 2001)? Might the motoneuronal drive
to a muscle even be increased up to supra-maximal levels, i.e. become so strong that
some (minor) decline of MN activity would produce no decline in force? The most
straightforward method for answering such questions would be to evoke the maximum

tetanic force by direct electrical stimulation and compare this force with whatever was produced reflexly or voluntarily (e.g. Fig. 9.3A) (Bigland-Ritchie *et al.* 1983b). However, such tetanic stimulations are often very painful. A more subject-friendly technique serving the same purpose, referred to as of 'twitch interpolation' (Fig. 8.6), was introduced by Merton (1954b) and developed further by others (e.g. Belanger and McComas 1981; Gandevia 2001).

Experimental measurements from various laboratories indicate that, in several muscles at least, forces close to the maximum tetanic force may be elicited voluntarily. However, the experiments also indicate that this is typically only just possible; the maximum is reached only in a certain percentage of a series of repeated trials (Fig. 8.6B). This is also indicated by the common occurrence of a large short-term variability of force during the maintenance of a MVC (e.g. from second to second), i.e. there is usually no saturation of force at the MVC (Gandevia 2001). Interestingly, this variability is larger for some muscles than for others; for example, it is larger for index finger abduction than for thumb adduction (Zijdewind and Kernell 1994b). Thus, the voluntary command levels of the CNS are apparently somehow dimensioned such that they often just reach, but never exceed, the amount of drive needed for a truly maximum contraction (Gandevia 2001). In some muscles and subjects, the maximum evocable force is reached occasionally (Fig. 8.6B), and in others the MVC is consistently somewhat lower than the MEF (cf, Belanger and McComas 1981). Interestingly, the maximum limit for voluntary activation can be shifted upwards by training, including by imaginary efforts performed without producing actual contractions (Yue and Cole 1992; Zijdewind *et al.* 2003). One of the possible effects of such training sessions, with or without contractions, might be to increase the facilitation of 'booster-PICs' or 'plateau currents' via the activation of descending monoaminergic systems (Chapter 7, section 7.5). One might expect that such 'setting systems' would also show a diurnal variation in their activity, which would be reflected in a corresponding variation in MVC forces. There is indeed a diurnal variation of MVC force, which is larger in the evening than in the morning (Gauthier *et al.* 1996; Martin *et al.* 1999); however, surprisingly, this force variation was found to depend on changes in muscle properties and not on central factors (Martin *et al.* 1999).

Near-maximum voluntary contractions have a number of particular characteristics: as mentioned above, the force tends to be unstable, and forces tend to 'irradiate' beyond the immediate target muscles, even to the extent that muscles are activated in contralateral limbs (Dimitrijevic *et al.* 1992; Zijdewind and Kernell 2001). Thus muscle coordination becomes disturbed. Both characteristics become progressively more evident as the MVC is prolonged during an increasing degree of fatigue. The 'irradiation' phenomena might reflect the effects of booster-PICs, emerging during extreme efforts and increasing the excitabilities of MNs and upstreams command systems.

8.4.4. Modification of recruitment and rate gradation properties

There are indications that the balance between rate and recruitment gradation might differ between different tasks for the same MN pool (Mottram *et al.* 2005). Theoretically, such task-related differences would also be expected to occur because mechanisms are available for synaptically evoked changes in both recruitment and rate gain. This will be discussed using the simple pool model of Fig. 8.5 (see caption for details). As is apparently the case in 'real' MN pools (Chapter 7, section 7.2.5), the various pool members received fractions from the same kinds of synaptic input, i.e. an increased pool input would not only recruit more cells but would also cause an increased rate of firing in MNs that were already recruited. In the model in Fig. 8.5, the various pool members differed in intrinsic excitability, requiring different intensities of current to start firing. Each pool member received the same fraction of the synaptic drive, and initially they all had the same slope for their frequency–current relation (f–I slope, 'rate gain'). In such a model, the 'recruitment gain' might be quantified as the ratio of the increase in number of recruited MNs to the increase in mean pool excitation current. In the model pool of Fig. 8.5A, an 8 nA increase in mean pool excitation increased the number of recruited MNs from 1 to 5, i.e. the recruitment gain was equal to 0.5 cells/nA. Compared with the 'control case' in Fig. 8.5A, recruitment gain is doubled in Fig. 8.5B, and both recruitment and rate gains are doubled in Fig. 8.5C.

The recruitment gain depends on the distribution of MN excitabilities and synaptic inputs across the pool (Kernell and Hultborn 1990). An additional excitatory or inhibitory input to the MN pool would alter recruitment gain if its distribution across MNs of different intrinsic excitability differed from the distribution of the synapses that were already active (Kernell and Hultborn 1990). For instance, compared with an input like that for Ia afferents (Fig. 7.6B), a synaptic system delivering more excitatatory current to high-threshold than to low-threshold MNs would decrease the differences in recruitment threshold within the pool and thus cause an increase in recruitment gain (also referred to as 'threshold compression' (Burke 2004)). This might happen, for instance, for inputs to spinal MNs from skin afferents or from descending rubro- or corticospinal tracts (Burke *et al.* 1970; Kanda *et al.* 1977; Dum and Kennedy 1980b; Garnett and Stephens 1981; Heckman and Binder 1993b; Nielsen and Kagamihara 1993). Effects on recruitment gain would not only be produced by driving systems with particular synaptic distributions, but this gain might also be 'preset' by suitable distributions of a steady background excitation and/or inhibition (Kernell and Hultborn 1990). There is a great degree of variation with regard to how synaptic currents are distributed across MNs of different intrinsic excitability (Fig. 7.6B), i.e. there is ample scope for synaptic effects on recruitment gain.

The rate gain may be increased by MN-modifying synaptic effects. The best known example is the decrease in AHP conductance caused by serotonin (5HT), resulting in an increase in f–I slope (Fig. 7.7; see Chapter7, section 7.5.2). MNs receive a rich 5HT innervation, i.e. there is also ample scope for synaptic effects on rate gain.

The very simple model versions in Fig. 8.5 show that, for instance, the force range covered by recruitment gradation might be decreased by an increased recruitment gain (Fig. 8.5B versus Fig. 8.5A), increased by an increased rate gain (Fig. 8.5C versus Fig. 8.5B), and left unchanged with a net increase of overall pool gain if both recruitment and rate

gain are increased (Fig. 8.5A versus Fig. 8.5C). This illustrates some aspects of the potential flexibility in MN pool control. It still remains to find out experimentally how these
various possibilities are used in motor behaviour; for further calculations, using more
sophisticated and 'life-like' pool models, see Heckman and Binder (1991b, 1993a,b),
Fuglevand et al. (1993), Heckman (1994), and Taylor and Enoka (2004). It should be
stressed that, over the whole possible range of force production, rate gradation is by far
the most powerful mechanism. For instance, with a twitch:tetanus ratio of about 0.2 and
a minimum steady MN firing rate causing almost no twitch fusion (cf. Figs. 6.8C,D and
8.1B,C), barely recruited muscle fibres would only deliver a mean force of about 10 per
cent of their maximum tetanic tension. The remaining 90 per cent would only be mobilized using rate gradation.

8.5. Renshaw inhibition: a system for synaptic 'pool feedback'

Skeletal MNs have central as well as peripheral targets. The known central effects, via
axon collaterals and Renshaw cells, seem to be of particular relevance for the control of
MN pools.

8.5.1. MN recurrent collaterals

Before they emerge from the spinal cord, most axons of alpha MNs give off one or more
side branches which make synaptic contacts with other cells of the CNS. The intraspinal
courses of these 'recurrrent collaterals' have been traced following intracellular HRP
staining of individual identified MNs (Cullheim et al. 1977; Cullheim and Kellerth
1978a,b,c). Apparent synaptic boutons, formed by the terminals of such collaterals, are
found within about ± 1 mm from the parent cell body (Cullheim and Kellerth 1978b),
i.e. at distances much smaller than the total length of a typical MN pool (Fig. 5.2D). Most
of the collaterals give off terminals to a ventromedial region within the grey matter of the
spinal cord (Fig. 8.7A); this is the region containing the inhibitory interneurones referred
to as 'Renshaw cells' (see further below). Individual MNs show systematic differences in
their number of axon collaterals, and with regard to muscle unit type these numbers are
ranked such that FF > FR > S (Cullheim and Kellerth 1978a), i.e. MN categories with
large muscle units and many terminals to muscle fibres (Table 3.1) also have many
intraspinal axonal branches. Interestingly, these differences are also very clear between FF
and FR MNs which, in the cat, typically show no significant differences in soma or axon
diameter (Fig. 6.7A and Table 6.1).

8.5.2. MN connections to MNs

A small number of collaterals from MN axons have terminals within the same region as
the MNs (Fig. 8.7A), and EM studies have shown that such terminals apparently have
conventional synaptic connections to MNs (Cullheim et al. 1977, 1984). The function of
these connections is obscure; they are not specific for MNs with particular types of muscle fibres. It cannot be excluded that these connections have slow 'trophic' effects rather

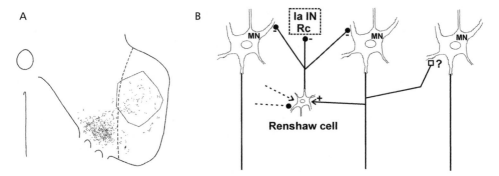

Figure 8.7 Intraspinal targets of MNs: Renshaw cells and other MNs. (**A**) Observations of sites of probable synaptic connections for recurrent MN collaterals in cat lumbar spinal cord. MNs were intracellularly labelled with HRP; axons and their collaterals were reconstructed. Distribution in the L7 ventral horn of 734 axon collateral swellings (dots), interpreted as synaptic boutons in light microscopy. The swellings originated from collaterals of 19 triceps surae alpha MNs. The broken line shows the medial border of the motor nuclei, as estimated from Romanes (1951). The circumscribed area within the motor nuclei shows the extent of the triceps surae motor nucleus, as defined by the positions of 63 retrogradely labelled motoneurones after HRP injection in the triceps surae muscle. (Reproduced with permission, from Cullheim *et al.* 1977) (**B**) Simplified scheme showing the destinations of intraspinal axon collaterals from MNs: Renshaw cells and other MNs. The synaptic effects on other MNs are still unknown. Renshaw cells become excited by motoneuronal cholinergic axon terminals, and this will cause inhibition in MNs of the same and other (mainly synergic) pools as well as in at least two categories of segmental interneurones (Ia IN, Ia interneurones mediating reciprocal inhibition; Rc, other Renshaw cells); in addition to these two categories of segmental neurones, Renshaw cellls also inhibit cells of origin of the ventral spinocerebellar tract. The excitability and activity of the Renshaw cells may be influenced by segmental afferents and descending fibres from the brain (interrupted lines).

than acute actions of conventional synaptic kinds. Furthermore, cholinergic terminals might conceivably have a modifying effect on MN membranes; such actions have been seen in turtle MNs after the *in vitro* activation of muscarinic receptors (Alaburda *et al.* 2002; Hornby *et al.* 2002a).

8.5.3. MN connections to Renshaw cells

In the rat spinal cord, each Renshaw cell receives about 67 cholinergic terminals from MN axon collaterals (Alvarez *et al.* 1999; see also Lagerback *et al.* 1981a). Under optimal conditions, a single Renshaw cell can even be weakly activated by the collaterals of a single MN (Van Keulen 1981). However, single Renshaw cells are normally driven by the combined input of many MNs from nearby portions of the input MN pools. In the craniocaudal direction along a MN pool, the Renshaw cell activation effects decrease relatively rapidly with distance from a given activated MN axon (Van Keulen 1981; Hamm *et al.* 1987). Individual Renshaw cells are influenced by MNs from several different pools of, typically, synergistic muscles (Eccles *et al* 1961). As synergist MNs also tend to lie within similar regions of the ventral horn (Chapter 5, section 5.4.1), the selection of input MNs for a given Renshaw cell may partly be a question of proximity.

When activated simultaneously by all its recurrent collateral inputs (e.g. using electrical stimulation of a ventral root), Renshaw cells deliver a high-frequency burst with an initial rate close to 1000 Hz and a duration of about 40 ms (cat) (Eccles *et al*. 1954). However, this does not mean that such bursts represent normal types of Renshaw cell activity; when activated more asynchronously during motor programs they fire in phase with the activating MNs (fictive locomotion) (Pratt and Jordan 1987), and they may fire spontaneously in a decerebrate animal (Cleveland *et al*. 1981).

The excitation produced in Renshaw cells by MN collaterals is mediated by ACh acting partly on muscarinic receptors (Eccles *et al*. 1954). At these excitatory synapses, the synaptic current evoked by a single presynaptic spike is apparently relatively long-lasting, greatly exceeding the duration of the axon spike. Thus the synaptic effects of MN axons on Renshaw cells are markedly different from the brief nicotinic effects at the motor endplate (cf. brief downward transients in Fig. 4.2B,C).

In addition to the effects of recurrent MN collaterals, the activity of Renshaw cells may also be modulated (facilitated or inhibited) by several supraspinal and segmental inputs (reviewed by Baldissera *et al*. 1981).

8.5.4. Inhibitory connections from Renshaw cells to MNs

In reponse to a synchronous activation of its ventral root (i.e. activation of many recurrent collaterals and Renshaw cells), a MN receives a postsynaptic inhibition with a time course reflecting the long-lasting burst of the Renshaw cells. The duration of this compound R-IPSP is typically about 40 ms and its peak is reached quickly after its onset. In cat MNs, the synchronous R-IPSP is typically briefer than the AHP; i.e. it does not interfere with AHP duration measurements.

The compound R-IPSP is produced by the simultaneous action of many Renshaw cells, each activated by the collaterals of many (largely synergistic) MNs. The IPSP produced in a MN by single spikes of an individual Renshaw cell is very weak, on average only about 0.013 mV (Van Keulen 1981). When activated by all the motor axons of a given MN pool, the R-IPSP tends to be larger in slow-twitch than in fast-twitch MNs, i.e. it is typically greater in high-resistance than low-resistance cells (Friedman *et al*. 1981; Hultborn *et al*. 1988a,b; cf. Eccles *et al*. 1961). However, these differences seem largely to reflect differences in MN input resistance. At a membrane potential corresponding to the threshold for spike initiation, the R-IPSP current is very similar in high- and low-resistance MNs (Hultborn *et al*. 1988a; Lindsay and Binder 1991) (see Fig. 7.6B). MNs tend to be most effectively inhibited by collaterals from their own and synergist pools.

The R-IPSPs are generated by an increased Cl^- conductance (Eccles *et al*. 1954; Burke *et al*. 1971a), and this postsynaptic effect is apparently produced by a co-release of the transmitters glycine and GABA at the terminals of the Renshaw cells (cf. Ornung *et al*.

1994). Hence the R-IPSP may be partly blocked by a glycine antagonist (e.g. strychnine) and partly by a GABA-A antagonist (e.g. picrotoxin) (Cullheim and Kellerth 1981). However, the R-IPSPs are less readily influenced by injected Cl⁻ than is the case for the IPSPs of reciprocal Ia inhibition, i.e. the Renshaw inhibition seems to be generated by electrotonically more remote synapses (Burke *et al.* 1971a). A dendritic localization of these synapses was indeed also confirmed by other measurements (anatomy, Fyffe 1991; impedance determinations, Maltenfort *et al.* 2004). The axons of individual Renshaw cells may travel for considerable distances within the white matter of the spinal cord (Jankowska and Smith 1973), providing MNs and other targets with a large number of inhibitory connections via intermittent side branches (van Keulen 1979; Lagerback and Kellerth 1985).

8.5.5. Inhibitory connections to other target cells

In addition to inhibiting MNs (gamma MNs are also inhibited), the Renshaw cells provide inhibitory connections to other Renshaw cells (weak connections) (Ryall 1981), the inhibitory interneurones which are responsible for reciprocal Ia inhibition (Chapter 2, section 2. 8.2) (Hultborn *et al.* 1968), and cells of the ventral spinocerebellar tract (for further references, see Windhorst 1996). In lightly anaesthetized animals, the Ia inhibitory interneurones often display a spontaneous discharge, producing a continuous inhibitory input to their target MNs. Thus, if these cells are inhibited by Renshaw cells, their target MNs will become disinhibited ('recurrent facilitation') (Hultborn *et al.* 1971). Hence, activity in recurrent MN collaterals will produce not only inhibitory effects in some MNs but also, in other MN populations, a facilitation due to a decrease in tonic inhibition.

8.5.6. Functional role of recurrent inhibition and Renshaw cells

Because of its unique organizational features, Renshaw inhibition has attracted much experimental attention. At a cellular level, the Renshaw cell loop is probably one of the best known interneuronal circuits in the CNS. However, the functional meaning of this circuit is still obscure; we do not know what types of disability would occur if the Renshaw cells were absent. When considering their function(s), it is important to remember that some MN pools lack recurrent collaterals, for example short muscles of the digits (Cullheim and Kellerth 1978b) and the long digital flexor (FDL, McCurdy and Hamm 1992) (reviewed and discussed by Illert and Kümmel 1999). A few of the different (but not mutually exclusive) hypotheses for the functions of the Renshaw cell inhibition of MNs are briefly discussed below (for further alternatives and details, see Windhorst 1996).

Whatever their other functions, control of pool gain will certainly represent one aspect of the effects of Renshaw cells (Hultborn *et al.* 1979). When Renshaw cells are active, part of the excitatory current driving a discharge would become 'neutralized' by recurrent inhibition. This kind of pool control would act on both the two gain dimensions of the pool, recruitment gradation as well as rate gradation, and both aspects would become affected to the same degree as long as the Renshaw inhibitory input was distributed across the MN pool in the same manner as the excitation driving the discharge (Kernell 1976). The size of the Renshaw effect on pool gain might turn out to be relatively modest. In anaesthetized cats, the total inhibitory current generated by a repetitive activation of the ventral root amounted to only about 1–2 nA (<1 nA in Fig. 7.6B) (Lindsay and Binder 1991; see also Hultborn et al. 1988a; Maltenfort et al. 2004), which is only a small fraction of the current needed for recruitment and for covering the whole range of repetitive firing in a fast-twitch MN (cf. Fig. 6.2B). It is not known whether the Renshaw inhibitory effects might become significantly more impressive under other functional conditions (without anaesthesia? other biological 'settings'?).

Renshaw inhibition will, of course, 'limit' discharge rate in the general sense that, for a given level of excitation, the rate of a MN will be lower with than without this inhibition. However, this does not mean that Renshaw inhibition would necessarily decrease the amount of rate gradation that happens in parallel with recruitment; a stabilization of discharge rate during ongoing recruitment would only take place under very particular (and unrealistic) conditions of Renshaw cell distribution across single MN pools (Kernell 1976). Thus the Renshaw inhibition is not a strong candidate for explaining why some MNs seem to reach saturated rates while total pool response increases (cf. Fig. 8.4A,C).

When using MNs firing at low rates for the production of a smooth and continuous contractile force (e.g. in posture), it is important for the smoothness of the maintained force that the various cells of the same pool show low levels of synchronization. It has been suggested that Renshaw inhibition would contribute to the desynchronization of MN discharges (Maltenfort et al. 1998).

8.6. Pathophysiological issue: imitating the action of motoneurone pools in functional electrical stimulation

In patients with a complete interruption of the spinal cord, limbs from segments caudal to the lesion cannot be reached by commands from the CNS. Hence these patients are paralysed in their lower (and sometimes also upper) limbs, even though they still possess muscles which are innervated and potentially useful, for example for standing and walking. Therefore much effort has been invested in trying to help these patients to activate their muscles using external electronic stimulators as a replacement for normal motor commands (**functional electrical stimulation** (FES)). This has proved to be difficult, partly because of the sheer number of muscles that would ideally have to be controlled using implanted electrodes and stimulator connections. Another difficulty concerns muscle coordination and corrective motor behaviour, which requires the use of some kind of sensors, possibly including signals from the patient's own sensory afferents (Hoffer et al. 1996; Jensen et al. 2002). Furthermore, there are problems specifically related to the muscle activation itself when delivered via a single pair of electrodes to each whole muscle nerve. Such contractions will show large oscillations, with largely unfused twitches, if FES is given at low rates (cf. Fig. 3.1B,D). On the other hand, contractions produced by stimulation rates fast enough for a high degree of twitch fusion will be prone to fatigue, which has proved to be a major problem in FES (Scott *et al.* 2005). In normal motor control, large force oscillations and undue fatigue reactions are avoided because a single muscle is operated by a whole population of MNs, which can activate their muscle fibres asynchronously at low rates (Wise *et al.* 2001). Several different technical solutions for FES have been considered and employed to try and solve this 'twitch-dilemma', separately stimulating different portions of the axonal supply to the target muscle(s) (for further details and references see: Mortimer 1981; Andrews 1992; Veltink and Alsté 1992). However, such techniques are complex to use and have not yet reached a refinement similar to that of the natural voluntary drive.

Chapter 9

Short-term plasticity: fatigue and potentiation

9.1. General issues

One of the complexities in the control of behaviour lies in the fact that the functional properties of neurones, synapses, and muscles often change as a result of preceding use. In the short term (minutes to hours), such changes are typically rapidly reversible and may be expressed as either a net increase or, potentially more disturbing, a net depression of input–output relations. Phenomena of this kind are well known in the neuromuscular system, and they are often denoted by descriptive terms like 'potentiation' or 'facilitation' for enhancement and 'fatigue' or 'depression' for decline. Both polarities of time- and use-dependent change are frequently present for components within as well as outside the CNS, and 'facilitation' and 'depression' are also important concepts in the study of higher mental or sensory functions.

In this book, 'motor potentiation' and 'motor fatigue' are used as descriptive terms for an increase or decrease in neuromuscular input–output relations, from organizational levels including the whole motor system (e.g. joint torque per 'unit' perceived effort) to levels of subcellular components (e.g. cross-bridge force per unit activating Ca^{2+}).

9.2. What do we mean by fatigue?

When we say that we get 'tired' or 'fatigued' during some kind of motor performance (e.g. running, carrying a heavy suitcase, etc.), we typically mean that we have to use an increasing amount of effort to maintain the function. Ultimately, it might even be impossible to continue; we become 'exhausted' (state of 'task failure'). However, becoming exhausted does not usually mean that we lose consciousness and fall down, but we might, for instance, interrupt a whole-body kind of activity like running or cycling on the basis of a conscious decision that, considering the exorbitant effort and other unpleasant details (e.g. pain), we can no longer 'stand it' and cannot continue (Kayser 2003). It may be important and of protective value that this decision is taken before the peripheral machinery has been overloaded to the point of becoming useless. By giving up while the muscles can still provide useful amounts of force and work, physical activities can be decreased in an orderly way (e.g. stepping to the side of the road and finding a suitable resting place before lying down).

The characteristics of exhaustion in motor behaviour differ depending on the total volume of muscle mass used. In strenuous whole-body exercise, the moment of exhaustion might be determined by experiencing an insufficiency of the respiratory and circulatory supply systems rather than by reactions related to the target muscles themselves. The physiology of the supply systems and related issues concerning the energy metabolism of muscle tissue are, rightly, highly important in texts dealing with exercise physiology. In the present review, the analysis will be focused on less generalized types of motor excercise in which the overall capacity of the respiratory and cardiovascular systems do not form the limiting factors (e.g. forces exerted by single muscles or limbs).

The motor activities of everyday life do not normally make us 'tired'; we can move light things around, stand and sit for whole days, and walk about at a leisurely pace for hours without feeling fatigued or exhausted. Thus there appears to be a threshold below which motor fatigue does not occur. This 'fatigue threshold' has been assessed, for various muscles, by measuring for how long (e.g. up to 1 h) subjects can maintain steady forces at various levels before becoming exhausted. In the original investigation, this 'fatigue threshold' was reported to be at about 15 per cent of MVC (Rohmert 1960), but there is some variation between different subjects and muscles (Ulmer et al. 1989), as would be expected considering intermuscular and inter-individual variations in fibre type composition (Chapter 3, section 3.6.1). In long-lasting contractions, even the maintenance of forces as weak as 2.5 per cent MVC may cause signs of fatigue (e.g. leg extensors, post-contraction decrease of MVC force) (Kouzaki et al. 2002). Above threshold level, endurance time decreases for increasing loads in a non-linear fashion. At 50 per cent MVC the endurance time is often as brief as about 1–2 min (Zijdewind et al. 1995), and at 75 per cent MVC exhaustion may occur after less than 0.5 min. Above the 'fatigue threshold', the sense of exerted effort increases continuously with time until it reaches its maximum perceived value just before the muscle fails and/or the subject 'decides' to become exhausted.

Psychophysical experiments have indicated that the 'sense of effort' does not primarily depend on sensory inputs from the periphery (although such inputs might influence the process), but is mainly related to the intensity of cortical commands needed for continuing with the function (feedback loops with 'corollary discharges' inside the CNS) (Fig. 9.1A) (reviewed by McCloskey 1981; Jones 1995; Gandevia 2001). Thus, an increased sense of effort might result whenever there is a decrease of input–output gain at any of the many stages between the cortical 'will' to move and the intramuscular cross-bridges producing the mechanical results. The behaving individual perceives the increased effort and will typically not be able to pinpoint at which central and/or peripheral stage(s) the input–output problems appeared. For instance, if major portions of the central command system (e.g. the corticospinal tract) have become destroyed after a stroke, the performance of a very weak finger movement may be possible only at the cost of an enormous degree of effort (Brodal 1973).

In accordance with the view that the sense of effort largely reflects the intensity of central commands, there is often a linear relation between EMG and sense of effort in submaximal endurance tests (cf. Fig. 9.1B) (Jones and Hunter 1983). However, the level of EMG does not translate directly into a relative measure of effort; in constant-effort

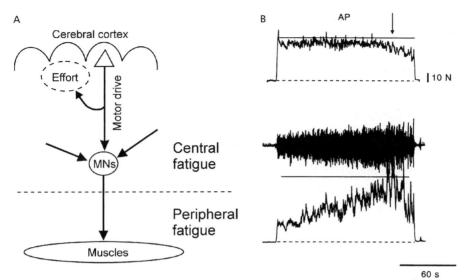

Figure 9.1 Fatigue, motor drive and sense of effort. (**A**) Scheme illustrating functional entities of importance in relation to subjectively experienced motor 'fatigue'. See text for further comments. (**B**) Illustration of commonly seen EMG reactions during a submaximum voluntary holding task. Recordings of thumb adduction force (top panel) and surface EMG from thumb adductor muscle, adductor pollicis (AP) (lower panels). The middle panel shows the EMG and the bottom panel shows the same signal after rectification and smoothing (rsEMG). The force of an initial maximum voluntary contraction (MVC) had been measured before this test contraction. In the illustrated experiment, the subject was instructed to maintain 50 per cent of the MVC for as long as possible. A progressive increase in EMG activity is seen, continuing for as long as the constant submaximum force could still be maintained. (Reproduced with permission, from Zijdewind and Kernell 1994a.)

contractions there is a gradual decline of both force and EMG (Solomon *et al.* 2002). In a voluntary contraction, it is often difficult to separate the subjective sense of effort from that relating to the level of exerted force; some subjects seem capable of doing this while others cannot (Jones 1995).

From an experimental point of view, it is convenient to make a distinction between 'central' and 'peripheral' components of motor fatigue (Fig. 9.1A). Peripheral components are those that may be assessed using electrical stimulation of peripheral motor nerves or muscles. Thus the peripheral components include the motor axon, the neuromuscular junction, and the muscle fibres. Central components include the CNS portions of the MNs (soma, dendrites, and initial portion of axon) and all the parts of the brain and spinal cord that are involved in determining the intensity and distribution of commands to the MNs. A complicating factor in this definition is that some 'central' components include a peripheral trajectory; part of the excitation arriving at the MNs comes via the 'gamma loop', including the gamma MNs, their axons, and the muscle spindle afferents with their central synapses, including those landing directly onto alpha MNs. Furthermore, other muscle afferents may also be of importance in motor fatigue (see section 9.6.3). A major issue in the analysis of motor fatigue concerns the relative contributions of central and peripheral mechanisms.

9.3. **Peripheral versus central fatigue**

Simple tests for fatigue can be performed using voluntary contractions of only one muscle or a synergistic muscle group (e.g. elbow flexors, knee extensors, index finger abductor). Such tests are easily performed in humans, but not in animals because the procedures normally require precise verbal instructions and complex visual feedback. There are two main types of such tests.

1. MVC tests: the subject contracts the target muscles as strongly as possible during a specified time (often about 1–2 min). Typically, there is a considerable loss of force during the test period.

2. Submaximal endurance tests: the subject maintains a specified force (typically given as a percentage of an initial MVC) for as long as possible (Fig. 9.1B). If brief MVCs are interspersed during such a test (Fig. 9.2A,B), they are typically found to drop with time, suggesting that the muscle gradually becomes weaker. Hence the constant target force can often only be maintained by activating the muscle with more MNs and/or at higher MN firing rates, which shows up as an increased EMG signal (Fig. 9.1B). Finally, the MVCs approach the target force, which can then no longer be continued; the point of 'exhaustion' has been reached (Fig. 9.2A,B).

In voluntary fatigue tests, the force of an MVC depends on the maximum evocable force of the muscle as well as on the maximum achievable degree of voluntary muscle activation. As has already been discussed in Chapter 8, section 8.4.3 (see Fig. 8.6), the maximum realized degree of voluntary muscle activation can be approximately determined using interpolated electrical stimulation. Electrical pulses are applied to the 'motor point' of the target muscle (i.e. at a low-threshold region on the skin overlying the muscle), and the size of the electrically induced increase in force during an MVC is measured. The test pulses are generally given singly or in pairs, evoking, if anything, short-lasting muscle 'twitches' (twitch interpolation technique) (Merton 1954b; Gandevia 2001). If the MVC were as strong as the maximum evocable force of the muscle (i.e. the maximum force that could be evoked with tetanic stimulation), no interpolated twitch should be visible. The greater the voluntary activation deficit, the larger is the interpolated twitch (Fig. 8.6).

In the example shown in Fig. 9.2, the submaximal target contraction was at 30 per cent MVC, interrupted by brief MVCs and pauses. This contraction could be maintained for about 9–10 min, and during this period the interspersed MVCs declined almost linearly with time (Fig. 9.2B) and there was also a nearly continuous increase in perceived effort (Fig. 9.2C). On average, the MVC decline was partly due to central fatigue because there was an evident increase in size of the MVC-superimposed twitches (Fig. 9.2D); this reaction was very variable between the different subjects (see large error bars). However, these central factors were typically responsible for only a relatively small portion of the

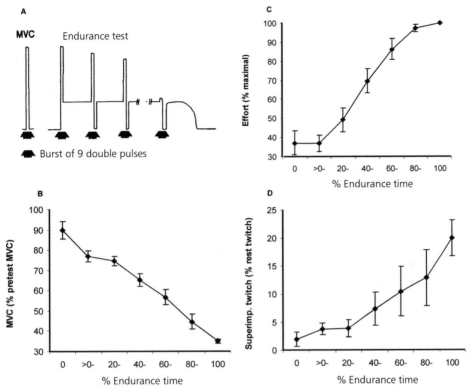

Figure 9.2 Example of a voluntary fatigue test. Test for fatigue in voluntary contraction of intrinsic hand muscle (first dorsal interosseus, FDI) in normal human subjects (*n* = 7). (**A**) Schematic illustration of test procedure. Measurements were made of the abduction force of the index finger. Before the endurance test, initial measurements were made of the size of the maximum voluntary contraction (pretest MVC) and of test contractions ('twitches') evoked at rest by pairs of supramaximal electrical stimuli to the skin overlying the muscle (pulse interval, 11 ms). The endurance test consisted of 30 s cycles of (i) maintained contraction at 30 per cent of pretest MVC, (ii) a test MVC (about 4 s), and (iii) a 3–4 s rest period. Parts (i)–(iii) were repeated until the subject failed to maintain 30 per cent pretest MVC for 5 s or more. Before, during, and after each test MVC, superimposed double-pulse stimulations were applied to the skin above the FDI ('twitch interpolation'). The arrows indicate the timing of these sequences of double pulses. (**B**)–(**D**) Plots of various test parameters versus time, normalized relative to the total endurance time (mean endurance time, 582 ± 248 s (SD)). (**B**) Sizes of test MVCs, normalized (per cent) relative to pretest MVC. (**C**) Degree of perceived effort on a scale from 0 to 10. (**D**) Sizes of interpolated twitches normalized (per cent) in relation to test twitches evoked at rest. (Data from Zijdewind *et al.* 1998.)

drop in MVC during the fatigue test; most of the force decrease was due to peripheral mechanisms. This is often the case in various kinds of human voluntary contractions, and in some experiments and subjects almost no central fatigue was seen (Fig. 9.3A) (Merton 1954b; Bigland-Ritchie *et al.* 1983b). On the other hand, central fatigue may be very substantial in some contraction categories; this is the case for the voluntary activation of diaphragma units during forced air expulsion (up to 50 per cent central fatigue) (Bellemare and Bigland-Ritchie 1987). The recovery from central fatigue of the type seen in tests like Fig. 9.2 is relatively fast; reactions to interpolated twitch stimuli becoming almost normal within 5–10 min. Furthermore, starting a new fatigue test in one hand immediately after testing the other hand had very little effect on central fatigue levels in the second test (Zijdewind *et al.* 1998). The mechanisms involved in central fatigue will be discussed briefly in a later section.

9.4. Manifestations of peripheral motor fatigue

Peripheral motor fatigue can be studied in voluntary contractions (Fig. 9.2) as well as in contractions evoked by peripheral electrical activation of the muscles. Studies of the responses to electrical muscle activation have shown that the choice of stimulation frequency is important for both the fatiguing contraction and subsequent test contractions.

If a muscle nerve is stimulated continuously for, say, 1 min at the rate needed for maximum tetanic tension, force and EMG responses will drop relatively quickly. Such high rates, if maintained for longer times, apparently cause a block to occur somewhere along the chain of events from nerve to muscle action potential. After such 'high-frequency fatigue' (HF fatigue), the recovery of tetanic force may be relatively fast. For instance, in the experiments of Bigland-Ritchie *et al.* (1979), a force decline was seen during the repetitive stimulation of human muscle at 80 Hz. When the rate of stimulation was decreased to 20 Hz, the decline stopped and within a few seconds the force adjusted itself to a *higher* level. Over a period of about 1 min, the largest accumulated force × time area was obtained by a stimulation frequency which started at rate close to that needed for maximum force and then gradually decreased to a much lower value (Bigland-Ritchie *et al.* 1979; Marsden *et al.* 1983). Interestingly, similar changes in MN discharge rate occur during strong voluntary contractions (see sections 9.6.1 and 9.6.2, and Fig. 9.3B).

In muscles that are fatiguing in response to a long-lasting series of partly fused contractions, the post-fatigue recovery may be faster for the maximum tetanic force (high-rate test stimulation) than for twitches or partly fused contractions evoked by lower rates of repetitive stimulation. Initially during a fatiguing contraction, twitches and T–f relations become slower (leftward shift of T–f relation, Fig. 9.3C,D) (Bigland-Ritchie *et al.* 1983b) and lower rates are then needed for the same relative force, which helps to counteract neuromuscular transmission problems. However, in later stages, during the contraction or afterwards, the T–f relation may shift to the right; higher stimulation rates will then be needed for the same relative force (cf. Fig. 6.8D) (Edwards *et al.* 1977; Jami *et al.* 1983; Powers and Binder 1991a). This 'low-frequency fatigue' (LF fatigue) may partly be caused by processes that also cause simultaneously recorded twitches to become smaller and faster (Powers and Binder 1991a), but other factors are also of importance; the rightward shift of the T–f curve in LF fatigue might also take place in the presence of a slower post-tetanic relaxation (Fuglevand *et al.* 1999). LF fatigue typically needs a very long time for recovery, from several hours up to more than a day. As this kind of fatigue may be present together with a fully recovered tetanic force, it should be due to processes involved in excitation–contraction coupling. The existence of LF fatigue was first shown after voluntary exercise (Edwards *et al.* 1977); it appears also after clearly submaximal contractions (Jami *et al.* 1983; Powers and Binder 1991a). In humans, the condition is often associated with muscle pain and it has been suggested that it may be partly caused by fibre damage leading to a heterogeneous distribution of active sarcomeres within single fibres (Jones 1996). Interestingly, the shift in T–f relation does not in itself appear to cause much inconvenience for persons with LF fatigue (Jones 1996); they can apparently easily adjust their command levels to fit the altered muscle properties.

Fatiguing contractions not only cause changes in muscle force, but also produce characteristic alterations in both the major aspects of muscle speed. Changes in twitch speed and T–f relations are commented upon above. In addition, there may be a marked decrease in the muscle's maximal speed of shortening, which will aggravate the loss of maximum power already caused by the decreased force (for normal force–velocity and power–velocity relations, see Fig. 3.3) (Hatcher and Luff 1988; de Haan *et al.* 1989; De Ruiter and De Haan 2000). This type of fatigue also has a slow recovery time (>5 h) (Hatcher and Luff 1988).

In peripheral motor fatigue, the decrease in muscle force need not be maximum just after the end of the fatigue-provoking contraction, but the fatigue (e.g. LF fatigue) may continue to increase for some time afterwards (delayed fatigue) (Jami *et al.* 1983; Lannergren *et al.* 1989).

9.5. Components of peripheral motor fatigue

9.5.1. Energy metabolism and metabolites

As was noted in an earlier chapter, intramuscular ATP should never be completely depleted place because that would lead to a dangerous stiffening of the muscles, i.e. rigor mortis (Chapter 2, section 2.5.3). Accordingly, fatiguing muscles do not stop working because of fuel shortage (Vollestad *et al.* 1988), but rather because of mechanisms that appear to have developed in order to prevent ATP stores from running out; peripheral fatigue includes mechanisms with a protective value. After exhausting fatigue tests of muscles *in vitro*, using electrical activation, ATP levels may indeed show a substantial drop but they always remain safely above the levels that would lead to rigor. Mechanisms for excitation–contraction coupling and force generation all decline in efficiency for other reasons, probably because of actions of ions and/or molecules that increase in concentration as a consequence of the contractile activity itself (i.e. negative feedback). Which are the main candidate molecules?

Low-level motor activity, such as that needed for maintaining posture or for a gentle walking pace, does not cause fatigue and these kinds of contractions must be continuously supplied with energy from oxidative metabolism, using oxygen and fuel (fat, glucose) delivered via the circulation. Fatigue problems potentially arise for high or suddenly increasing levels of activity for which the energy needs would not be covered by continuous delivery resources. Essentially, this means that problems arise at times when the circulation and/or the intra-fibre oxidative mechanisms cannot work rapidly enough to supply the contracting muscle. The ATP will then have to be provided via the phosphocreatine (PCr) system (small energy buffer) and by the anaerobic metabolism of glucose, mainly from stored glycogen. Under taxing conditions, there is a marked rise in the concentrations of inorganic phosphate (P_i), lactate, and H^+ ions (i.e. lower pH). In addition, there is a less dramatic increase in ADP and there may be a slight decrease in ATP. Lactate and H^+ ions also enter the circulation, i.e. their potential effects are not restricted to the exercising muscle cells themselves. As a result of the action potentials evoked in the muscle fibres, there is also an increase in intracellular Na^+ concentration and, more importantly, a large relative increase in K^+ concentration just outside the surface and T-tubular membranes.

Intense muscle activity also has an effect on the energy stores of the muscle fibres themselves; it might result in a depletion of glycogen from the active cells (cf. Fig. 3.10D). It has been known for many years that this has an effect on exercise endurance. In bicycle ergometry (Hultman 1967), the time to exhaustion was positively correlated with the muscle glycogen content. Rebuilding glycogen stores takes several days.

9.5.2. Muscle circulation

Oxidative metabolism requires an effective circulation and blood perfusion. The local circulation is also very important for 'washing out' undesirable accumulations of various metabolites in the extracellular space (e.g. K^+ and H^+ ions). In muscle, the circulatory needs increase substantially in the transition from rest to activity, and, correspondingly, in intermittent contractions muscle blood flow may increase by a factor of 10 because of various neuronal and biochemical mechanisms (including vasodilatory effects of metabolites from working muscles). However, muscle fibres also have the somewhat impractical property of exerting a sideways pressure as they contract. In strong contractions, this increase in intramuscular pressure may be large enough to decrease or even completely cut off muscle blood flow. The relative contractile force at which these complications occur is very different for different muscles, as it depends on their size and architecture (Sejersted and Hargens 1995). The interference of muscle contraction with muscle circulation constitutes an inescapable and deplorable factor which promotes fatigue in strong maintained contractions.

9.5.3. Cross-bridge interactions

The fatigue-associated decrease in maximum shortening velocity provides clear evidence for effects directly at the level of actin–myosin interactions. The loss of maximum force (Fig. 9.3A) may also be partly due to effects directly at the level of the cross-bridges.

According to the classical explanation, muscle fatigue is caused by lactic acid formation and the associated acidification during intense muscle activity. However, this view is oversimplified; fatigue can take place without acidification, and under normal conditions pure acidification does not lead to muscle fatigue. The earlier conclusions were largely based on experiments performed on isolated muscles that were kept at room temperature rather than at normal mammalian body temperature; *in vitro* preparations are easier to maintain at low temperatures. At low temperatures, H^+ ions indeed have a pronounced depressing effect on cross-bridge interactions (maximum shortening speed, maximum force). However, almost none of these effects of H^+ ions exist at normal mammalian body temperatures (reviewed by Westerblad *et al.* 2002). In addition, the released lactate can be directly used as a fuel in oxidative processes elsewhere, including the brain (Pellerin 2003; Dienel 2004).

Another metabolite which may play an important role in fatigue is inorganic phosphate (P_i). The concentration of P_i increases markedly during fatiguing muscle contractions (reviewed by Westerblad *et al.* 2002). However, in this case also the effects on cross-bridge interactions are relatively slight at temperatures approaching mammalian body temperature. For instance, at 30°C, P_i had no effect on shortening velocity and little effect on the maximum force of fast muscle fibres of the rat (Debold *et al.* 2004). It is still unclear precisely which metabolic events cause the depression of Ca^{2+} release and cross-bridge interactions in fatiguing muscle at mammalian body temperature. Perhaps combinations of metabolites have stronger effects than the same metabolites tested individually.

9.5.4. Excitation–contraction coupling and Ca^{2+} kinetics

A fatigue-associated decrease in action-potential-elicited Ca^{2+} release from the SR has been directly measured in mammalian muscle fibres (Westerblad and Allen 1991); the fatigue-associated drop in force occurs more or less in parallel with a drop in intramuscular Ca^{2+} release. In addition, there is a decrease in the Ca^{2+} sensitivity of the myofilaments (presumably at troponin C) and a decreased re-uptake of Ca^{2+} ions into the SR (presumably important for the slowing of fatigued twitches). These multiple effects are probably partly caused by various metabolites that accumulate during fatigue. However, the classical candidates for such actions (P_i, H^+) apparently have little or no effect when tested close to normal body temperature (see discussion of metabolites in section 9.5.3) (Westerblad *et al.* 2002; Debold *et al.* 2004). Paradoxically, the released Ca^{2+} itself might cause an inhibition of further Ca^{2+} release (Westerblad *et al.* 2000).

9.5.5. Sarcolemmal and T-tubular action potentials

During the course of fatiguing contractions, the muscle fibre action potentials may become broader and smaller (extra- or intracellular recordings). However, these changes may occur without being directly related to changes in force production (Lüttgau 1965; Lannergren and Westerblad 1986). The depression and slowing of the action potentials are partly effects of changes taking place in the T-tubuli; activity has less effect on sarcolemmal action potentials after detubulation (Lannergren and Westerblad 1987). The sarcolemmal action potential itself does not necessarily have direct contraction-controlling tasks; its main function is to propagate along the muscle fibre and activate spikes diving

⁻own into the T-tubuli. However, theoretical considerations have suggested that, in the fast-twitch fibres of mammals, the sarcolemmal action potential might also be of importance for full activation (Fuglevand 1995). Muscle fibres from different types of units show different EMG reactions during fatigue tests; there is often a more pronounced EMG decline in units which also show a marked decline in force (Clamann and Robinson 1985; Enoka *et al.* 1988). Experiments with chronic stimulation have indicated that fatigue-associated EMG reactions may be dissociated from the force reactions (see Figs 11.1B and 11.2) (Kernell *et al.* 1987a), i.e. the EMG decline, if present, may not have caused any of the force decline.

As a result of action potential generation, intense muscle activity leads to an accumulation of extracellular K^+ ions; locally, the concentration may even be doubled (Hnik *et al.* 1976; Vyskocil *et al.* 1983). This causes a positive-going shift in the resting membrane potential and a decrease in sarcolemmal spike amplitude; such changes would influence the EMG but they would not necessarily endanger excitation–contraction coupling. However, K^+ ions accumulating in the small volumes of narrow T-tubuli would less rapidly diffuse away and they might have a strong influence on local K^+ concentrations, which might potentially reach levels impeding the inward spread of excitation within the muscle fibres (Sejersted and Sjogaard 2000). This may be an important reason for decreased excitation–contraction coupling in muscle fatigue.

The effects of the accumulating K^+ ions are counteracted by the electrogenic Na–K pump, which becomes very active in contracting muscle (Hicks and McComas 1989; reviewed by Clausen 2003). The activity of this pump counteracts a K^+-generated depolarization, both by removing extracellular K^+ ions and by the hyperpolarizing electrogenic nature of its activity, pumping three Na^+ ions out for every two K^+ ions pumped in. The actions of this pump are probably the reason for the 'potentiation' of M-wave size (EMG amplitude) which may sometimes takes place during fatiguing contractile activity (cf. Fig. 11.2). The presence of different degrees of 'EMG fatigue' for different muscle unit categories (Clamann and Robinson 1985; Enoka *et al.* 1988) might depend on differences in the balance between ion fluxes and pumping capacities for different fibre types (reviewed by Clausen 2003).

9.5.6. Neuromuscular junction

In the limb muscles of normal subjects, the neuromuscular junction (NMJ) seems to have a sufficiently large margin of safety to guarantee continued transmission even during prolonged strong contractions (Bigland-Ritchie *et al.* 1982). However, transmission failure may occur in contractions evoked at higher activation rates than those used in voluntary contractions (e.g. when using electrical stimulation, HF fatigue). Furthermore, some muscles may be particularly sensitive to NMJ transmission failure; this seems to be the case for the diaphragm, particularly in young animals (Kuei *et al.* 1990; Fournier *et al.* 1991). In certain pathological situations, NMJ failure may have a major impact (Chapter 4, section 4.5). It should be noted that the presence or absence of neuromuscular block cannot be well judged using EMG recordings; changes in the amplitude of the compound muscle action potential (M wave) might also be caused by changes in action potential configuration and conduction speed of the muscle fibres themselves (cf. Fig. 11.2).

9.5.7. Motor nerve

Peripheral motor nerve fibres may conduct action potentials continuously at frequencies far exceeding those needed for motor functions, i.e. under normal circumstances a conduction block along non-branched axons would be highly improbable. However, inside (or close to) the target muscle the axon subdivides into tens to hundreds of terminals, and conduction may be more difficult at those branching points because of a potentially increased membrane load (Zenker and Hohberg 1973). It is clear that branch blocks of conduction may occur (*in vitro* experiments, Krnjevic and Mildedi 1958; model calculations, Luscher and Shiner 1990; sensory axons, tissue culture, Luscher *et al.* 1994), although this does not seem to happen normally (Bigland-Ritchie *et al.* 1982), but perhaps only under particularly taxing conditions, such as during repetitive discharges maintained at high rates by electrical stimulation.

9.6. Motoneurone-associated components of central motor fatigue

9.6.1. Motoneurone activity in maintained maximal contractions

During a maintained MVC, there is a drop not only of force, but also of mean MN spike frequency (Fig. 9.3). However, this drop of MN firing rate does not necessarily cause a drop in force but it might, paradoxically, instead serve to optimize force production by minimizing the risk of a block of action potential transmission, i.e. by counteracting high-frequency fatigue (see section 9.4). Simultaneously with the drop in MN firing rate, there is also typically a slowing of the muscle twitch and force-gradation speed, i.e. the T–f curve temporarily shifts to the left (Fig. 9.3C,D). Correspondingly, in some cases the fall of force and MN firing rate in a maintained MVC are not (for some time) associated with signs of a decreased degree of central activation, i.e. there might be no concomitant increase in the size of interpolated twitches or tetanic contractions (Fig. 9.3A) (Bigland-Ritchie *et al.* 1983b). In such cases there is, as it were, a good match between the slowing twitch speed of muscle and the slowing discharge rate of the MNs (Bigland-Ritchie and Woods 1984). This match has been termed 'muscle wisdom' (Marsden *et al.* 1983), although the 'wisdom' might be more motoneuronal than muscular and must concern both. MVC-associated decreases in MN-pool activity do not always or only represent this kind of fatigue-preventing 'wisdom', but they are apparently often large enough actually to contribute to the force decrease (Fuglevand and Keen 2003), i.e. to produce substantial degrees of central fatigue (Gandevia 2001). For instance, this will always be the case if units are de-recruited, which happens in prolonged maximal MVCs (Grimby *et al.* 1979, 1981; Peters and Fuglevand 1999), possibly simply as a result of decreasing central drive. Furthermore, although there seems to be some kind of parallel behaviour between the

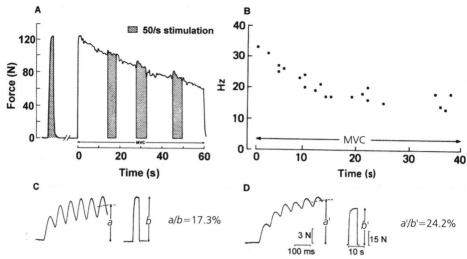

Figure 9.3 Parallel slowing of muscle contraction and MN discharge. Experiments on human adductor pollicis. (**A**) Force versus time during 60 s MVC with superimposed periods of 50 Hz tetanic transcutaneous stimulation of the ulnar nerve. The stimulation caused almost no extra force, i.e. this muscle remained maximally activated throughout the contraction. (**B**) Discharge rates of single units during 40 s of MVC. (**c**),(**d**) Unfused tetanic contractions evoked by 7 Hz electrical stimulation after a 5 s MVC (*a*) and after a 60 s MVC (*a′*). Note post-contraction muscle slowing and more effective force summation following the 60 s MVC. Records *b* and *b′* show near-maximum tetanic contractions (50 Hz stimulation, note different calibration) before and after the 60 s MVC, demonstrating weakening. ((**A**), (**c**), and (**d**) reproduced with permission, from Bigland-Ritchie *et al.* 1983b; (**b**) reproduced with permission, from Bigland-Ritchie *et al.* 1983a.)

slowing of muscle contraction and MN firing rates during MVCs, there is nothing to suggest that there is a direct continuous feedback from muscles reporting their current *T–f* speed to the MNs. For instance, changing the *T–f* speed of a muscle by cooling it or changing its length does not produce any corresponding alterations in MN discharge rates during voluntary contractions (Bigland-Ritchie *et al.* 1992a,b).

9.6.2. Role of late spike-frequency adaptation of motoneurones

The drop of MN firing rate during maintained MVCs in humans has a time course and amplitude very similar to the drop of MN firing rate seen during late spike-frequency adaptation in cat MNs that are stimulated with relatively weak intensities of steady injected currents (compare Fig. 9.3B with Fig. 6.3A; see also Chapter 6, section 6.5.5) (Kernell and Monster 1982a,b; Sawczuk *et al.* 1995; Spielmann *et al.* 1993). In cat MNs, the late adaptation is more prominent for discharges with a high than with a lower starting rate. Mainly for this reason, very little late adaptation is present in cat MNs of slow-twitch muscle units (Fig. 6.3B; fast and slow units compared for stimulations with the same supra-threshold current intensity) (Kernell and Monster 1982a). Correspondingly, slow starting rates and very little drop in firing frequency were seen in maintained MVCs of the predominantly slow extensor hallucis longus (Macefield *et al.* 2000). In 'virtual' MVCs, performed after anaesthetic block of the motor nerve, the starting rates of MN discharges were also slower than normal and there was little drop of rate with time (Macefield *et al.* 1993); similar effects were also seen after a separate block of the (assumed) gamma MN fibres (Bongiovanni and Hagbarth 1990). The decreased frequency drop in the virtual MVCs might have been due to the slow starting rates and/or to the fact that all peripheral reflexes from the target muscle were interrupted by the anaesthetic nerve block (see further below). The slow starting rates after block of peripheral nerves were presumably caused by the lack of normally available MN excitation from muscle afferents.

In the intracellular experiments of Kernell and Monster (1982a,b) concerning late adaptation in cat MNs, the standard test currents were only 5 nA above the threshold for rhythmic firing, i.e. they were generally covering only a small portion of the adapted primary range of firing (cf. mean *f–I* relation for 'steady firing' in Fig. 6.2B); larger amounts of adaptation would have been expected with stronger currents (Kernell and Monster 1982b). The mean starting rate in Fig. 9.4A was 24.5 Hz, which would produce a mean force of only about 12 per cent P_0 in such fast-twitch cat units (Kernell *et al.* 1983b; Binder-Macleod and Clamann 1989). During such discharges (Fig. 9.4A), the resulting contractile forces were also recorded from the respective muscle units (Fig. 9.4B). For the fast-twitch units illustrated in Fig. 9.4A,B, the mean force dropped during the initial 4 s, but then stayed almost constant for about 13 s while the MN spike frequency continued to drop. This temporary force stabilization was probably caused by slowing and potentiation of the muscle units in combination with other factors underlying a hysteresis of its *T–f* relation (Binder-Macleod and Clamann 1989). However, at times longer than about 17 s from the start, force again dropped continuously and at about 45–60 s from the start the tension generated by the adapting discharge approached that predicted by the MN firing rates and the non-fatigued *T–f* relations. The final similarity between the real adapting and the calculated non-fatigued force values (Fig. 9.4B) suggests that, at these weak force levels, there was not yet much peripheral fatigue. These experiments on hindlimb MNs and muscle units of cats suggest that the late spike-frequency adaptation of MNs might cause a substantial amount of central fatigue while transiently adding a little additional 'muscle wisdom' to the process, i.e. the decreasing firing rate counteracts high-frequency fatigue while still generating rather more force than that predicted from the 'acute' *T–f* relation; the 'wisdom' component corresponds, in a way, to the separation between the two curves of Fig. 9.4B (Kernell and Monster 1982a). The MVC-associated drop of firing rate in humans is probably, at least to a significant extent, reflecting intrinsic MN membrane properties; if not, one must assume that human MNs have membrane properties that are drastically different from those of cats or rats. However, there is also strong evidence implying additional effects of inhibitory reflexes and of a decreasing central drive (see below).

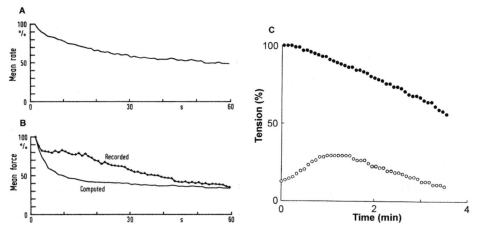

Figure 9.4 Potentiation of force during repetitive activation. (**A**), (**B**) Late phase of spike-frequency adaptation and effects of time-dependent muscle properties for fast-twitch motor units of cat medial gastrocnemius muscle. (**A**) Plot of mean spike frequency versus time for five GM MNs with fast-twitch muscle units during intracellular stimulation with steady current at 5 nA above the threshold for rhythmic firing (cf. Fig. 6.3). (**B**) Plot of mean contractile force ('Recorded') versus time for the respective muscle units during the discharges in (**A**). Forces and spike frequencies for each unit normalized relative to values obtained for second number 2 of the same discharge, i.e. after the initial phase of spike-frequency adaptation (100 per cent rate, 24.5 Hz). The force values of the 'Computed' curve were calculated from the recorded firing rates of (**A**) using the relationship between muscle tension and stimulus rate in fast-twitch gastrocnemius units, as determined with 1 s constant-frequency trains of stimulation (for each train, the mean force was measured at 0.5–1.0 s). Note that the effects of the adaptive decline in rate (**A**) are only partly compensated by muscle properties (**B**), i.e. by the combined effects of muscle slowing, potentiation. and *T–f* curve hysteresis (cf. Chapter 3, section 3.3.4.3). (Reproduced with permission, from Kernell and Monster 1982a). (**c**) Whole lumbrical muscle of cat activated by supramaximum stimulation of the plantar nerve. Bursts of repetitive stimulation (burst duration 0.36 s) given at intervals of 2.45 s. Maximum amplitude of contraction produced by each burst plotted against time after the first stimulus in the series. The stimulus rate was high enough to produce fused contractions (121 Hz) for every second burst (filled circles), and low enough to give incompletely fused contractions (30 Hz) for the intervening bursts (open circles). The amplitude of contraction is expressed as a percentage of that evoked by the initial high-frequency burst of stimulation. (Reproduced with permission, from Kernell *et al.* 1975.)

9.6.3. **Role of peripheral reflexes**

If a maintained MVC is performed with ischaemic muscles, a drop of motoneuronal spike frequency and a slowing of muscle isometric speed (*T–f* relation) take place in parallel as normal, but there is no recovery of the MN firing rates until the blood supply is allowed to return (Bigland-Ritchie *et al.* 1986; Woods *et al.* 1987). Such findings suggest that these ischaemic muscles apparently send some signals to the MNs that keep their firing rates supressed. However, as these MNs probably also share the property of late frequency adaptation, it is interesting to speculate about how the effects of this intrinsic property might have been combined with the inhibitory reflex effects. Possibly, the MN late adaptation might have been a major cause of the frequency drop during the MVC while there was a gradual rise in the reflex inhibition. At the end of the MVC, the inhibitory (nociceptive?) reflex might have grown sufficiently strong to keep the MNs firing at a lower maximum rate than would normally have been the case. Further experiments are needed to test these assumptions.

The afferents responsible for MN inhibition during (ischaemic) contractions probably include the thinnest myelinated fibres and the unmyelinated ones (groups III and IV), many of which are nociceptive and others are supposedly chemoceptive, signalling the presence of molecules that tend to increase in concentration during muscle activity (including, presumably, various metabolites). The intramuscular concentration of such molecules will remain high until circulation is restored. Interestingly, pain afferents might conceivably play an important role in this context. The performance of contractions under ischaemia is a very efficient way of evoking pain (Mills *et al.* 1982). Nociceptive reflexes may be very powerful suppressors of MN activity, and their actions might be exerted at spinal as well as supraspinal levels. Such reflexes might well make important contributions to central fatigue by limiting MN activation and also by having central effects that would tend to limit endurance time (i.e. facilitating the decision to stop with the exercise). Pain is often mentioned as a factor of importance in exhaustion (Kroon *et al.* 1986).

In addition to potentially MN-depressing reflexes, there are also important MN-facilitating effects of activity in peripheral muscle afferents. The best known are the excitatory effects of the afferents from muscle spindles, some of which are directly monosynaptically linked to the MNs. These excitatory effects are particularly intriguing because an (unknown) portion of the central commands to alpha MNs is normally relayed via the 'gamma loop'. For many central inputs, alpha and gamma MNs are activated more or less in parallel ('alpha–gamma linkage') (Granit 1975), and therefore, paradoxically, a voluntary isometric muscle contraction is often accompanied by an increased discharge in the homonymous spindle afferents (e.g. Edin and Vallbo 1990). As long as these spindle afferents keep on firing, they will contribute to the total excitatory (background) drive of the alpha MNs. This afferent discharge gradually declines during a maintained constant-force voluntary contraction, and it has been suggested that a similar decline during a maintained MVC would produce a decreasing MN drive that would contribute to the gradual drop of MN firing rate (Macefield *et al.* 1991; Hagbarth and Macefield 1995). Experiments with 'virtual' MVCs, performed after peripheral anaesthesia of the nerve to the target muscle, indicate that the excitatory contribution from (spindle) afferents is not unimportant for the total MN drive (Macefield *et al.* 1993; cf. Bongiovanni and Hagbarth 1990). The mean MN discharge rates recorded for the human tibialis anterior muscle (ankle dorsiflexor) during an MVC were 28.2 Hz in the control situation and only 18.6 Hz after anaesthetic block of the common peroneal nerve (Macefield *et al.* 1993). Part of this effect may have been due to the interruption of other afferents than those of the muscle spindles (e.g. skin, joints, etc.). Furthermore, the normal presence of peripheral kinaesthetic and other sensory feeback ('feeling' the positions, movements, and possible strains in one's limbs) might be important for generating the central drive itself.

9.6.4. Role of other sources of motoneurone excitation

A major portion of the central motor fatigue is probably dependent on a decrease of the motoneuronal drive from the brain caused by processes inside the brain as well as in the spinal cord (e.g. effects of preceding activity on the function of cortico-motoneuronal synapses (cf. Petersen *et al.* 2003)). Much of the experimental analysis concerning the brain-related aspects of fatigue is done using various methods for brain stimulation and recording (e.g. electroencephalography and magnetic electrocorticograms, functional magnetic resonance imaging (fMRI), transcranial magnetic stimulation (TMS) (reviewed by Mills 1991; Gandevia 2001). There are also intriguing problems concerning the possible interactions/associations between motor and mental aspects of fatigue (Mosso 1904; Lorist *et al.* 2002; van Duinen *et al.* 2005). However, further discussion of these interesting fields of research falls outside the scope of the present book.

9.7. Neuromuscular features alleviating motor fatigue

In preceding chapters, fatigue has been mentioned in several contexts concerning the neuromuscular organization. It might be useful to summarize a number of these features in the present fatigue-dedicated chapter. Thus in voluntary contractions the occurrence of motor fatigue will be counteracted by several factors including the following:

1 The speed match between MNs and their muscle fibres, causing barely recruited MNs to discharge at rates eliciting only slight degrees of twitch fusion (Fig. 6.8).

2 The fact that single muscles are commanded by MN populations (Fig. 8.1), such that weak muscle contractions are produced by many weak muscle units firing asynchronously with each other at slow rates. Such an asynchronous multi-unit drive of a muscle is not only good for force stability and endurance, but it is also more 'effective' than synchronous stimulation in the sense that somewhat lower rates will be needed for a particular force (Rack and Westbury 1969; Wise *et al.* 2001). Furthermore, the relatively stable force seen with an asynchronous drive means that the use of metabolically expensive shortening contractions is minimized.

3 The intra-pool distribution of MN excitability (cf. Fig. 6.7B) implies that fatigue-resistant units will generally be more easily recruited than more fatigue-sensitive ones; this will counteract fatigue in long-lasting postural contractions.

4 The recruitment thresholds seem to be more closely spaced among the low-threshold (i.e. fatigue-resistant) units than among higher-threshold ones (Henneman *et al.* 1965; Gustafsson and Pinter 1985b; Bakels and Kernell 1994). This means that, at the

lower end of the recruitment trajectory, only modest increases in discharge rate will take place in parallel with recruitment, which would promote endurance.

5 The high initial f–I slope just after the abrupt onset of MN activation (Fig. 6.2B) favours the appearance of initial brief impulse intervals in brisk contractions. In a series of intermittent muscle contractions, less fatigue will generally be caused by activating impulse trains containing initial 'doublets' (cf. Fig. 3.1E) than by constant-frequency trains (e.g. Binder-Macleod and Barker 1991; Bigland-Ritchie *et al.* 2000; reviewed by Binder-Macleod and Kesar 2005).

6 The late phase of frequency adaptation in MNs might have a dual role. In some situations it might help to match the spike frequency driving the muscle to a progressive slowing of contractile speed (cf. Fig. 9.3). In other situations the late adaptation might be large enough to necessitate an increase in central drive in order to maintain a constant force output, i.e. this motoneuronal adaptation might itself be a cause of (substantial) central fatigue (Fig. 9.4A,B) (cf. Fuglevand and Keen 2003).

7 Because of the normal checkerboard distribution pattern of muscle fibres belonging to different units and types (Fig. 3.10), neighbouring muscle fibres will contract out of phase with each other and, for low-level contractions, active and inactive fibres will be intermingled. During weak contractions, this kind of organization is beneficial for capillary perfusion inside the muscle (Fuglevand and Segal 1997). However, strong contractions of whole muscles may cause partial or complete occlusion of the local blood supply (see section 9.5.2).

8 Most joint torques can be produced by several different combinations of muscle actions. In long-lasting voluntary submaximal contractions, it has repeatedly been demonstrated that the distribution of activity between synergists tends to shift around, resembling to some extent the way in which a standing or sitting person fights fatigue by intermittent changes of posture. Evidence for such 'synergist rotation' has been seen in maintained voluntary contractions of, for instance, knee extensors (Sjogaard *et al.* 1986; Kouzaki *et al.* 2002), back muscles (van Dieen *et al.* 1993), and jaw muscles (Hellsing and Lindstrom 1983). Furthermore, phenomena of a similar nature apparently take place even within single muscles, for example regional shifts of activity within an intrinsic hand muscle (Zijdewind *et al.* 1995) and 'rotation' of motor unit activity in the human trapezius (Westgaard and de Luca 1999). The multi-unit contractile entities controlled by the CNS do not necessarily coincide with anatomically defined 'muscles' (cf. Fig. 8.2).

9.8. **Motor potentiation and facilitation**

It is a common observation in sports physiology that bodily achievements may be improved by doing some initial 'warming up' exercises. Part of the effect of such introductory movements seems to be what the name suggests—increasing the temperature of the muscles and thereby increasing their speed and power (see section 9.8.2) (Sargeant 1987). The introductory movements might also be associated with purely central effects, such as the facilitation of 'plateau currents' (section 9.8.3), possibly in combination with a mental rehearsal or calibration of the coordinative aspects of the tasks ahead. However, local muscle mechanisms may also contribute: various cellular components of the neuro-muscular system will achieve an increased output for the same input after a (limited) period of preceding activity (section 9.8.1). During early periods of physical exertion, these potentiating effects will merge with those of the more long-lasting manifestations of fatigue. The phenomenon of 'delayed fatigue' is probably caused by the sum of a short-lasting potentiation and a more long-lasting fatigue (cf. Jami *et al.* 1983; Lannergren *et al.* 1989).

9.8.1. **Muscle potentiation**

In submaximal and partly fused contractions, or in single twitches, muscle force is commonly highly dependent on the duration and intensity of the preceding muscle activation. The safety margin of neuromuscular transmission is normally high enough to guarantee a 1:1 transmission (Chapter 4, section 4.4), and the 'acute' use-dependent changes in contractile force (timescale, seconds to minutes) primarily reflect contractile characteristics of the muscle fibres themselves (for comments on endplate and EMG potentiation see Chapter 4, section 4.4.3, and section 9.5.5 above). Submaximal contractions may become potentiated ('twitch potentiation') by preceding activity, whereas maximal tetanic contractions, which are evoked by saturating degrees of Ca^{2+} release (Chapter 2, section 2.5.3), are then either unchanged or depressed. Thus the twitch potentiation is likely to reflect effects on the excitation–contraction coupling mechanisms within the muscle fibres (Jami *et al.* 1983). The intramuscular kinetics of Ca^{2+} ions is of great interest in this context (as is also true for muscle fatigue). In addition, phosphorylation of myosin light chains is apparently also of importance for potentiation (Sweeney *et al.* 1993).

Potentiation and depression of muscle contractions depend on different mechanisms and both phenomena may be present simultaneously. This is demonstrated by the very simple experiment illustrated in Fig. 9.4 c, in which a small muscle of the cat's foot is alternately activated by high- and low-rate trains of repetitive pulses (Kernell *et al.* 1975; see also Rankin *et al.* 1988). The high-rate trains gave a near-maximal contraction, and their peak forces decline with time, i.e. from the start of this experiment there was a gradually increasing degree of fatigue. However, the low-rate trains, which gave only partly fused contractions, elicited gradually increasing peak forces (potentiation) during roughly the first minute, and a progressive depression only became apparent later for these weaker contractions. Thus, with regard to the submaximal contractions, there was a 'delayed' fatigue reaction, apparently due to the fact that the net result depended on the sum of depressing and potentiating effects with different time characteristics.

The net potentiation of force in ongoing submaximal contractions may be very dramatic, leading to a marked and progressive increase of tension (e.g. Kernell *et al.* 1975, Fig. 2D; Jami *et al.* 1983 several cases illustrated). During Burke-type fatigue tests of fast cat muscle units, the potentiation behaviour has consequences for the calculations of a fatigue index (Chapter 3, section 3.3.5.2). As the contractile potentiation of muscle is present for submaximal contractions, it also has a marked effect on the relation between muscle force and activation rate; the T–f curve shifts towards the left (Fig. 6.8D) (Kernell *et al.* 1975). Potentiated twitches do not only become larger, but they also often acquire a slower time course (increase of twitch contraction and half-relaxation time). The shift of the T–f curve partly reflects this slowing in the time course of potentiated twitches.

9.8.2. **Effects of temperature**

The temperature of limb muscles may be much lower than the normal body core temperature of 37–38°C. For instance, even under comfortable conditions of 27°C ambient temperature, thigh muscles were only about 34°C at 2 cm depth, and under cold external conditions (15°C) this temperature dropped to about 31°C (Webb 1992; cf. Sargeant 1987). Less massive muscles, such as intrinsic hand muscles, might easily become even colder, probably below 20°C, when working outside on a cold day. On the other hand, the temperature in a working muscle might increase to well above the normal core temperature of 37 °C. Thus there is considerable scope for temperature effects in muscle physiology. As changes of muscle temperature belong to the relatively rapid after-effects of motoneuronal muscle activation, such issues are included in this chapter.

Warming a muscle from, say, 25°C to 37°C makes it much faster and somewhat stronger. Particularly at temperatures close to normal mammalian core temperature, the temperature dependence of maximum tetanic force is variable and slight. More marked effects, in a speeding-up direction, are seen for the force–velocity relation and for isometric twitch speed (Ranatunga 1982; de Ruiter *et al.* 1999; De Ruiter and De Haan 2000). The increased speed of the force–velocity relation means that there is also an increase in maximum power (Fig. 3.3C,D) which, in sports performance, is perhaps even more important than the maximum speed itself. However, at the shortening speeds used in actual movements, slow units seem to profit more than fast units from the increased power on warming up (Fig. 3.3D, vertical line) (Jones *et al.* 2004). This is of interest in relation to the fact that slow fibres also tend to be more centrally (i.e. more 'warmly') placed within a limb than faster fibres of the same muscle (Fig. 3. 11); thus the common kind of fibre type regionalization might help to optimize mechanical power production when muscles are warmed up during motor activity.

The effects of warming a muscle do not cause an enhancement of input–output relations for all aspects of muscle function. Twitches become more rapid and, as a result, the warmed-up muscle shifts its T–f curve to the right (Ranatunga 1982). Hence the warmed-up muscle might need a higher MN spike frequency (i.e. presumably a more intense central drive) for generating a given ratio of its maximum output force. This effect might be partly compensated by twitch potentiation (see section 9.8.1) and, to a limited extent, by slight temperature-related changes in maximum tetanic force.

9.8.3. Use-dependent facilitation of motoneuronal 'plateau' currents

As has been described in preceding chapters, MN membranes contain voltage-gated channels which, when sufficiently depolarized, may be induced to generate self-stimulating persistent inward currents (PICs) or 'plateau currents', which add to the synaptic or injected current driving a discharge (Figs 6.5 and 6.9) (Chapter 6, section 6.7). The activation and deactivation kinetics of these mechanisms is known to be comparatively slow (Svirskis and Hounsgaard 1997). In humans, there is a gradual increase in contractile force in response to repeated muscle activation over a period of several seconds (Collins *et al.* 2002; Gorassini *et al.* 2002); it seems likely that these potentiating effects are indeed (partly) dependent on the moblization of plateau currents, which might play a role in the 'warming up' seen in sports and which might be needed for achieving a maximum motor output.

9.9. Clinical and applied aspects of fatigue

It should be noted that the present chapter is largely restricted to fatigue phenomena that concern the MNs and their muscle fibres. Thus much of the wide and complex research field concerning fatigue falls outside the scope of this book. In addition the MN and muscle aspects, 'fatigue' is also very much as issue concerning complex CNS functions and mental mechanisms, and these kinds of fatigue probably dominate in medical practice. Subjectively experienced 'fatigue' is one of the most common complaints reported by patients and it is an important symptom in neurological diseases, including multiple sclerosis, Parkinson's disease, and many others (reviewed by Chaudhuri and Behan 2004). In some cases, it is the dominating symptom (e.g. chronic fatigue syndrome (Jason *et al.* 2005)).

An increased neuromuscular fatiguability is sometimes caused by specific known causes. At the level of the NMJ this is true for myasthenia gravis and the Lambert–Eaton syndrome (both dealt with in Chapter 4, section 4.5). At the level of the muscle, diseases are known in which pathological changes result in an increased fatigue sensitivity despite an almost normal muscle mass (reviewed by Jones *et al.* 2004). These diseases are not very common; they include mitochondrial myopathies and disorders of glycogen metabolism (e.g. McArdle's disease, Tauri's disease). Furthermore, fatigue is often a problem in any disease that causes a weakening of the neuromuscular system, for example because of MN death (reviewed by Thomas and Zijdewind 2006); higher levels of motor drive and more 'effort' are then needed to performing normal daily tasks.

In addition to the clinical relevance of fatigue studies, knowledge about neuromuscular aspects of fatigue is also important for the analysis of work situations (ergonomics) (Nussbaum *et al.* 2001; Vieira and Kumar 2004). Furthermore, various manifestations of neuromuscular fatigue are important subjects for further investigation in contexts where a maximal use of neuromuscular resources is essential (e.g. rehabilitation and sports science) (Lieber 2002; Jones *et al.* 2004). In these various contexts, it is also important to realize that motor fatigue also has a potentially deteriorating effect on simultaneously performed cognitive functions (Lorist *et al.* 2002; van Duinen *et al.* 2005).

Chapter 10

Denervation and reinnervation

10.1. General issues

Physiology concerns life processes that take place on greatly varying timescales. So far in this book we have dealt with events occurring within periods from milliseconds to hours, i.e. processes which can easily be studied during a normal working day. This kind of 'acute physiology' dominates classical textbooks. However, many equally important processes, typically involving changes in the functional properties of various cells and tissues, take place over periods of days, weeks, or months. Such processes are more difficult to study, and they can only be appropriately analysed after the 'acute physiology' has been reasonably well understood. This chapter and the two that follow all deal with various aspects of 'long-term physiology'.

In the present chapter, a description will be given of the various processes and cellular adaptations taking place in association with muscle denervation and reinnervation. Studies of injury reactions and repair processes are important in themselves, but they also help us to understand the normal long-term interactions between MNs, muscles, and other cells (including other neurones). Mechanisms which may be involved in such cellular adaptations, including various long-term effects of neuromuscular usage on cell properties, will be dealt with further in Chapter 11.

10.2. Reactions of motoneurones to transection of their axons

The various motoneuronal changes in response to axotomy provide important illustrations of the very high degree of plasticity in adult differentiated nerve cells (Table 10.1).

10.2.1. Changes in the cell body: chromatolysis and changed RNA synthesis

The long axonal and dendritic extensions of nerve cells have to be supported by a continuous supply of products from the biochemical 'factory' in the cell body (see Chapter 2, section 2.4.6, axoplasmic transport). Therefore, if one of these extensions is interrupted, the distal portion degenerates and dies (Wallerian degeneration) (Waller 1850). In mammalian neurones, there are no healing processes available whereby severed central and distal portions can be reunited; repair can only take place by new outgrowth from the proximal stump of the axon. Once it has become injured, the biochemical processes of a neurone have to be adapted from those appropriate for a 'transmitting state' to those needed for a 'growth and connection state'. This alteration of neuronal task and

Table 10.1 Changes of MN properties after axotomy

Structure	Changed property	Direction/type of change	Reference
Soma cytochem	rough endoplasmic reticulum	reorganized ('chromatolysis')	R15
—	SDH activity	↓	R4
Connections	Ia-EPSP size and time course	smaller & slower	R6, R12
—	Ia-EPSP frequency modulation	more negative	R14
—	morphol of synapses soma (EM)	removed (stripping)	R1, R3
—	gap junctions	↑permeable	R5
—	axonal extensions	↑from soma (spinal MN)	R9
		↑from dendrite (neck MN)	R17
SD membr	threshold current	↓	R6, R7, R11, R21
—	input resistance	a/ ~; b/↑	a/ R6, R11; b/R7, R20
—	R_m, τ_m	↑	R7, R20
—	AP overshoot	↑	R13, R21
—	DD hump	↑	R7
—	AHP conductance	↓	R7, R21
—	f–I slope (repetitive firing)	a/ ↑↑; b/ ↑	a/ R10; b/ R7
Dendrites	extent, area	a/ ↓ (spinal); b/ ↑ (neck)	a/ R2, R8#, R19, R20#; b/ R16
—	high excitability, local APs	↑	R6, R7, R10, R11, R18

Examples of the many changes that may take place in alpha MNs after transection of their axons. *Abbreviations*: *cytochem*, cytochemical properties; *Ia-EPSP*, monosynaptic EPSP elicited in MNs by stimulation of Ia afferents from muscle spindles; *SD membr*, soma-dendrite membrane (membrane properties as seen with intracellular recording from soma); R_m, membrane resistivity; τ_m, membrane time constant; *AP*, action potential; *DD*, delayed depolarization; *AHP*, after hyperpolarization; *f–I slope*, slope of relation between discharge rate (y) and stimulating current intensity (x); *extent, area*, total dendritic extent or total dendritic or cell area (# for electrophysiological estimate). *Cited references*: R1 (Blinzinger and Kreutzberg 1968), R2 (Brannstrom *et al.* 1992a), R3 (Brannstrom and Kellerth 1998), R4 (Chalmers *et al.* 1992), R5 (Chang *et al.* 2000), R6 (Eccles *et al.* 1958b), R7 (Gustafsson 1979), R8 (Gustafsson and Pinter 1984a), R9 (Havton and Kellerth 1987), R10 (Heyer and Llinas 1977), R11 (Kuno and Llinas 1970b), R12 (Kuno and Llinas 1970a), R13 (Kuno *et al.* 1974), R14 (Mendell and Munson 1999), R15 (Nissl 1892), R16 (Rose and Odlozinski 1998), R17 (Rose *et al.* 2001), R18 (Shapovalov and Grantyn 1968), R19 (Sumner and Watson 1971), R20 (Yamuy *et al.* 1992a), R21 (Yamuy *et al.* 1992b).

functional context may lead to (temporary) changes in many of the neuronal characteristics. Some of these alterations are visible using the optical microscope and were described more than 100 years ago by Nissl (1892), who studied facial MNs after injury to their axons; within a few days, the cell bodies became larger and the prominent granular material in their cytoplasm (**Nissl bodies**) became less strongly stained by aniline dyes; this process is known as chromatolysis, a term introduced by Marinesco in 1894 (see LaVelle and LaVelle 1987).

Electron microscopy (EM) has shown that the Nissl bodies of nerve cells, which are conspicuous in large MNs, correspond to multilayered sheets of rough endoplasmic reticulum (rER) with many attached ribosomes (e. g. Johnston and Sears 1989). After axotomy, these sheets are broken up into numerous smaller units, which leads to the apparent dissolution of the Nissl material, i.e. to the signs of chromatolysis under the optical microscope. This reorganization of the rER is associated with an increased RNA synthesis and a raised nucleolar and somatic content of RNA. Characteristic EM changes and the alteration in RNA metabolism are typically also seen in axotomized cells which fail to show the coarser optical microscopy signs of chromatolysis (e.g. intercostal gamma MNs (Johnston and Sears 1989)). For both spinal MNs and corticospinal neurones, the classical optical microscopy signs of chromatolysis are less clearly present in small cells than in larger ones (Romanes 1964). The reaction was previously widely used in neuroanatomy for spotting cells that are connected to particular peripheral nerves or central fibre tracts (e.g. MNs reacting after section of motor nerves (Romanes 1951)). In this context, it was a forerunner of the use of retrograde tracer substances that emerged in the 1970s.

After axotomy, the resulting change in mRNA (and protein) synthesis is not purely quantitative, but the process apparently (and expectedly) includes a change in the selection of activated genes. Thus there is rise in mRNA for tubulin and actin and an increased synthesis of the regeneration-associated protein GAP-43 (Tetzlaff et al. 1988, 1989, 1991). Tubulin and actin are important for axonal transport and growth cone functions and thus may be of direct relevance for the regeneration process. The precise function of GAP-43 is still uncertain. Other proteins, including the neurofilament protein, are downregulated after axotomy (Tetzlaff et al. 1988). Moreover, there is decreased transport of AChE along the proximal stump of the motor axon (O'Brien 1978).

Cytological and mRNA-associated responses may be seen a few days after axotomy, with the swelling of the soma tending to precede the rise in nucleolar RNA production. However, this swelling may be a temporary change; in MNs surviving for a long time after axotomy, the cell bodies rather tend to be smaller than normal (Vanden Noven et al. 1993).

10.2.2. **Rate of motoneurone survival**

Neurones may die if their axons are cut. The risk of this happening strongly depends on the type of neurone. For instance, axotomized facial MNs of mice often die but those of the hamster typically survive (LaVelle and LaVelle 1987). Moreover, the number of surviving cells is markedly greater in adult than in young animals, and the chance of survival increases with the distance of the lesion from the soma. For example, cutting the sciatic nerve caused the death of many or all the MNs in newborn rats (Schmalbruch 1988), particularly if reinnervation of the muscle was prevented (Kashihara et al. 1987); in adult rats the MN death was more limited (Ma et al. 2001).

10.2.3. **Shrinkage of proximal axon diameter**

The diameters of myelinated axons become smaller in the proximal stump of a cut nerve and, partly as a result of this, their conduction velocities are decreased and extracellularly recorded spikes become smaller. For instance, in the common peroneal nerve of rabbits, a distal section caused a proximal decline of extracellular spike amplitude within a few days, and by 80 days spike size was less than 20 per cent of the original value (Gordon *et al.* 1991b). The relative shrinkage of axon size is greater for large than for smaller axons. In alpha motor axons of the cat medial gastrocnemius, the average conduction speed was 94 m/s for controls and 77 m/s for axons that were still unconnected to muscle after 18 months (Foehring and Munson 1990).

In myelinated fibres, the shrinkage and associated slowing of the proximal axon is one of the most predictable consequences of axotomy, and is seen in many different kinds of cell. It is apparently mainly caused by a downregulation of the neurofilament protein gene and by a change in the transport of this protein along the axon (reviewed by Titmus and Faber 1990). As well as affecting axon diameter, axotomy may also lead to the elimination of some of the intraspinal axon collaterals (Havton and Kellerth 1990, 2001).

10.2.4. **Dendrites**

Damage to an axon apparently has consequences for a neurone's maintenance of all its extended processes, including the dendrites. However, the nature of these changes may be drastically different for different MNs. Morphological studies have shown that the dendrites of axotomized spinal MNs retract (Sumner and Watson 1971; Brannstrom *et al.* 1992a) and, correspondingly, electrophysiological measurements have suggested a change in the same direction, i.e. a decrease in anatomical dendritic length, particularly in MNs of fast-twitch muscle units (Gustafsson and Pinter 1984a; cf. Gustafsson 1979). The changes may be substantial; at 12 weeks following a permanent axotomy of spinal MNs, their dendritic membrane area had decreased by 36 per cent (Brannstrom *et al.* 1992a). On the other hand, axotomized neck MNs may show considerable growth of their dendrites (Rose and Odlozinski 1998). Furthermore, in MNs the damage to the peripheral axon apparently induces a compensatory mechanism leading to the differentiation of central structures acquiring the morphological and molecular characteristics of axons; such new axon-like processes might emanate from the soma (spinal MNs) (Havton and Kellerth 1987) or from portions of the dendritic tree (neck MNs) (Rose and Odlozinski 1998; Rose *et al.* 2001; MacDermid *et al.* 2004). Following reinnervation of muscle, spinal MNs regain their normal dendritic area, although long-lasting changes remain in dendritic arborization patterns (Brannstrom *et al.* 1992b).

Dendrites are normally densely covered with synaptic connections. Hence the retraction and subsequent expansion of dendrites is likely to be associated with the loss and subsequent new acquisition of thousands of synaptic connections. Hardly anything is known about the consequences and details of such drastic synaptic changes in association with axotomy.

10.2.5. **Motoneuronal activation properties**

In its normal adult state, the main short-term task of a neurone is to process information ('transmitting' state), i.e. to dispatch action potentials along its axon in response to the sum of synaptic messages received across its soma and dendrites (see Chapters 6 and 7). Hence it is not surprising that many of the properties of importance for signalling functions may become affected when a MN is switched from a 'transmitting state' to a 'growth and connection state' by axotomy. Some of these changes in the membrane and synaptic properties of axotomized MNs are summarized in Table 10.1. Three things are obvious from this overview.

1 Most of the parameters involved in motoneuronal signal processing may indeed become affected by axotomy, i.e. these various properties are readily malleable even in adult neurones.

2 Some of the changes are highly context dependent, taking place to different extents (or even in different directions) for different groups of MNs (e.g. average expansion of dendrites in neck MNs and average retraction in spinal MNs; see Table 10.1, Dendrites).

3 The changes are not restricted to the MNs themselves but also, directly or indirectly, involve their connections from other central neurones. Changes in central connectivity are not limited to those associated with the dendritic retraction or expansion, but drastic alterations may also take place in membrane regions close to the soma where synaptic boutons become dislocated from the MN membrane as a result of the actions of microglia (Blinzinger and Kreutzberg 1968; Brannstrom and Kellerth 1998). With regard to the monosynaptic input from Ia afferents of muscle spindles, this 'synaptic stripping' removes, in particular, Ia EPSP components with a rapid time course, presumably associated with Ia synapses close to the soma. The remaining compound Ia EPSPs become smaller and slower than normal (Kuno and Llinas 1970a). However, these changes in EPSP time course may not be due only to 'synaptic stripping' at the soma because EPSP alterations of this kind are also seen before there are any changes in Ia fibre connectivity (Mendell *et al.* 1976). Additional factors which might play a role include changes of motoneurone membrane properties and a partial detachment of synaptic boutons before their total disconnexion.

Remarkably, not only the size and time course of the EPSPs change, but also their responses to repetitive activation become more similar to patterns normally seen in MNs of slow muscle units (Fig. 7.4c), i.e. a gradual depression rather than facilitation is seen during a train of repetitive stimulation (Mendell and Munson 1999). This suggests the presence of retrograde effects on presynaptic elements of axotomized MNs (see also Chapter 11, section 11.4.3.2).

Older studies of spinal reflexes had shown that the discharges evoked by stimulation of muscle afferents tended become more dispersed in time for axotomized MNs than for normal cells. Correspondingly, in the first intracellular analysis of axotomized MNs it was noted that the Ia EPSPs were slower and smaller than normal, the electrical excitability of the MNs was higher, and EPSPs often evoked small spike-like 'partial responses' which seemed to emanate from the dendrites (Eccles *et al.* 1958b); for later reports on 'partial responses', see Table 10.1. Not only the dendrites but also the membrane close to the soma show an increased excitability after axotomy (lower threshold current for evoking action potentials). This increase in electrical excitability seems to be partly due to an increased input resistance and partly to a lowered voltage threshold for spike initiation, as caused by changes in the voltage dependence of the Na^+ permeability system. The increased electrical excitability (including, possibly, dendritic 'partial responses') would be expected to cause an increase in the rhythmic 'gain' of the MN, i.e. in the slope of its relation between spike frequency and activating current (f–I slope). The f–I slope would also be expected to increase if the AHP current became weaker and/or shorter lasting (Chapter 6, section 6.6.2). In one study, the observed increase of f–I slope was moderate and seemed well explained by the observed changes in AHP current (Gustafsson 1979). In another report, which may have concerned another sample of spinal MNs (not identified with regard to original target muscle), very large increases in f–I slope were found which might have reflected a lowering of spike threshold (Heyer and Llinas 1977).

From some points of view, axotomized MNs seem to become 'dedifferentiated'; differences tend to decrease between cells that originally innervate fast units and those originally innervating slow ones (e.g. converging values of R_m, AHP duration, and Ia EPSP modulation).

10.2.6. Signals and mechanisms

Most of the reactions of MNs to axotomy are reversible; more or less normal properties recover once the appropriate targets are reinnervated (see further below). Thus the MN reactions to axotomy may be due to the lack of trophic factors normally brought, by retrograde transport, to the cell body from the muscle fibres. Target-derived neurotrophins are known to be essential for the survival of many types of neurone during development (cf. Bartlett *et al.* 1998). In addition, parts of the initial reaction to axotomy might be triggered by the lesion itself (e.g. by leakage of substances from the extracellular fluid, or the effects of cytokines and other molecules associated with inflammatory reactions). Experimental attempts have been made to counteract the 'chromatolytic' reactions of MNs by providing their cut motor axons with known neurotrophic substances of various kinds (see Chapter 11, section 11.4.6). Thus application of the neurotrophic factor NT-3 to cut nerves has been shown to restore the depressed Ia EPSP amplitude (Munson *et al.* 1997b), and a similar application of glial-cell-derived neurotrophic factor (GDNF) caused an increase in the conduction velocity of motor axons after they had been slowed down by axotomy (Munson and McMahon 1997). Furthermore, NT-3 and NT-4/5 seem to be important for the maintenance of normal conduction velocities along intact as well as distally transected motor axons (Munson *et al.* 1997c). Factors with these beneficial effects on MNs are apparently also delivered by other tissues than muscle; the input resistance, rheobase, and axonal conduction velocity of MNs all normalized to values typical for 'slow' MNs after regeneration of the motor nerve fibres into a cutaneous nerve (Nishimura *et al.* 1991).

The post-axotomy reactions in the soma take place earlier the closer to the soma the axon had been damaged. For rat hypoglossal MNs, the speed of this apparent retrograde signal transmission was 4–5 mm/day (Cragg 1970), which is slow compared with the rate of retrograde axonal transport (about 50 mm/day or more) (Chapter 2, section 2.4.6). In other reports the calculated rate of retrograde signalling was as high as 140 mm/h (i.e. 3360 mm/day), a speed far exceeding that seen for normal transport processes (calculated from the accumulation of transported phospholipids in rat sciatic nerve after crush-injury (Dziegielewska *et al.* 1980). Different retrograde signals might be involved, having an influence on different neuronal functions.

10.2.7. Effects of muscle paralysis

MN reactions very similar to those caused by axotomy can be elicited by the injection of botulinum toxin (BoTx) into the target muscle (Watson 1969). BoTx causes muscle paralysis as a consequence of a block of the exocytosis needed for transmitter release (reviewed by Meunier *et al.* 2002). The axotomy-like effects of BoTx have been interpreted as suggesting that chromatolytic reactions of MNs appear as a consequence of a decreased retrograde transport of molecules normally generated during muscle activity. However, it should be remembered that, at terminal nerve endings, there is a balance between exo- and endocytosis (Chapter 4, section 4.3.3); as a consequence of exocytosis, vesicular membrane will be added to the cell membrane and this 'extra' membrane is recycled into the cell by a corresponding amount of endocytosis (Royle and Lagnado 2003). Thus a block of exocytosis would, secondarily, be expected to result in decreased endocytosis and a decreased amount of axonal uptake of extracellular material (e.g. 'trophic' molecules secreted by the muscle fibre).

10.3. Peripheral reactions to loss or damage of motor axons

Motor nerve fibres may become interrupted or lost because of axonal damage, neuronal disease, or ageing (Fig. 12.2). It is well known that skeletal muscles become atrophic if their motor nerve supply is interrupted for a prolonged period. Ultimately, the denervated muscle cells may die.

Denervation leads to drastic alterations of electrophysiological properties in the muscle fibres. Thus denervated muscle fibres provide an interesting model system for studying how membrane properties of importance for signal processing are controlled. Many of the effects of MNs on muscle fibres are activity dependent; these aspects will be dealt with further in Chapter 11, section 11.3.

10.3.1. Electrophysiology

10.3.1.1. Distal axons

The distal portion of a cut motor axon may remain electrically excitable for several days after the lesion. In the rat, all axons of a cut nerve had become inexcitable after about 80 h, but in humans and baboons some nerve fibres may continue to be able to conduct action potentials for as long as 200 h (reviewed by McComas 1996). Microscopically, one of the earliest changes in the axons is a retraction of myelin at the nodes of Ranvier, which may occur at sites as far as 20 mm from the injury as soon as 1 h after the lesion. Close to the lesion, degenerative changes within the axon cylinder are already evident at 24 h (e.g. breakup of microtubuli, endoplasmic reticulum, and neurofilaments). The myelin sheath and the axon will eventually disintegrate. Schwann cells multiply and reach a maximum about 15–25 days after the lesion.

10.3.1.2. Neuromuscular junctions

If the nerve is cut distally, close to the neuromuscular junctions (NMJs), endplate transmission and the spontaneous quantal release of ACh (mEPPs) may continue to function almost normally for about 8 h (rat diaphragm) (Miledi and Slater 1970). Once the neuromuscular functions have started to deteriorate (i.e. after 8 h or more), the process is rapid and only a few hours are required for a disruption of the endplate structure. Transmission fails abruptly and mEPPs stop appearing. Presynaptic neuronal components of the NMJ disintegrate and are removed. Postsynaptic structures also change (e.g. disappearance of postsynaptic folds (Matsuda *et al.* 1988)), but major aspects of the postsynaptic molecular organization are more persistent (e.g. endplate AChRs, basal membrane molecules).

In a denervated muscle, the time of occurrence of neuromuscular failure and alterations in muscle fibre membrane properties are delayed in proportion to the length of the distal nerve stump (Harris and Thesleff 1972). Such a length-dependent delay is also found with regard to the degeneration of the distal nerve itself, and the breakdown of nerve terminals close to muscle fibres may cause denervation-associated membrane changes to appear (e.g. spike resistance to tetrodotoxin (TTX), fall of membrane potential) (see below). This is also the case for the degeneration of terminals without synaptic connections to the muscle fibres (Arancio *et al.* 1992).

10.3.1.3. Muscle fibres

Relatively soon after denervation, several characteristic changes take place in the electrophysiological properties of twitch muscle fibres. All these changes are reversible, and normal properties return on reinnervation. Roughly in their order of appearance these changes include the following.

1 The resting membrane potential becomes less negative, i.e. less depolarization will be needed to reach the threshold. This effect is very fast and changes have been reported to take place within 2–3 h of cutting the motor nerve (Albuquerque *et al.* 1971; Bray *et al.* 1976). The changes start to appear at the endplate and proceed from there in both directions. They are largely caused by decreased activity of the Na—K pump and its associated electrogenic action (Bray *et al.* 1976). Ultimately, the decrease in membrane potential amounts to about 20 mV.

2 The membrane permeabilities for K^+ and Cl^- ions decrease (Klaus *et al.* 1960; Thesleff 1963). There is an increase in resting membrane resistivity and a drop in

membrane capacitance; for instance, in rat soleus muscle R_m increased from 766 to 2291 Ω cm^2, and C_m dropped from 3.6 to 2.7 μF/cm^2 (Westgaard 1975).

3 Sensitivity to extracellular ACh increases for extrajunctional membrane portions. Normally only regions close to the endplate have a high ACh sensitivity. Starting 24 h after a distal denervation, the ACh-sensitive region expands from the endplate towards the ends of the fibre (Axelsson and Thesleff 1959). These changes result from the insertion into the extrajunctional membrane of newly synthesized ACh receptor molecules of the 'fast' turnover type (fAChR) with a half-life about 1 day (Berg and Hall 1974, 1975; Szabo *et al.* 2003). Compared with the 'slow' sAChRs of normal adult endplates (half-life 6 days, Berg and Hall 1975; half-life 10 days, Szabo *et al.* 2003), the fAChR ion channels have longer open times per channel (Sakmann and Brenner 1978). Structurally, the two AChRs differ in one of their four subunits (Brenner *et al.* 1990). The normally very high concentration of AChRs at the original endplate remains for a long time after denervation.

4 Muscle fibre action potentials can still be elicited using direct electrical stimulation. However, the action potentials change their properties: their rate of rise decreases and their duration increases, their overshoot becomes smaller, and the conduction velocity becomes slower (at least partly a consequence of the slower and smaller spikes). Furthermore, the action potentials become insensitive to the blocking action of TTX, i.e. new types of Na$^+$ permeability channels are being inserted into the membrane. These changes start about 36 h after distal denervation (Harris and Thesleff 1972; Sellin and Thesleff 1980). The TTX-resistant Na$^+$ channels are of type SkM2, and those normally present are of type SkM1 (Kallen *et al.* 1990; Yang *et al.* 1991). Compared with SkM1 channels, those of type SkM2 show a smaller maximal current and a slower onset of inactivation (reviewed by Yoshida 1994).

5 During the first 2 weeks following denervation, the endplate concentration of AChE drops by more than 50 per cent (Guth *et al.* 1981). This drop is particularly marked for the asymmetric isoform A12, and there is even a transient increase in isoform A4. Moreover, in fast but not in slow muscle there is also a transient increase in the globular isoform G4 (Sketelj *et al.* 1992).

6 After about a week, denervated muscle fibres may start to generate spontaneous discharges of action potentials (fibrillation potentials). These potentials are readily recognizable in EMG recordings; fibrillation potentials appear independently of each other in individual muscle fibres and therefore they are smaller and faster than the multifibre motor unit action potentials of a normally innervated muscle. In patients, the discharge rate of fibrillation potentials is often around 0.5–3 Hz. In rat diaphragm kept in organ culture (Purves and Sakmann 1974a,b), only about a third to a quarter of all the fibres were active at any one time. Each fibre had periods of activity of 21–22 h alternating with more prolonged silent periods. This was a self-limiting kind of activity cycle: pauses were shortened by preceding inactivity (e.g. by block of action potentials) and lengthened after increased activity (e.g. caused by chronic

stimulation). The fibrillation action potentials remain sensitive to TTX, and this activity cannot be blocked by curare, i.e. ACh plays no role in the appearance of the fibrillation potentials. The activity typically starts close to the old endplate (although other trigger sites also occcur), and seems to be generated as a result of the properties of voltage-sensitive Na^+ permeability sites in the denervated muscle membrane. There are intriguing differences between different muscles and animal species with regard to the amount of fibrillation after denervation (Robinson *et al.* 1991).

10.3.1.4. Effects of actinomycin D

Several of the denervation-elicited changes in muscle fibre activation properties can be prevented by treatment with actinomycin D, which blocks RNA synthesis (Grampp *et al.* 1972). This includes the expansion of ACh sensitivity and the appearance of TTX-insensitive action potentials and spontaneous fibrillations. These various changes are dependent on the appearance of new types of protein as a result of altered DNA transcription.

10.3.2. Atrophy and degeneration

Following denervation there is a rather rapid loss of contractile material and other components from the muscle fibres. The fibres become thinner (denervation atrophy) and after a few weeks the whole muscle has already become much lighter and weaker. The atrophy can be detected 3 days after denervation, and 60–80 per cent of total muscle mass may be lost after 2 months (Sunderland and Ray 1950). The extent of denervation atrophy is much the same in slow- and fast-twitch fibres of the same muscle. After a few days, many of the nuclei will move from their normal subsarcolemmal position towards the centre of the fibres, i.e. to sites typically seen in unripe muscle fibres (myotubes) (Chapter 12, section 12.5). In late atrophy (e.g. after more than 6 months (Schmalbruch *et al.* 1991)), some fibres may consist mainly of rows of nuclei surrounded by a thin layer of cytoplasm. Ultimately, after many months, some fibres (or parts of fibres, i.e. some of the nuclei) may die, while new thin fibres appear to arise from satellite cells. As long as even severely atrophic fibres remain present, most of the intramuscular consequences of denervation are reversible on reinnervation. Much of the atrophy can also be counteracted with chronic electrical activation (Hennig and Lomo 1987; Schmalbruch *et al.* 1991).

10.3.3. Denervation hypertrophy

In some denervated muscles, the atrophy may be preceded by a transient stage (often 1–2 weeks) of increased muscle fibre diameter (denervation hypertrophy). This atypical reaction has been reported for the denervated hemidiaphragm, and the hypertrophy then apparently depends on the stretching of denervated muscle fibres caused by contractions in the half of the muscle that is still innervated (cf. Chapter 11, section 11.3.2.1; Miledi and Slater 1969). A similar explanation might be valid for the hypertrophy seen in denervated external eye muscles, which might also be passively stretched by eye movements generated by muscles which are still innervated (Asmussen and Gaunitz 1981a).

10.3.4. Contractile and related biochemical properties

10.3.4.1. Force

After denervation, the maximum tetanic force drops even more than muscle mass because of a decrease in specific tension (Finol *et al.* 1981; al-Amood *et al.* 1991). This weakening may be partly due to a greater atrophy of contractile than of non-contractile muscle tissue.

10.3.4.2. Speed

The time course of the isometric twitch initially tends to become slower after denervation in all muscles, although there may be a reversal of this slowing later on (Finol *et al.* 1981; al-Amood and Lewis 1989). In denervated slow muscle fibres, the relative content of fast myosin increases and that of slow myosin decreases (Gauthier and Hobbs 1982). However, increases in isotonic shortening velocity may be weak or absent, and there is even a progressive slowing of shortening speed in the extensor digitorum longus (fast muscle) of the guinea pig (al-Amood and Lewis 1989). Thus, to some extent, the various muscle fibre types tend to converge in their speed-related properties. However, they do not ultimately become identical. The change in shortening speed may reflect changes in myosin composition, while alterations of isometric speed may predominantly depend on changes in structures involved in intracellular Ca^{2+} dynamics (Chapter 3 section 3.3.2).

10.3.4.3. Endurance and metabolic properties

In the context of denervation, fatigue resistance has been less well investigated than the contractile properties of speed and force. However, also in this respect, slow and fast muscles apparently tend to converge in properties after denervation: following denervation, the normally fatigue-sensitive EDL became more fatigue resistant whereas the normally fatigue-resistant soleus muscle became somewhat more fatigue-sensitive (rat, Westgaard and Lomo 1988). Most kinds of metabolic enzyme activity decrease and the normally occurring histochemical differences between different types of muscle fibres become increasingly vague. Red fibres become paler, losing their myoglobin. After some time, conventional histochemistry can no longer be used to identify fibres of (originally) different types (Hogan *et al.* 1965; Romanul and Hogan 1965; Gundersen *et al.* 1988).

10.3.5. Responses to electrical stimulation of whole muscles

It has long been known that, compared with normally innervated muscles, denervated muscles (e.g. in patients) require longer stimulation pulses for transcutaneous electrical activation applied via electrodes on the skin covering the muscle. These alterations in neuromuscular properties are used as a diagnostic sign of muscle denervation in clinical neurophysiology, typically (previously) quantified as an increased **chronaxie**, i.e. the minimum pulse duration needed for muscle activation at twice the threshold intensity (threshold first measured with very long pulses). For instance, if a muscle is stimulated with very long pulses of threshold intensity and pulse duration is gradually shortened, the pulse will still be effective down to durations below 1 ms in a normally innervated muscle, whereas in a denervated muscle pulse intensity may have to be increased for durations below 10–100 ms (e. g. Lenman and Ritchie 1977). Such changes of duration requirements are not primarily dependent on altered properties of the muscle fibres themselves but on the fact that, in normal muscles, transcutaneous stimulation has its lowest-threshold effect on the intramuscular nerve fibres, i.e. this type of stimulation normally activates the muscle fibres via their motor endplates. Only after degeneration of the intramuscular nerve fibres does electrical stimulation become dependent on the electrical excitability of the muscle fibres themselves. Muscle fibres have a larger specific membrane capacitance and longer membrane time constants than myelinated nerve fibres (Chapter 4, section 4.4.1); hence stimulation intensity can be kept low only if pulse duration is relatively long.

10.4. **Muscle reinnervation**

Several recovery conditions have to be satisfied for the restoration of muscle function after nerve damage:

(a) the nerve fibres must be able to grow out far enough to reach their appropriate destinations.

(b) along their outgrowth trajectory, motor axons have to make the correct path selections for reaching their 'own' muscle

(c) inside muscles, axons have to establish functionally adequate and well-matched connections with their target cells, the muscle fibres

(d) general muscle properties that were changed after denervation have to revert to their normal state (e.g. muscle fibre bulk, force and activation properties).

These different aspects of muscle reinnervation are discussed below.

10.4.1. **Motor axon growth**

The importance of recovery condition (a) is self-evident. Inside the mammalian CNS, regenerative axonal outgrowth is generally only possible for very short distances; after lesions, large-scale restoration is impossible. However, in the peripheral nervous system, all axons seem capable of long-distance outgrowth. Very soon after an axon has been transected, it develops growth cones at its tip and starts elongating. This transformation apparently takes place using locally available molecules; the latency is too short to allow for a preceding transport of the essential components from the cell body (Sjoberg and Kanje 1990). Growth cones are highly specialized structures (Alberts *et al.* 2002) containing large concentrations of microtubules which are used as a dynamic cytoskeleton. The growth cone sends out multiple extensions into the immediate environment. Some of these extensions are rapidly retracted and others remain and expand in diameter and length, 'pulling' the growing axon along. Typically, one regenerating axon may initially extend several parallel branches along the same or different trajectory(ies). In the phase of 'ripening', after connecting to a target, many of these parallel branches will gradually disappear, leaving only few main branches (typically only one) in the peripheral nerve.

The direction taken by an outgrowing axon, and the speed of this process, is stongly dependent on both biochemical and physical properties of surrounding structures and tissue components. In culture, growing axons will extend along grooves in the floor of the culture chamber. In the body, the direction of regeneration may be guided by inserted tubes of various materials (e.g. transplanted blood vessels or artificial material). Outgrowth over longer distances is well guided by nerve sheaths containing surviving Schwann cells, which are highly effective in providing the optimal surroundings for nerve regeneration. In the distal nerve stump, the Schwann cells become arranged into long rows, known as 'bands of Büngner', and axons grow out along those bands. Schwann cells produce a large number of 'trophic' substances and adhesion molecules which have an effect on the nerve, including NGF, BDNF, CNTF, *N*-cadherin, N-CAM, laminin, tensacin, and L1/NILE (Bunge *et al.* 1990; Richardson 1991). On the other hand, Schwann cells are themselves influenced by the outgrowing axon, which stimulates Schwann cell mitosis and promotes an upregulation of Schwann cell synthesis of myelin and basal lamina components. If Schwann cells are denervated for long periods of time (weeks to months), their ability to promote axonal outgrowth becomes progressively diminished (Sulaiman and Gordon 2000). Interestingly, this decline takes place without any loss of the myelinating capabilities of the Schwann cells (Sulaiman and Gordon 2000).

The speed of axonal outgrowth is initially low and increases gradually during the first 3 days. Thereafter, its speed is often around 2–3 mm/day, which is likely to reflect the velocity of the slow axonal processes for bulk transport (Hoffman and Lasek 1980). Attempts to increase the speed of nerve outgrowth by various kinds of physical or biochemical treatment have had mixed and partly contradictory results. In such studies, it is important to differentiate between the delay before regeneration starts and the speed of axon outgrowth; in the rat femoral nerve, electrical stimulation shortened the delay without changing the speed of outgrowth (Al-Majed *et al.* 2000; Brushart *et al.* 2002; methods for promoting axonal outgrowth reviewed by Gordon *et al.* 2003). The initial stages of regeneration and the associated slow component of axonal transport are accelerated if a nerve lesion is succeeded, 2 weeks later, by a second more proximal lesion (McQuarrie 1978; McQuarrie and Jacob 1991).

10.4.2. Path selections of regenerating motor axons

With regard to recovery condition (b) it should be realized that individual cranial nerves or spinal roots each deliver axons to many different peripheral nerves, and that each single nerve is itself typically a multi-user cable, containing axons for many different ultimate destinations (different skin regions, and different muscles and muscle portions). During development, outgrowing motor axons navigate within this complex 'road map' with great precision, enabling MNs of a given central location (and correspondingly preprogrammed functions) to connect with their own peripheral muscle (portion) (see Chapter 12, section 12.6). For an outgrowing motor fibre, there are generally at least three major levels of path selection:

(i) going to muscle rather than to skin or other tissues;

(ii) going to the correct muscle among those served by the same nerve or root;

(iii) choosing where to go and what to innervate within the selected target muscle.

In all instances considered below, nerves were regenerating after complete interruption (i.e. they were cut, not crushed).

Selection (i) It has long been known that there are differences between cholinergic and sensory regenerating axons with regard to their possible innervation targets. Sensory axons will not make synapses onto muscle fibres, and motor axons will not make appropriate mechanosensitive connections with skin or other tissues (although skin may have a retrograde 'trophic' effect on the motor nerve and its MN (Nishimura *et al.* 1991). Even in the adult, regenerating motor axons make a somewhat better than random choice between the cutaneous and muscular side branches of a nerve (Brushart 1988; Brushart 1993). If tested in a T-maze situation with a choice between a tube with skin tissue components and a tube with muscle tissue components, most motor axons turn towards the muscle side (Jerregard *et al.* 2001). The molecular basis for these selections is still uncertain.

Selection (ii) In neonatal animals, the capability of making correct intermuscular path-selections is not perfect (some selectivity, Gerding *et al.* 1977; negative results, Ito *et al.* 1994), but it is still at least partially present (Aldskogius and Thomander 1986; Hardman and Brown 1987; DeSantis *et al.* 1992), and this is also true for some adult non-mammalian vertebrates (e.g. axolotl) (Wigston and Sanes 1982). This capability appears to be almost completely lost in adult mammals. In a choice between the original 'own' and a 'foreign' branch of a motor nerve, adult regenerating motor fibres seem generally to make a random choice (Weiss and Hoag 1946; Bernstein and Guth 1961; Brushart and Mesulam 1980; Gillespie *et al.* 1986; Thomas *et al.* 1987; Bodine-Fowler *et al.* 1997). As a result, after reinnervation following the regeneration of a mixed transected nerve, MNs innervating single muscles are now distributed along a wide region of the ventral horn, covering many different motor nuclei (Brushart and Mesulam 1980). Shortly after reinnervation, single MNs may send collaterals into several different nerve branches; in the longer term, only the collaterals to one muscle tend to remain (guinea pig facial MNs, 12–13 weeks) (Ito and Kudo 1994).

Selection (iii) Two apparently independent kinds of topographical order normally exist within muscles: slow and fast muscle fibres tend to be unevenly distributed ('fibre type regionalization') (Fig. 3.11), and the intramuscular destination tends to differ between rostral and more caudal MNs within the spinal cord ('cord-to-muscle topography') (Fig. 5.6). Both these aspects of intramuscular organization tend to recur after reinnervation, even in adults. With regard to the cord-to-muscle topography, the degree of post-reinnervation recovery has been tested for two axial muscles (diaphragm, serratus). The tendency for a return of the normal innervation patterns was weak but significantly present, and this tendency was stronger in young animals than in adults (Laskowski and

Sanes 1988). With regard to fibre type regionalization, the tendency for a post-reinnervation recurrence of normal patterns is strongly present, regardless of whether the motor
axons grow into the muscle via their original or another path (Fig. 10.1) (Wang and
Kernell 2002; see also Foehring *et al.* 1987a; Parry and Wilkinson 1990; Rafuse and
Gordon 1996b; Wang *et al.* 2002). The precise orientation of the recovered fibre type
regionalization is partly dependent on the orientation of the muscle within the limb
(Fig. 10.1D, intralimb molecular gradients?) (Wang and Kernell 2002). Within slow-fibre
regions, the fine-grain distribution of type I fibres was changed after reinnervation
(Fig. 10.1A,B), displaying a considerable amount of type grouping (section 10.4.3.2)
(Wang *et al.* 2002; Wang and Kernell 2002). Hence the restored type I fibre regionalization (Fig. 10.1C,D) did not depend on a cell-to-cell recognition between slow MN axons
and originally slow muscle fibres. Hoh (1975) noted that, in the rat hindlimb, soleus MN
axons provided reinnervation more efficiently and faster to the slow soleus muscle than
to a fast muscle (EDL), whereas the MN axons of EDL were non-selective. Such differences between slow and fast MN axons might have reflected preferences with regard to
different kinds of 'muscle space', analogous to those underlying the restoration of intramuscular fibre type regionalization after reinnervation.

It should be stressed that capacities for appropriate axonal path selections can only be
well tested after a complete interruption of the nerve (i.e. nerve cut or macerated). If the
nerve fibres are made to regenerate after a nerve crush, they will typically find their way
back to their original muscles (Bodine-Fowler *et al.* 1997), probably because they are
then growing along their original fascicles and Schwann cell bands.

10.4.3. Recovery of functionally adequate connections

With respect to recovery condition (c) there are two subconditions. The connections
should be such that:

(i) the target cells can indeed become activated by the axon (i.e. recovery of neuromuscular transmission);

(ii) the properties of the target cells of a given motor axon are, or will become, well
matched to the activity patterns of their MN (e.g. with regard to speed, tension–
frequency relation, force, endurance, and related biochemical properties).

10.4.3.1. Recovery of neuromuscular transmission

Regenerating axons recognize the site of the old endplate. When arriving there, they stop
growing (Rich and Lichtman 1989) and then very rapidly establish a functioning contact
with synaptic transmission. The old endplate site is recognized by the growth cone
because of the persistent presence of marker molecules in the basal lamina (McMahan
et al. 1980; McMahan and Slater 1984; reviewed by Sanes 1983). Furthermore, the growth
cone is actively guided towards the endplate site by extensions of Schwann cells (Son and
Thompson 1995; Son *et al.* 1996). Motor growth cones spontaneously release ACh already
before making any synaptic contact (Hume *et al.* 1983; Young and Poo 1983). When arriving

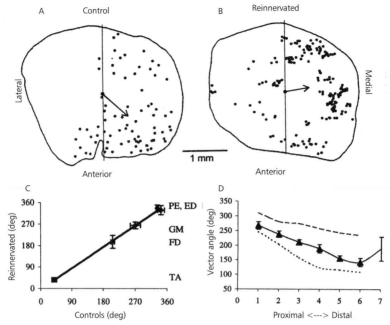

Figure 10.1 Recovery of type I fibre regionalization after reinnervation. Experiments on hindlimb muscles of rats. (**A**), (**B**) Drawings of cross-sections from extensor digitorum longus (EDL) muscles on (**A**) normally innervated side and (**B**) experimental side where EDL had become reinnervated after section and resuture of the sciatic nerve. Muscle outline and positions of all type I fibres (slow) indicated; both muscles from same animal. Arrow drawn from 'centre of mass' for whole muscle section to that for only the type I fibres ('type I fibre vector'). Anteroposterior line drawn through muscle centre. Note that most of the type I fibres are on the medial side in both case (**A**) and case (**B**). Marked 'clumping' of type I fibres after reinnervation ('fibre type grouping') can be seen in (**B**). (**C**) Post-reinnervation reappearance of a normal direction of type I fibre regionalization. The direction of regionalization was measured by determining the direction of the type I fibre vector ('vector angle'; see arrows in (**A**) and (**B**)). After section and resuture of the sciatic nerve, this was done at different proximo-distal levels for five different muscles in each of five rats (survival time 21 weeks). In the diagram, average vector angles ± SE for control muscles are plotted versus averages for corresponding reinnervated muscles (ED, extensor digitorum longus; PE, peroneus longus; GM, gastrocnemius medialis; FD, flexor digitorum longus; TA, tibialis anterior. Note the strong similarity between experimental and control values ($r = 0.998$, $P < 0.001$). Vector angles were zero for medial, 90° for posterior, 180° for lateral, and 270° for anterior directions. ((**A**)–(**C**) Reproduced with permission, from Wang et al. 2002.) (**D**) Effects of muscle rotation on the direction of type I fibre regionalization after reinnervation. Experiments on GM muscles after self-reinnervation by their own nerves (survival time 21 weeks). The distal tendon and much of the muscle was rotated around its length axis at the time of nerve section and reconnection. Plot of mean type I fibre vector angle ± SE versus proximo-distal level along the muscle. The experimental values are compared with two sets of normally innervated controls: (a) GM muscles with a normal intralimb position (upper broken line); (b) GM muscles that had been rotated 21 weeks beforehand (lower dotted line). Note that the reinnervated and rotated values fall between the two sets of controls. Only the reinnervated GM muscles had any type I fibres at the most distal level. (Reproduced with permission, from Wang and Kernell 2002.)

at the endplate site, this release is enhanced by signals from the muscle. After being rein-nervated, postsynaptic folds again develop under the nerve endings. During reinnerva-tion, each single endplate initially tends to be contacted by several axons, but only one of these connections will ultimately remain (reviewed by Jansen and Fladby 1990; Sanes and Lichtman 1999). Thus, to some extent, the adult reinnervation processes re-enact the events seen during the perinatal development of the neuromuscular system (Chapter 12).

If reinnervation takes place after a simple transection and resuture of a motor nerve, the muscle fibres are predominantly contacted at the site of the old endplate and inner-vation at other sites ('ectopic' endplates) is scarce. However, such ectopic endplates may be induced to appear using particular procedures, for example by inserting a cut motor nerve into a target muscle which is later denervated or kept inactive (for further details, see Lomo 2003).

10.4.3.2. Recovery of matching properties between MNs and their muscle fibres: fibre type grouping

Experiments have shown that reinnervating MNs of different kinds (e.g. slow versus fast) have strong and differential influences on muscle fibres with regard to their contractile properties (e.g. speed, endurance) and their associated bio/histochemical characteristics (e.g. myofibrillar ATPase, myosin type, metabolic enzymes). Physiologically, this was first clearly demonstrated in the classical cross-reinnervation experiments of Buller et al. (1960b) (Fig. 10.2A). The nerves to a slow hindlimb muscle of the cat (soleus) and a pre-dominately fast muscle (flexor digitorum longus) were sectioned and cross-united. After an appropriate time for axon regeneration and 'ripening', the contractile properties of both muscles were tested under isometric contractions. The fast muscle had become very much slower and the slow one had clearly become faster (Fig. 10.2A). Corresponding changes in isometric contractile speed were also seen in the tension–frequency curves (e.g. in the rates needed for generating 50 per cent of maximum force). No such changes in contractile speed occurred on self-reinnervation (Fig. 10.2B), i.e. the effects were not unspecific consequences of reinnervation but they were dependent on the identity of the reinnervating MNs. These experiments have since been repeated many times, confirmed, and extended, and measurements have also been performed at the level of single motor units (Bagust et al. 1981; Lewis et al. 1982; Dum et al. 1985a,b; Foehring et al. 1987a; Gordon et al. 1988). The change in contractile speed concerns not only the isometric twitch but also the maximum rate of force increase (decreased in cross-reinnervated fast muscle) (Buller and Lewis 1965a) and the maximum shortening speed (Close 1969; Luff 1975; Buller et al. 1987; Thomas and Ranatunga 1993). In addition to the change in speed, alterations in endurance have also been observed; for example, fast units inner-vated with a slow nerve became more fatigue resistant (Dum et al. 1985a), and extensor muscles innervated with a 'fast' peroneal nerve became more fatiguable (Gordon et al. 1988). However, in some cases this parameter was not altered (Edgerton et al. 1980). There are often marked changes in muscle fibre histochemistry (Romanul and Van der Meulen 1966; Chan et al. 1982; Reichmann et al. 1983; Dum et al. 1985a,b). For most types of physiological measures, the changes of an originally fast muscle to a slower and more fatigue-resistant one are more drastic and complete than the changes in opposite directions for an originally slower muscle; this is particularly evident for the highly specialized soleus muscle. Thus, after reinnervation with slow soleus MNs, many of the type II fibres of a fast muscle will acquire the properties characteristic for the slow type I fibres. For cross-reinnervated soleus muscle fibres some changes in the opposite direction take place, but typically are more sparing and less complete (Luff 1975; Dum *et al.* 1985b; Foehring *et al.* 1987a), although in some species and experimental situations a large proportion of slow soleus fibres may indeed acquire fast-type histochemical properties (e.g. 90 per cent of fibres converted in the rabbit soleus innervated by the peroneal nerve (Reichmann *et al.* 1983)). The size relations and normal fibre type compositions of the respective 'crossed' muscles are of importance for the efficiency and completeness of the conversion caused by a cross-reinnervation experiment (for further details, see Buller *et al.* 1987; Thomas and Ranatunga 1993).

It is clear from the fact that fast (F) versus slow (S) cross-reinnervation is possible that regenerating motor nerve fibres are prepared to innervate any denervated muscle fibre,

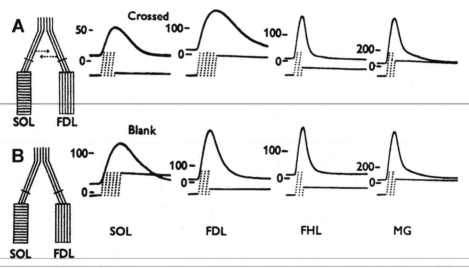

Figure 10.2 Change of muscle speed after cross-reinnervation of fast and slow muscles: experiments on kittens. (**A**) The nerves to the slow soleus (SOL) and the faster flexor digitorum longus (FDL) muscles were sectioned and cross-resutured on the left side at the age of 21 days. (**B**) On the control side, the soleus and FDL nerves had been severed and rejoined (self-reinnervation). Measurements of isometric muscle properties were made 30 days later. The illustrated isometric twitch contractions are clearly changed for both cross-reinnervated muscles: SOL is faster than the self-reinnervated control, and FDL is much slower. Muscles with unchanged innervation had the same contractile speed in both limbs (FHL, flexor hallucis longus; MG, medial gastrocnemius). Twitch contraction times (time to peak, ms) were indicated by a decade-counter device (lower beam at twitches). Tension scales in grams. Weight of kitten, 0.85 kg. (Reproduced with permission, from Buller *et al.* 1960b.)

irrespective of their initial functional type. F and S axons seem to be capable of grabbing whichever fibre happens to be in their way (provided that they are in the 'right' intramuscular region; see section 10.4.2). The muscle fibres then tend to become transformed into the type matching the reinnervating MN. Thus, for a given axon, one might expect many of the reinnervated muscle fibres to lie close to each other and to be of the same histochemical type. This is often the case after cross- as well as self-reinnervation (i.e. reinnervation by original nerve). This **fibre type grouping** (Kugelberg *et al.* 1970) is particularly striking for the less common fibre type within a muscle; in a normally innervated muscle the least common fibre type seldom lies close to other fibres of the same type (e.g. type I fibres in Fig. 3.10A; cf. Fig. 10.1A versus Fig. 10.1B). The appearance of fibre type grouping is an important diagnostic sign of partial or complete muscle reinnervation (see also discussion of sprouting below). However, the extent to which (self- or cross-)reinnervation gives rise to fibre type grouping varies with the experimental circumstances. Fibre type grouping is promoted by having few motor axons reinnervating a muscle and by suturing the regenerating nerve to the muscle fascia instead of to a peripheral nerve stump (Rafuse and Gordon 1996b). Under some experimental circumstances, fibre type grouping might not be increased at all after reinnervation (Unguez *et al.* 1996); thus the absence of fibre type grouping cannot be used as a (clinical) sign that there has been no regeneration of motor nerve fibres.

In normally innervated muscle units, histochemical properties tend to be very similar across all the muscle fibres of the same unit (rat, Nemeth *et al.* 1981; cat, Nemeth *et al.* 1986; Unguez *et al.* 1993). After reinnervation, this homogeneity is sometimes much less striking; also, after very long recovery times, some muscle fibres may persist in having histochemical characteristics that are widely different from the average for other fibres of the same muscle unit (Unguez *et al.* 1993; 1995). Thus the degree to which individual muscle fibres may have their properties 'reset' by an innervating MN may apparently differ considerably across the fibre population of a single muscle; the different fibres seem to be provided with individual differences in their 'adaptive range' (cf. Chapter 11, section 11.3.6.3; Westgaard and Lomo 1988).

Initially after the reinnervation of a muscle, normally existing relationships between the properties of motor axons and those of their muscle units are lost (e.g. axonal conduction velocity or extracellular spike size versus muscle unit twitch or tetanic force (Gordon and Stein 1982b)). After a period of several months the force-related relationships return, largely because of a restoration of the correlation between axonal size and the number of innervated muscle fibres which is normally present (Gordon and Stein 1982b; Gordon *et al.* 1986b, 2004). In a self-reinnervated muscle, such processes of recovery are less efficient if the number of motor axons falls below 50 per cent of normal, and if the ingrowing axons are not allowed to follow their original nerve sheath (suture of proximal nerve stump to muscle fascia) (Rafuse and Gordon 1998).

In humans, a recovery of the normal relationship between motor unit force and recruitment threshold (Chapter 8, section 8.2.1) is restored after reinnervation provided that the motor axons innervate their original muscles or close synergists (Thomas *et al.* 1987). At the level of single cat MNs, systematic measurements have been made of the input resistance R_{in}, the threshold current for evoking action potentials I_{rh}, and the time course of the after-hyperpolarization (AHP$_h$, time taken for a decline to half-maximum amplitude). Normally, these parameters are ranked in a characteristic way across the population of MNs with different contractile types of muscle units; for AHP$_h$ S > FR ≈ FF; for R_{in}, S > FR > FF; for I_{rh}, S < FR < FF (Table 6.1) (Zengel *et al.* 1985). After self-reinnervation (and a suitable period of recovery), muscle units classified on the basis of their contractile characteristics had MNs with the normally corresponding values for R_{in}, I_{rh}, and AHP$_h$, including the ratio I_{rh}/R_{in} (Foehring *et al.* 1986), and after cross-reinnervation this was true for MNs of the medial gastrocnemius which innervated the lateral gastrocnemius (Foehring *et al.* 1987b). In most cases, this matching of MN to muscle unit seems to recover because MNs cause appropriate changes to occur among their newly innervated muscle fibres (see discussion of fibre type grouping above). However, under some circumstances, changes in MN properties might be evoked by the muscle fibres, and the matching might then instead recover the other way around. Processes of this kind were suggested by the results of cross-reinnervation by MNs of a predominantly fast muscle (gastrocnemius medialis) to muscle fibres of a uniformly slow muscle (soleus). In this case, most of the cross-reinnervated soleus units remained slow and many of them were apparently innervated by originally fast MNs which had changed their properties in the direction of normal S-type MNs (changes included a slower time course of AHP) (Foehring *et al.* 1987b).

After cross-reinnervation, MNs tend to maintain their original activity patterns irrespective of the mechanical actions of their (new) muscle fibres (O'Donovan *et al.* 1985; Gordon *et al.* 1986a). The MN versus muscle unit matching of properties after slow versus fast cross-reinnervation is likely to be mainly caused by activity-dependent changes in the muscle fibres (see Chapter 11, section 11.3). However, in the almost complete absence of activity, slow versus fast cross-reinnervation has an added effect on muscle properties (Roy *et al.* 1996). For changes occurring in the MNs, the effects of retrogradely transported molecules would have to be considered. For muscle fibres as well as MNs, preset 'adaptive ranges' are likely to limit the possible extent of usage- and innervation-dependent adjustment of functional characteristics (Chapter 11, section 11.3.6.3).

10.4.4. Restoration and maturation of general muscle properties

As was mentioned in section 10.3.1.3, the denervation-elicited changes in electrophysiological muscle fibre properties are reversed by reinnervation, and the recovery of a normal neuromuscular transmission is relatively rapid. As long as the muscle fibres have not died, even a very severe post-denervation atrophy can be largely reversed by motor reinnervation. Furthermore, the motor nerve fibres will grow in diameter and myelin thickness after contacting their targets, with both axonal changes promoting an increased conduction velocity (for internodal distances, see Chapter 2, section 2.4.3). However, these various aspects of 'maturation' may take many months to complete (Gordon and Stein 1982a,b).

10.5. **Sprouting and collateral reinnervation**

In addition to the kinds of reinnervation that are associated with long-distance (extra-muscular) outgrowth of lesioned axons, there is also a local type of reinnervation which takes place within muscles. If part of the normal innervation is lost (e.g. due to MN death or loss of individual motor axons), denervated muscle fibres induce neighbouring nerve fibres to send out new side branches, thus providing them with innervation at their 'empty' endplates (reviewed by Tam and Gordon 2003). This phenomenon is called 'sprouting' or 'collateral reinervation', and it is known to occur in muscles as well as inside the CNS. New sprouts may appear in two different ways: from the terminals at an endplate ('terminal sprouts'), or from nodes of Ranvier in preterminal portions of intra-muscular axons ('nodal sprouts') (Fig. 10.3A).

Collateral reinnervation, as produced by sprouting, is commonly associated with a con-siderable degree of fibre type grouping. This is intuitively understandable; terminal sprouts from still innervated endplates will primarily establish contacts with muscle fibres in the immediate surrounding. After becoming reinnervated, these neighbouring muscle fibres will generally be induced to assume contractile and biochemical properties similar to those of the fibre with the sprout-generating terminal, i.e. they will be matched to their new MN

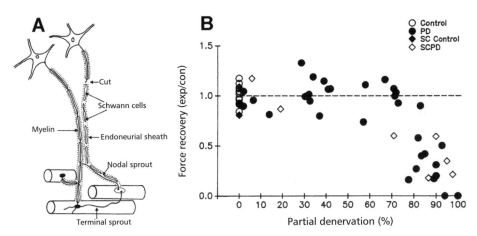

Figure 10.3. Sprouting and collateral reinnervation. (**A**) Diagram showing nodal and terminal sprouting of motor axons in skeletal muscle. Nodal sprouts must cross two endoneurial sheaths to gain access to the track to the denervated endplate. Terminal sprouts may have to run for some way on the surface of innervated fibres. (Reproduced with permission, from Brown 1984.) (**B**) Maximum tetanic force exerted by the tibialis anterior muscle of the rat 4–12 months after different amounts of denervation by sectioning of ventral root fibres. Forces are expressed as the ratio of the force exerted by the partially denervated muscle to that exerted by the intact con-tralateral muscle. Data for muscles from control animals (open circles), animals with a partially denervated muscle (filled circles), animals with a spinal cord transection (filled diamonds), and animals with both spinal cord transection and partial denervation (open diamonds). (Reproduced with permission, from Gordon *et al.* 1993.)

in the same way as was described above for reinnervation after cutting a nerve. Some studies of sprouting have shown unexpected crossed effects, apparently transferred via the spinal cord from the MNs on one side to homologous cells on the other (frog, Rotshenker 1979; mouse, Rotshenker and Tal 1985). Contralateral effects have also been noticed in experiments with cross-reinnervation (muscle histochemistry, Reichmann *et al.* 1983).

Collateral reinnervation is a very powerful mechanism in compensating for the effects of partial muscle denervation. Motor unit size might become increased by a factor of up to 5–8, and a muscle weakening due to MN loss might not become apparent until more than 80 per cent of all the MNs have disappeared (Fig. 10.3B) (Gordon *et al.* 1993). However, in a long-term perspective, MNs which maintain a very large number of target cells might be more vulnerable (see section 10.6.2, post-polio syndrome).

The appearance of sprouts might normally be actively inhibited by trophic substances of some kind which are released by innervated and active muscle fibres. Also in an innervated muscle, motor axons will generate sprouts if the muscle is paralysed using BoTx (Meunier *et al.* 2002). The intramuscular administration of NT-4 was reported to cause sprouting of intact adult motor nerves (Funakoshi *et al.* 1995).

10.6. **Pathophysiological issues**

10.6.1. **Nerve trauma and restoration of function**

In peripheral neurosurgery, the two major problems encountered after motor nerve injury are (a) how to enable the interrupted nerve to grow out towards the region containing the target muscles, and (b) how to enable the motor axons to make correct selections as to precisely which muscle to innervate.

With regard to problem (a), the classical approach has been to guide regenerating nerves towards the desired target region using nerve sheaths, which provide an ideal guiding structure and an appropriate Schwann-cell-generated biochemical surrounding for growing nerve fibres. If part of the original nerve sheath has become destroyed, the gap may be filled using the sheath of a less essential nerve from elsewhere, typically a skin nerve ('nerve transplantation'). For years, experimental attempts have also been made in various laboratories to guide regenerating nerves using tubes of synthetic materials (e.g. using biodegradable substances, Meek *et al.* 2001).

A special innervation problem exists in cases of spinal cord injury in which MNs have been destroyed. Muscles might then be rescued from denervation atrophy and death by providing new innervating MNs. Promising efforts in this direction are being made using embryonic spinal cord cells transplanted into the distal stump (sheath) of a peripheral nerve (rat, Thomas *et al.* 2000, 2003; mouse, MacDonald *et al.* 2003).

With regard to problem (b), no useful strategies have yet been found. Major peripheral nerves, which are easily damaged in accidents, normally supply motor axons to several muscles with different biomechanical functions. As was described above, regenerating nerve fibres of adult mammals are incapable of finding their way towards their 'own' muscle. Because of this navigational disability, there is often a disappointingly slight degree of recovery of normal motor functions after peripheral nerve damage, even if all muscles have been successfully reinnervated. Why is this such a major problem?

Inside the CNS, MNs are prewired with regard to their motor functions, and centrally generated activity patterns do not easily adapt to changes in the peripheral connections; for instance, flexor MNs largely continue to act as such even if connected to extensor muscles (O'Donovan *et al.* 1985; Gordon *et al.* 1986a). As long as the natural MN pools remain intact to serve as 'command units' for whole muscles (Chapter 5, section 5.4, and Chapter 8, section 8.2), changes in peripheral organization might to some extent be compensated for by motor learning. Thus a limited degree of improvement of motor coordination will occur with time after cross-connecting the tendons of flexors to extensors, with a different rate of adaptive success for different MN pools (Wiedemann *et al.* 1997). However, such motor learning is apparently (and expectedly) exceedingly dificult to achieve if the normal pool organization is disrupted, for example when MNs originally destined for a single muscle have become distributed across a whole group of muscles with different biomechanical functions. The motor control confusion will, of course, be further aggravated by problems of navigation in the regeneration of damaged sensory fibres.

10.6.2. Poliomyelitis and post-polio syndrome

In the virus disease poliomyelitis, muscle weakening and paralysis is caused by the death of MNs. Much of the resulting muscle denervation is compensated for by collateral reinnervation, and surviving patients often have muscles with very large muscle units, sometimes combined with a normal voluntary strength. In developed nations, vaccination schemes introduced in the 1950s have been highly successful and almost no new cases of polio are emerging in these countries. However, in survivors of acute paralytic polio, new symptoms have been found to occur several decades later (post-polio syndrome) (reviewed by Sunnerhagen and Grimby 2001). In addition to general complaints concerning issues such as muscle and joint pain and fatigue, there is also a progressively increasing weakness and muscle atrophy. These symptoms are more striking in patients who originally, just after the acute stage, showed the most remarkable recovery of force following an initial paralysis (Klingman *et al.* 1988). Thus the post-polio syndrome seems particularly prone to appear in patients who profited from a large degree of collateral reinnervation, presumably having exceedingly enlarged motor units. At least in the most rapidly progressive cases of the post-polio syndrome, measurements suggest a gradual decrease in the number of surviving MNs (McComas *et al.* 1993). Some of these MNs may have died because of mechanisms associated with ageing (Chapter 12, section 12.12). However, the post-polio syndrome might perhaps also be partly generated by some kind of very long-term 'stress' produced in MNs that have to support an abnormally large number of terminal nerve endings and muscle fibres (biochemical overload due to the requirements of too many peripheral targets?).

Chapter 11

Long-term plasticity

11.1. General issues

It is well known that the properties of muscles can be altered by training or disuse, i.e. by changing their activity patterns during weeks to months. Such slow processes (which also include adjustments taking place inside the CNS) are important for the adaptation of the neuromuscular system and the motoneuronal output to changing tasks. How are such slow adaptations influenced by activity patterns, i.e. what are the long-term effects of MNs on their own output parameters? This is a question of general relevance for many functions of the CNS and its various target structures. In Chapter 10, section 10.4.3.2, examples were given of how reinnervating slow and fast MNs can change the properties of muscle fibres such as to maintain an adequate MN versus muscle unit match (e.g. Fig. 10.2). We also know that slow and fast MNs have different daily amounts and frequency patterns of spike activity; compared with fast MNs, the slow MNs are active over a frequency range extending down to slower rates and during much longer periods of time per day (see Table 2.2, Chapter 6, section 6.9.3, and Chapter 8, section 8.2.5). Hence, the differences in activity between fast and slow MNs might be (partly) responsible for the differences in properties of their muscle fibres, i.e. these latter differences might be (partially) maintained because of differentiating kinds of natural 'training' of fast versus slow muscle fibres. Similarly, some of the effects of muscle denervation might be caused by the loss of normal patterns of activation. However, there is also a lively bidirectional traffic of molecules along axons, and MNs and muscle fibres might influence each other by molecular means, possibly independently of the action potential activity. Furthermore, many of the cell properties are set early in development. The neuromusclar system offers unique possibilities for investigating such various aspects of long-term interactions and plasticity.

11.2. Methods of studying use-related plasticity in the neuromuscular system

11.2.1. Voluntary training

Training is highly important in sport and revalidation, and bed rest may cause a great deal of physical weakness. The kinds of training to be dealt with in this book are mainly those of a simple non-skilled type, intending to improve basic qualities of muscle contractions such as the endurance or maximum force. There are qualitative differences in the results of different basic training patterns. Two major types are generally recognized: **endurance training** and **force training**. In either type of procedure, an improved physical performance might become noticeable within a few weeks and changes may proceed for several months of continued training (or even for several years for professional sportspersons or body-builders). Both types of training produce numerous biochemical and physiological changes within the neuromuscular system. Endurance training typically involves the production of submaximal muscle contractions for several hours per day (e.g. jogging or cycling). Force training involves maximal muscle contractions (e.g. weight-lifting), but the total daily training time may be considerably less than that for endurance training (cf. example in section 11.3.2.1) Endurance-trained athletes (e.g. marathon runners) have a great resistance to motor fatigue, but their muscles do not usually look particularly impressive (they may even seem more slender than normal) and they do not excel in force production. On the other hand, force-trained athletes have enlarged muscles of enhanced force, but do not necessarily show an increased resistance to fatigue. Voluntary training programmes are most easily applied in human experiments, but animal models have also been extensively used. Thus endurance training by running or swimming has often been used in animal studies (Jasmin *et al.* 1987; Nakano *et al.* 1997), and force-training programmes analogous to human weight-lifting have been implemented for cats and rats (Gonyea and Ericson 1976; Wirth *et al.* 2003; Hornberger and Farrar 2004).

11.2.2. Chronic electrical stimulation

During voluntary training activities, the different MNs and fibres of a muscle will be used to different extents because of the hierarchy of recruitment gradation (Chapter 8, section 8.2). When electrical stimulation is applied to a motor nerve, it is possible instead to activate all the units of a muscle in the same way. Therefore in studies of neuromuscular plasticity, results of artificial training programmes using 'chronic' electrical stimulation are often more easily interpreted than the results of natural training (see below). Furthermore, chronic stimulation can be given for longer times per day than is possible with voluntary training programmes.

For long-lasting chronic stimulation, the electrodes are either implanted or, in human experiments, attached to the skin (Salmons and Vrbova 1969; Rutherford and Jones 1988; Pette 2002). During the course of such investigations, it is important to certify that stimulation intensity is sufficient to activate all motor axons of the target nerve (Eerbeek *et al.* 1984); if not, the results will be more difficult to interpret. One of the concerns when using repetitive supramaximal electrical stimulation of peripheral nerves is that this treatment might cause pain and extra motor activity in the form of reflexes. In some investigations, such side effects were avoided by applying the stimulation to animals that had been deafferented on the experimental side (these animals had also been hemispinalized) (Eerbeek *et al.* 1984; Kernell *et al.* 1987a,b; see also Gordon *et al.* 1997). In the absence of chronic stimulation, experimental peroneus longus muscles of hemispinalized and deafferented animals retained a normal weight and maximal tetanic force after 10 post-operative weeks of observation. In response to Burke-type fatigue tests, they were slightly more fatigue sensitive than normal (probably because of their relative inactivity), and during brief high-rate bursts of activation they showed a normal persistence of force (Eerbeek *et al.* 1984).

When comparing the effects of different patterns of chronic stimulation, the amount of daily treatment can be quantified in two different ways: (a) in terms of the number of stimulation pulses delivered; (b) in terms of the total duration of time covered by the stimulation bursts (and, roughly, by the evoked contractile activity). Alternative (a) would be the optimal choice if each pulse had a similar effect on the muscle, independently of pulse rate. However, this is not the case for contractile muscle behaviour; the same total duration of contraction can be achieved at very different pulse rates (i.e. at different force levels), and contractile force is not directly proportional to pulse rate (Fig. 3.7A). As an alternative, daily amounts of chronic activation might instead be quantified in terms of the total time covered by activity per day (e.g. expressed as a percentage of 24 h) (Kernell *et al.* 1987b); this measure has the further advantage that it can be applied, for comparative purposes, to quantification of voluntary training programmes. In addition of the total daily duration of activity (and, perhaps, the daily distribution of activity periods) (Kernell *et al.* 1987b), pulse rate and the evoked contractile force are, of course, also interesting parameters in their own right (for further comments, see sections 11.3.2.1 and 11:3.3.3).

11.2.3. Muscle disuse due to decreased motoneurone input

Training programmes and chronic stimulation are typically employed in order to increase activity beyond a normal level. The opposite experimental situation, a decrease in motor activity, is most drastically achieved by a pharmacological block of the conduction of axonal action potentials (e.g. using TTX) (Spector 1985). For practical reasons (the capacity of implanted osmotic pumps for delivery of the blocking compound), such experiments are typically limited to time periods of about 4 weeks. In such experiments, the nerve should not be blocked with common local anaesthetics, such as procaine, which also inhibit fast intra-axonal transport mechanisms (Aasheim *et al.* 1974; Lavoie 1982).

An alternative non-pharmacological method for producing a marked long-lasting decrease in hindlimb MN activity in animals is to transect the spinal cord (**spinal transection** (ST)), typically at the low thoracic or upper lumbar level. In humans, a corresponding situation occurs in patients suffering from spinal cord injury at a cervical or thoraco-lumbar level. However, in chronic spinal cord damage, the MNs below the lesion may still be activated by various segmental reflexes (Zijdewind and Thomas 2001). From some points of view excitability is increased in chronic cases of spinal cord injury; even slight sensory stimuli will sometimes elicit relatively intense and transient spasms (e.g. evoked by slight touch or by a slight change in joint angles) (Thomas and Ross 1997).

Paradoxically, chronic spinal cord damage in humans may also be associated with the appearance of apparently spontaneous repetitive discharges in some of the MNs (Zijdewind and Thomas 2001) and, in subjects with incomplete lesions, voluntary MN discharges may be difficult to stop (Zijdewind and Thomas 2003). Similarly, in rats a low spinal transection leads to an increased reflex excitability and a tendency for plateau behaviour in MNs below the interruption (see section 11.4.2.2 for further details) (Bennett *et al.* 2004). In animal experiments, reflexes can be prevented by extending the operation such that, for a given portion of the spinal cord, all incoming channels from the periphery are removed by transection of the dorsal roots. Furthermore, the spinal cord can be transected both above and below the target segments. Such **spinal cord isolation** (SI) generally leads to almost complete MN silence which may be maintained for very long periods (Tower 1937; Steinbach *et al.* 1980; Pierotti *et al.* 1991). The ST and SI operations not only isolate MNs from synaptic input, tending to make them silent, but also partially denervate them, i.e. these MNs are deprived of biochemical influences from afferent, descending, or ascending fibres.

11.2.4. **Other models of neuromuscular disuse; changed muscle mechanics**

Muscles not only react to changed patterns of activation, but are also influenced by mechanical conditions such as their resting length, their predominant type of contraction with regard to concurrent length changes (concentric, isometric, eccentric), and the presence or absence of a load that resists shortening or promotes lengthening contractions. Long-term changes in muscle mechanics may play a role in all the training paradigms mentioned above as well as in various kinds of more specific disuse models, listed below.

1. Immobilization of joints (e.g. plaster cast) has been used in humans and animals as a method for discouraging motor activity. An important choice is whether immobilization occurs at a short, neutral, or long muscle length (see section 11.3.2.2). Immobilization may indeed lead to a considerable decrease in motor activity (e.g. Fuglevand *et al.* 1995), but typically not to a complete disuse (Fournier *et al.* 1983). However, the method is of interest for several reasons, including its relation to clinical plaster cast treatments of fractured limbs.

2. Space flight weightlessness (Ohira *et al.* 1992). Much of the normally ongoing motor activity is required for maintaining posture against gravity, which is removed by weightlessness during space flights.

3. Limb unweighting: in animals, limbs are unweighted using hindlimb suspension (Alford *et al.* 1987; Blewett and Elder 1993), and in humans unilateral lower limb suspension has been realized using a crutch (Berg *et al.* 1991). For antigravity hindlimb muscles, a somewhat similar unloading to that achieved in space flight weightlessness is achieved by using the methods for hindlimb unloading.

4. Human bed rest.

11.3. **Plasticity of muscle properties**

11.3.1. **Endurance-related properties**

11.3.1.1. Training and chronic stimulation may increase endurance

Endurance training and chronic electrical stimulation are both effective in producing increased endurance, as evaluated in fatigue tests lasting for a few minutes, for example using a 'Burke test', Fig. 11.1A). For a given training period, the extent of change seems largely dependent on the amount of chronic activation or voluntary training per day. For instance, in cat fast muscle (peroneus longus (PerL)), stimulation for 5 per cent of total time per day was sufficient for a substantial improvement of fatigue resistance, whereas stimulation for only 0.5 per cent of total time was insufficient (Fig. 11.1A,B; see also Table 11.2 below) (Kernell *et al.* 1987a). Also, for rat denervated soleus muscle, the fatigue resistance was significantly correlated with the total daily amount of chronic stimulation but not with the pulse rate of this treatment (Westgaard and Lomo 1988).

During chronic stimulation or voluntary endurance training, many changes in the muscle fibres happen more or less in parallel, including alterations in the sarcoplasmic reticulum (SR) and in enzymes for energy metabolism (Table 11.1) (reviewed by Pette and Staron 2000; Pette 2002). Thus, the activity of oxidative enzymes might show a 3- to 14-fold increase after stimulation for 2–5 weeks (e.g. succinic dehydrogenase (SDH), malate dehydrogenase, citrate synthase) and glycolytic and high-energy phosphate transfer enzymes might show a decrease (e.g. P-fructokinase, lactate dehydrogenase) (Henriksson *et al.* 1986). Compared with fatigue-sensitive fibres, fatigue-resistant fibres are normally better provided with enzymes for oxidative energy metabolism. However, the increased activity of oxidative enzymes is not the immediate cause of the increased endurance, as tested with a Burke-type fatigue test. During a period of chronic stimulation, endurance is improved before there are any significant changes in selected oxidative enzymes (e.g. SDH, Fig. 11.1) (Kernell *et al.* 1987a; Simoneau *et al.* 1993), i.e. the improved endurance was likely to have been a consequence of changes in excitation–contraction coupling processes (for further discussion concerning fatigue and metabolism, see Chapter 9, section 9.5.1). In contrast with the effects of voluntary endurance training, involving long-duration exercise at moderate force, high-intensity sprint training primarily causes an increase in the activity of key enzymes involved in glycogenolysis and anaerobic glycolysis (Roberts *et al.* 1982).

Chronic stimulation influences the electrophysiological behaviour of muscle during fatigue tests. In the cat PerL muscle, there is normally a decline of M-wave amplitude during a Burke-type fatigue test. This behaviour is drastically changed after even small daily amounts of chronic stimulation: following treatment for only 0.5 per cent of total time per day for 4 weeks, the EMG depression changed into a moderate degree of EMG potentiation (Fig. 11.2) (Kernell *et al.* 1987a). This small daily amount of chronic stimulation was insufficient for a significant improvement in muscle endurance (Fig. 11.1B). Thus the normal drop in M-wave amplitude during the fatigue test

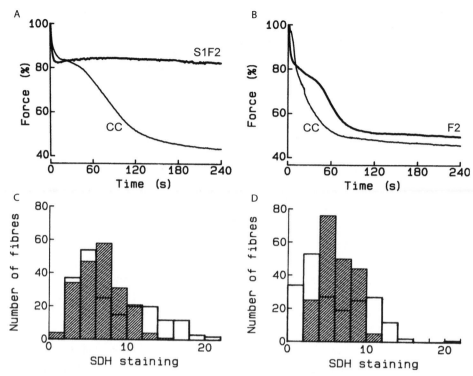

Figure 11.1 Effects of different daily amounts of chronic stimulation on fatigue resistance. Data for peroneus longus muscles (PerL) of cats. Plots of force versus time during Burke-type fatigue tests consisting of 0.33 s test bursts of stimulation at 40 Hz, repeated once every second for 4 min. Peak forces of successive bursts are joined by straight lines. Forces are given as percentages of maximum value for same fatigue test. Bold lines: data for chronically stimulated PerL muscle. Thin lines: data for contralateral PerL (control, CC) of same animal. (**A**) Animal treated for 8 weeks with chronic stimulation covering 5.5 per cent of total daily time (pattern S1F2: equal number of spikes at 10 Hz and 100 Hz, respectively). (**B**) Animal treated with chronic stimulation covering 0.5 per cent of daily time (pattern F2: 100 Hz bursts). Fatigue resistance was clearly improved by pattern S1F2 (equal effect after only 4 weeks), but hardly at all by the small daily amounts of pattern F2. (**C**),(**D**) Histograms showing the distribution of SDH staining intensity (optical density, per cent) among PerL muscle fibres subjected to chronic stimulation (hatched histograms) and their contralateral controls (open histograms): (**C**) stimulation pattern S1F2 (same muscles as panel **A**); (**D**) pattern F2. These types of relatively light chronic treatment have not yet caused any clear increase of SDH activity. (Reproduced with permission, from Kernell *et al.* 1987a.)

(Fig. 11.2A,B, Right) was presumably reflecting changes in the sarcolemmal action potential rather than a block of NMJ transmission. It is interesting to note that one of the early marked effects of chronic stimulation is an increase in the sarcolemmal concentration of the Na–K-ATPase, i.e. the Na–K-pump (Green *et al.* 1992), which would help to maintain normal ionic concentration gradients and action potential amplitudes during activity

Table 11.1 Changes in muscle fibre composition caused by large daily amounts of chronic low-frequency stimulation (fast to slow conversion)

Biochemical parameter	Functional relevance	Quantitative change	Isoform change
Membrane properties			
Na/K-ATPase (pump)	Membrane potential, AP conduction (sarcolemma, T tubules)	↑	
E/C coupling			
T-tubular volume	AP conduction (T tubules)	↓	
DHPR, RyR	Ca^{++} channels in triads	↓	
troponin-C (TnC)	with Ca^{++} → myosin-actin interactions		fast → slow
troponin-I (TnI)	regulation myosin-actin interactions		fast → slow
troponin-T (TnT)	—"—		1f/2f → 3f → 1s/2s
parvalbumin	Ca^{++} buffer	↓	
Ca^{++}-ATPase SR (pump)	Ca^{++} sequestering	↓	SERCA1a → 2a
calsequestrin	Ca^{++} sequestering	↓	
phospholamban	modify Ca^{++} ATPase	↑	
Myofilament composition			
myosin heavy chain (MHC)	shortening velocity, energy requirements		IIb → IIx → IIa → I
myosin light chain (MLC)	—"—		fast → slow
myosin ATPase activity	—"—	↓	
Metabolism			
oxidative enzymes (e.g., CS, MDH, SDH, etc.)	ATP production (oxidative)	↑	
glycolytic enzymes (e.g., LDH, PFK, etc.)	ATP production (anaerobic)	↓	
Protein management			
ubiquitin–proteosome system	catabolic processes	↑	
muscle mass	force	↓	

Examples illustrating the wide extent and complexity of the changes caused in skeletal muscle fibres by chronic stimulation.(list not complete). The alterations are quantitative as well as (in many cases) qualitative in the sense that stimulation causes a change of isoforms. *Abbreviations: AP*, action potential; *CS*, citrate synthase; *DHPR*, dihydropyridine receptor; *LDH*, lactate dehydrogenase; *MDH*, malate dehydrogenase; *PFK*, phophofructokinase; *RyR*, ryanodine receptor; *SDH*, succinate dehydrogenase; *SR*, sarcoplasmic reticulum; *triad*, contact region between T tubulus and SR. For further information and references, see Salmons and Henriksson (1981), Pette and Vrbova (1999), Pette and Staron (2000), Gardiner (2001), and Pette (2002).

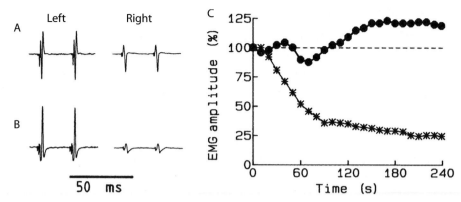

Figure 11.2 Effects of chronic stimulation on EMG behaviour. Peroneus longus muscle of cat, treated for 4 weeks with 100 Hz chronic stimulation covering 0.5 per cent of daily time (pattern F2). (**A**), (**B**) Compound muscle action potentials (M waves) evoked by muscle nerve stimulation during fatigue tests in control muscle (Right) and in muscle treated with chronic stimulation (Left). The Burke-type fatigue test consisted of 40 Hz bursts of 0.33 s duration, repeated once every second. Potentials in (**A**) were from the initial test burst and those in (**B**) from a test burst 2 min later (in all cases, the last two M waves of the respective burst; constant EMG amplification within each test). There was a marked decline in M-wave amplitude for the control muscle (Right) but not for the experimental one (Left). This is further illustrated in panel **c**, which shows the relative peak-to-peak amplitudes of M waves during the fatigue test for the experimental muscle (upper curve) and its contralateral control (lower curve). Plotted values refer to the last spike of each burst and amplitudes are normalized (per cent) relative to the initial burst of each test. The marked differences in EMG endurance (**c**) were not associated with any corresponding differences in force-endurance (cf. Fig. 11.1**B**, data for same muscles). (Reproduced with permission, from Kernell *et al.* 1987a.)

(cf. Hicks and McComas 1989). The existence of these types of EMG plasticity should be kept in mind when using EMG measurements for the indirect assessment of muscle fatigue during training procedures.

11.3.1.2. Effects of decreased activity

Severe muscle inactivity lasting for months or years after spinal transection or isolation (see section 11.2.3 above) causes changes in direction largely opposite to those of endurance training. Fatigue resistance and oxidative enzyme activities decrease and glycolytic enzyme activities may increase; the extent of the enzyme changes may vary with fibre type (Castro *et al.* 1999). This has been found in experimental animals (e.g. cat SI, enzyme activities, Jiang *et al.* 1991; endurance, Roy *et al.* 2002) as well as in patients with spinal cord injury (enzymes, Martin *et al.* 1992; Castro *et al.* 1999; endurance, Stein *et al.* 1992). The reactions after a shorter-lasting TTX block of the motor nerve (4 weeks or less) are similar but less marked (St-Pierre *et al.* 1988; Michel *et al.* 1994); however, in this case glycolytic enzymes might also show a decrease.

11.3.2. **Force and bulk**

11.3.2.1. Training and chronic stimulation may cause muscle fibres to grow or shrink

Force training requires the performance of strong contractions (resistance training). The resulting increase in maximum muscle force is largely dependent on fibre hypertrophy, and in human training programmes lasting about 20 weeks mean cross-sectional fibre areas may increase substantially; for example, triceps brachii, increase 15 per cent for type I and 17 per cent for type II (MacDougall *et al.* 1980), vastus lateralis, increase 14 per cent for type I and 32 per cent for type II (Hather *et al.* 1991). In addition to the fibre hypertrophy, some hyperplasia (i.e. increase in fibre numbers) might also occur after training (Giddings and Gonyea 1992; cf. Kernell *et al.* 1987b). Very limited daily amounts of actual training time are needed for a significant improvement in force and muscle bulk (Kraemer *et al.* 2002; Hornberger and Farrar 2004). For instance, Tesch *et al.* (2004) studied the improvement of knee extensor force in a one-legged training programme lasting 5 weeks (a total of 12 training sessions with 28 maximal concentric–eccentric contractions per session). The maximum voluntary extensor force was increased by 11–12 per cent, and the quadriceps volume by about 6 per cent. Each training session involved spending about 80 s in maximum contraction and an additional 70 s in actions at lower force (warm-ups). Hence, over the 5 weeks and 12 exercise sessions, the total amount of training time used for the performance of maximum and light to modest contractile activity amounted to approximately 16 min and 14 min, respectively. Even if we add both these durations, the total time of these training contractions corresponded to only 0.5 h/(5 × 7 × 24) h = 0.06 per cent of total time.

Muscle stretch may be an important factor in force training and body building. The fibre hypertrophy caused by maximum training contractions might partly be due to processes that are triggered by stretch- and deformation-sensing mechanisms in the muscle cells (Rennie *et al.* 2004). Correspondingly, one well-known method of producing hypertrophy of a muscle is simply to keep it stretched (Alway *et al.* 1989); however, compare absence of strengthening in stretched rat tibialis anterior (Pattullo *et al.* 1992). Similar results can be achieved for a weight-bearing muscle by removing or denervating its synergists ('overload') (reviewed by Goldspink 1999; Baldwin and Haddad 2001). In addition, the overload model may also cause the target muscle to be (temporarily) more active (Gardiner *et al.* 1986).

In most investigations of the effects of chronic stimulation on muscle properties, artificial 'training' was applied to experimental animals for large amounts of total time per day, often about 30 per cent or more. Muscles that are subjected to such large daily amounts of chronic stimulation typically become weaker (reviewed by Salmons and Henriksson 1981; see also Pette *et al.* 1975; Eerbeek *et al.* 1984; Kernell *et al.* 1987b; Gordon *et al.* 1997; Rafuse *et al.* 1997; Sutherland *et al.* 1998, 2003). This weakening can be accounted for, largely or completely, as being caused by a decrease in muscle fibre diameter, i.e. a loss of contractile material (Donselaar *et al.* 1987; Kernell *et al.* 1987b; Rafuse *et al.* 1997). Some people have been worried by this weakening and interpreted it as a sign of damage, analogous to the atrophy seen after inactivity and denervation. Intense chronic stimulation may indeed cause some damage and even fibre death, particularly in an initial stage and for fast glycolytic fibres (Maier *et al.* 1986; Schuler and Pette 1996), but in some muscles and under appropriate circumstances the incidence of such fibre damage may be very low, and it does not seem to be a necessary condition for other muscle effects of chronic stimulation (Lexell *et al.* 1992). It is highly likely that the weakening that cannot be accounted for as being due to fibre death (fibre loss) actually represents a type of physiological adaptation to a large daily amount of activity; perhaps the decrease in fibre diameter is useful for causing a decrease in intracellular diffusion distances. Muscles which have become weakened as a result of chronic stimulation typically seem quite healthy from other points of view, having a greater resistance to fatigue than fibres of normal non-treated muscles (Eerbeek *et al.* 1984). Furthermore, weakening is one of the most rapidly reversible effects of chronic stimulation; the muscle bulk and strength return after the end of stimulation about as fast as they declined at the onset of treatment (Brown *et al.* 1989; Kernell and Eerbeek 1991). It might be appropriate to refer to this weakening and the associated decrease in fibre size by a term like 'adaptive shrinkage' rather than using pathology-insinuating terms like 'atrophy'.

The degree of adaptive shrinkage seen after chronic stimulation depends not only on the daily amount of activation but also on the impulse rate of muscle activation during the treatment, i.e. presumably on the strength of the evoked contractions. Strong contractions, caused by higher pulse rates of chronic treatment, counteract weakening and fibre shrinkage (Eerbeek *et al.* 1984; Kernell *et al.* 1987b; Westgaard and Lomo 1988). The force-promoting effects of strong contractions were clearly demonstrated in experiments on the peroneus longus muscle of cats; chronic stimulation at 10 Hz for 5 per cent of total time caused a 30 per cent weakening and decrease in fibre area, whereas no weakening was seen after the same pattern plus extra interspersed bursts of 100 Hz (duration of stimulation 4–8 weeks) (Table 11.2) (Kernell *et al.* 1987b). In cat muscles of this kind, 10 Hz would cause largely unfused twitches and 100 Hz would cause near-maximal contractions. Similar force-promoting effects of high MN rates of firing were also observed in one study on humans (Rutherford and Jones 1988). Thus, in accordance with general exercise principles, strong training contractions are favourable for the maintenance (or increase) of muscle strength. Some human muscles might be less sensitive to the weakening effects of large daily amounts of activity. For instance, no weakening (but a significant slowing of isometric speed and improvement of endurance) was observed with chronic stimulation of the tibialis anterior muscle in patients with spinal cord injury (20 Hz, 50 per cent of total time) (Stein *et al.* 1992). However, the force-promoting effects of near-maximal activation (e.g. strength training) and the potentially opposite effects of large daily amounts of submaximal contractions (e.g. endurance training) correspond well to the consequences seen when training is stopped (detraining, section 11.3.5); the muscle fibre cross-sectional area then declines rapidly in strength and sprint athletes and in subjects who have recently undergone endurance training, whereas it may increase slightly in endurance athletes (reviewed by Mujika and Padilla 2001).

The fact that large amounts of slow impulse rates are prone to causing an adaptive shrinkage and weakening of limb muscles fits well with the fact that, also in normal untreated muscles, the fibres that are used during the longest accumulated times per day (type I fibres, S units) are generally thinner than those of faster and more phasically used units (e.g. type IIB fibres, FF units; Fig. 3.4).

In addition to the effects on muscle bulk and maximum tetanic force, chronic stimulation may influence the relative size of the twitch (the TwTet ratio). These effects also depend on the spike frequency of chronic stimulation; low rates (which tend to cause fibre shrinkage) promote a high TwTet ratio and high rates result in a smaller TwTet ratio (Eerbeek *et al.* 1984; Kernell *et al.* 1987b; Westgaard and Lomo 1988). These effects are independent of the effects on the twitch speed and the tension–frequency relation (Eerbeek *et al.* 1984; Kernell *et al.* 1987b).

11.3.2.2. Decrease in activity and absence of stretch makes muscle fibres smaller and weaker

The extent to which a relatively inactive muscle weakens and becomes atrophic partly depends on its length. Immobilization of a muscle will often cause it to become markedly atrophic if kept at a brief physiological length, while immobilization at a long physiological length might cause much less or no atrophy (Gallego *et al.* 1979; Spector *et al.* 1982). For instance, in animals subjected to a unilateral hemispinalization and deafferentation, the peroneus longus muscle was kept at a long length within its normal range of movement. These muscles were quite inactive and slightly more fatiguable than normal peroneus longus muscles, but their maximum force and muscle fibre sizes remained normal (Eerbeek *et al.* 1984; Donselaar *et al.* 1987). Hence, when studying the effects of inactivity caused by, for instance, TTX block of nerves or transection of the spinal cord, information about the muscle length is important for judging the possible causes of changes in bulk and force.

In many cases, the degree of muscle atrophy upon inactivity correlates with the normal muscle activity. Thus the largest degree of atrophy is often observed in those muscles and fibres for which the relative degree of disuse seems most prominent; for example, there is more atrophy for legs than for arms after bed rest (LeBlanc *et al.* 1992). Measurements indicate that arms are normally used more than legs (Kern *et al.* 2001), but much arm use might continue while lying in bed whereas leg use would then be largely absent. Correspondingly, disuse-related atrophy is typically larger in extensors (anti-gravity muscles) than in flexors (need not be weakened at all), and greater in muscles with a high percentage of the slow type I fibres (e.g. as seen after spinal cord transection) (Lieber *et al.* 1986a; Roy *et al.* 1999b); however, owing to possible changes in specific tension, even a substantial atrophy does not necessarily result in a decreased maximal tension

(Lieber *et al.* 1986b). After 6 months of spinal cord isolation, all fibre types had more similar small diameters (Roy *et al.* 1992).

The atrophy caused by a complete TTX block of motor nerves differs from that of other disuse models in that the muscle changes are as large (or even larger) for fast muscles and type II fibres as for slow muscles and type I fibres (St-Pierre and Gardiner 1985; Michel *et al.* 1994); in other models of disuse, small daily quantities of neural activity may perhaps occur which are sufficient for the maintenance of force and bulk in fast muscle fibres (see discussion in Gardiner 2001).

11.3.3. Speed and frequency gradation properties

Possible effects of activity on twitch speed were suggested by the results of Buller *et al.* (1960b) in their studies of cross-reinnervation between fast and slow muscles (Fig. 10.2). They demonstrated that this intervention produced no slowing of the cross-reinnervated fast muscles if performed in kittens which also had a transection of the spinal cord and hence possessed highly inactive muscles (Buller *et al.* 1960b). Long-term slowing effects of muscle activation on isometric twitch speed were first clearly demonstrated by Salmons and Vrbova (1969), who treated hindlimb muscles of adult cats and rabbits with chronic electrical stimulation for several weeks (Fig. 11.3A). In order to imitate, coarsely, the activity of slow MNs, they then activated fast mixed muscles continuously with the physiologically slow rate of 10 Hz. Other early experiments showed that the effects of chronic stimulation were not limited to the isometric aspects of speed, but there were also slowing effects on maximum shortening velocity (al-Amood *et al.* 1973). Furthermore, Lomo *et al.* (1974) added the important observation that long-term effects of activity on muscle properties would also be obtained in denervated muscles, i.e. these actions did not depend on chemical factors released by motor nerve fibres (for further comments and references, see section 11.3.6.2).

In general, muscles are pushed towards slower contractions when the daily amount of activity is increased, and towards faster contractions when daily activity is decreased. Such changes are seen for both the major aspects of speed: maximal unloaded shortening speed (highly dependent on myosin composition) and isometric twitch speed (highly dependent on Ca^{2+} kinetics and other aspects of excitation–contraction coupling (see Chapter 3, section 3.3.2)).

11.3.3.1. Training and chronic stimulation cause sequential changes of various speed-related properties

In chronic stimulation experiments, a slowing of twitch speed may be seen after only a few days (Fig. 3.6B), and in similarly short times changes also take place in many parameters of importance for excitation–contraction coupling: decreased number of T tubuli and volume of sarcoplasmic reticulum (Eisenberg and Salmons 1981), decreased concentration of the Ca^{2+} buffer parvalbumin, and decreased activity of 'fast' Ca^{2+}-ATPase (Ca^{2+} pump of SR, Fig. 3.6B (Klug *et al.* 1988)). On the other hand, a

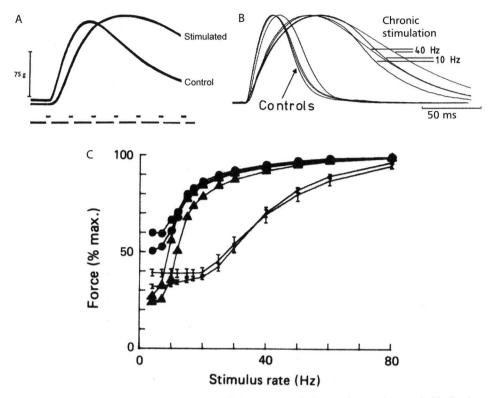

Figure 11.3 Effects of large daily amounts of chronic stimulation on isometric speed. (**A**) Slowing effects of chronic stimulation on rabbit tibialis anterior muscle: isometric twitch contractions of control muscle and muscle stimulated for 41 days. The chronic stimulation was given continuously at 10 Hz. Time mark: 10 ms intervals. (Reproduced with permission, from Salmons and Vrbova 1969.) (**B**) Similar slowing effects of 10 and 40 Hz patterns of chronic stimulation on isometric twitch contractions of cat PerL muscles. Controls: twitches from non-stimulated side of same four animals. The chronic activation covered 50 per cent of daily time for 8 weeks (pattern of 1 s on, 1 s off). In order to facilitate comparisons of time course, the twitches are displayed on a common time scale but with normalized amplitudes. (**c**) Contractile peak force (per cent of maximum) plotted versus rate of constant frequency test stimuli for muscles of panel **B** (triangles, 40 Hz chronic stimulation; circles, 10 Hz chronic stimulation). Data for rates above 80 Hz not shown. Average tension–frequency curves are also plotted for two groups of PerL muscles which had not been subjected to chronic stimulation (curves with vertical bars, means ± SE). Uppermost control curve at lower rates, mean for the four contralateral muscles of panel **B**; lowermost curve, mean for nine muscles from normal animals. The tension–frequency relation was similar in all the chronically treated muscles, despite the differences in relative twitch size. (Reproduced with permission, from Eerbeek *et al.* 1984.)

substantial increase in type I mATPase staining or slow MHC expression may take several weeks to appear for the same kind of chronic activation (reviewed by Pette 2002). This longer latency is caused partly by the sequential changes in MHC composition that precedes the appearance of slow type I myosin (see below), and partly by the relatively long turnover times of myosin molecules; mRNA changes appear much earlier than the changes in protein composition.

During ongoing muscle change, many fibres will display mixed MHC compositions. Normally there are few fibres with mixtures of type I MHC and varieties of type II MHC. During chronic stimulation, training, or disuse such mixtures become more common (reviewed by Pette and Staron 2000; Pette 2002). In muscles containing all four main types of mammalian MHC (e.g. fast limb muscles of rats), the changes in MHC composition take place in the sequence IIb → IIx → IIa → I. Thus, during initial periods of this process, the main effect might be a decrease in type IIb MHC and an increase in type IIx MHC, while later IIx may decrease and IIa increase. In addition to such MHC changes, there are also numerous other proteins which change from a 'fast' to a 'slow' isoform (Table 11.1) (Pette and Staron 2000; Pette 2002).

11.3.3.2. Different daily amounts of activity cause different degrees of slowing and MHC conversion: differences in 'adaptive threshold'

The extent of change in MHC composition, as investigated using (immuno-)histochemistry, is generally much less dramatic after voluntary training programmes than after large daily amounts of chronic stimulation. In the past it was sometimes even doubted whether voluntary training would cause any increase in the occurrence of slow myosin isozymes. Later experiments have proved that such changes may indeed occur. Rat muscles become both isotonically and isometrically slower when subjected to several weeks of compensatory overload (Roy et al. 1982), and there are also evident increases in the percentage of type I fibres (Oakley and Gollnick 1985). However, long-length muscle immobilization without increased activity may apparently cause an increased percentage of type I fibres without isometric signs of slowing (Pattullo et al. 1992). In human voluntary training, alterations of type I fibre frequencies take place, but the effects tend to be relatively slight. For instance, 15 weeks of high-intensity work raised the percentage of type I fibres by only about 6 per cent units (vastus lateralis, increase from 41 to 47 per cent) (Simoneau et al. 1985; cf. also Howald et al. 1985). This is in contrast with the findings that 8 weeks of chronic stimulation may change all the fibres of a fast mixed muscle to type I, expressing slow-type myosin (Rubinstein et al. 1978; Donselaar et al. 1987). When interpreting such differences between voluntary training and chronic stimulation, it should be remembered that most programmes of chronic stimulation involve daily amounts of activity which vastly exceed those of normal motor behaviour. Chronic stimulation patterns often cover about 30–100 per cent of total time, whereas in normal daily movements (albeit not during training) the most active units of fast mixed hindlimb muscles are active for only about 2–10 per cent of total time (Fig. 8.3, Chapter 8, section 8:2.5) (Monster et al. 1978; Hensbergen and Kernell 1997; Hodgson et al. 2001; Kern et al.

2001). For the least active units, normal activity periods might perhaps cover only 0.05 per cent or less of total time (Hennig and Lomo 1985; Hodgson *et al.* 2001).

In a fast mixed limb muscle of the cat (peroneus longus), some chronic stimulation patterns covering 5 per cent of total time per day cause only a rather modest increase in type I fibre composition (from 19 to 23 per cent), even though all muscle units received the same 'training' (10 Hz, 8 weeks, supramaximal nerve stimulation) (Kernell *et al.* 1987b). With 50 per cent of time covered by extra activity, 100 per cent of the peroneus longus fibres become type I (Donselaar *et al.* 1987). Such 'threshold differences' in the willingness of fibres to switch from type II to type I were systematically explored by Sutherland *et al.* (1998), who stimulated rabbit tibialis anterior muscles continuously for 10 months at 2.5 Hz, 5 Hz or 10 Hz. In their experiments, all fibres became type I following the 10 Hz treatment, but only about 15 per cent were converted to type I by the 2.5 Hz treatment. In the 5 Hz group, results were highly variable, with some muscles resembling the 10 Hz group and some the 2.5 Hz cases. These experiments indicate that, even for fibres of the same phenotype and within the same muscle, the threshold for a switch to type I may be very different. This is also indicated by the opposite type of experiment. A drastic decrease in MN activation for a few months causes many, but not all, of the type I fibres to switch to type II (see section 11.3.3.4). Thus, in addition to activity, other factors are also important for specifying muscle fibre speed (see section 11.3.6.3); fibres do not necessarily acquire the same properties by being activated with the same spike patterns (see also Gordon *et al.* 1997).

11.3.3.3. The speed-changing effects of chronic stimulation are not consistently related to pulse rate

In the original stimulation experiments of Salmons and Vrbova (1969), it was unclear whether the slowing effects were dependent on chronic muscle activation at low rates and/or for prolonged periods of time per day, both of which would be consistent with the discharge properties of slow MNs. In their experiments on rabbits some evidence was obtained in favour of an importance of spike frequency; slow rates (5–10 Hz) but not faster ones (20–40 Hz) counteracted the speeding-up of tenotomized soleus muscles (Salmons and Vrbova 1969). However, the interpretation of these findings is complex, partly because the tenotomized soleus muscles often showed a considerable degree of atrophy (cf. McMinn and Vrbova 1967).

The idea that pulse rates would be important for the speed-changing effects of activity received considerable support from the experimental findings of Lomo *et al.* (1974), who studied the effects of chronic stimulation on the denervated slow soleus muscle of the rat. In the absence of stimulation, the twitch of the denervated soleus muscle initially slowed down (Fig. 11.4A, Dn). Treatment with slow rates (10 Hz) made the muscle remain as slow as the normal soleus (Dn + 10), and treatment with 100 Hz bursts caused the muscle twitch to become considerably faster (Fig. 11.4A, Dn + 100). In later experiments further evidence was found for truly frequency-related effects: the slowing influence of low-rate chronic stimulation could be partly counteracted by additionally superimposed bursts of high rates (Westgaard and Lomo 1988; see also Eken and Gundersen 1988). No such frequency-specific effects on contractile speed were found in corresponding experiments on the innervated peroneus longus muscle of the cat (compare 10 Hz with 10 + 100 Hz in Table 11.2) (Kernell *et al.* 1987b); thus the 'adaptability properties' might be preset in different ways for the denervated rat soleus and the innervated peroneus longus of the cat (see also discussion of adaptive ranges in section 11.3.6.3). Findings from other experiments on rat denervated soleus muscles (Al-Amood and Lewis 1987) have suggested that the rates of stimulation might be less important than the duration of the contractile periods. When different animals were treated with different spike rates but constant burst durations and burst intervals, no consistent relation was found between the speeding-up effects and spike rate.

These various experiments and those of others (Sréter *et al.* 1982) also showed that, when given in sufficient daily amounts, fast-rate stimulation may have a slowing effect on muscle that equals that of physiologically slow rates (Fig. 11.3B) (Eerbeek *et al.* 1984). Correspondingly, for large daily amounts of stimulation, both slow and fast rates converted all fibres into slow type I (mATPase, 50 per cent of time covered with activity, 10 Hz versus 40 Hz) (Donselaar *et al.* 1987). For peroneus longus muscles that had first been slowed down by large daily amounts of chronic stimulation, subsequent speeding-up was not promoted by additional 100 Hz bursts given during the recovery phase (Fig. 11.4B) (Kernell and Eerbeek 1991). Thus, in a normally innervated fast hindlimb muscle, the slowing effects of chronic stimulation seemed to depend mainly on the daily duration of additional activation; impulse frequency did not play an important role in this context. Other aspects of chronic activation patterns, including differences in train length, interval between stimulation trains, intervals between groups of stimulation trains, and the presence of initial doublets, might also be of importance for the effects (Lomo *et al.* 1974; Kernell *et al.* 1987b; Eken and Gundersen 1988; Westgaard and Lomo 1988; Lopez-Guajardo *et al.* 2000).

11.3.3.4. Lack of activity makes many slow fibres faster, but does not make muscles homogeneous in fibre type composition

Whatever the role of spike frequency, lack of activity generally tends to make an innervated slow muscle faster, with regard to the time course of its isometric twitch, its maximum shortening velocity, and its myosin composition (Spector 1985; Pierotti *et al.* 1991; Graham *et al.* 1992). However, even after 8 months of spinal cord isolation, allowing very little MN activity, only 38 per cent of cat soleus fibres were classified as fast, and more than 60 per cent of the fibres were still slow (cat soleus is normally 100 per cent slow) (Roy *et al.* 1996). In rat soleus, 12 per cent of the fibres still contained type I MHC after a very long survival period (up to 360 days) after spinal transection (rat soleus is normally about 85–90 per cent slow) (Talmadge *et al.* 1999); many of the remaining fibres were IIa + IIx hybrids and very few contained type IIb MHC. Thus even a long-lasting lack of activity does not produce a muscle of uniform myosin composition.

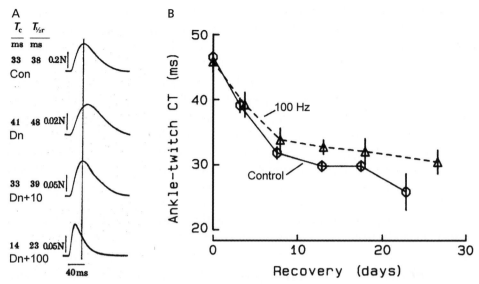

Figure 11.4 Varying effects of fast-rate chronic stimulation. (**A**) Isometric twitch contractions evoked by direct electrical stimulation of rat soleus muscle: Con, curarized but otherwise normal muscle; Dn, denervated for 39 days; Dn + 10, denervated and stimulated intermittently at 10 Hz for 36 days; Den + 100, denervated and stimulated intermittently at 100 Hz for 39 days. The 100 Hz stimulation was given with the same total number of stimuli per day as the 10 Hz treatment. Measured values for contraction time T_c and half-relaxation time $T_{1/2\,r}$ are noted beside each twitch. There is evident speeding up of the muscle treated with 100 Hz (lowest row). (Reproduced with permission, from Lomo et al. 1974 (added labels)) (**B**) Speeding up of ankle dorsiflexor muscles (eight cats) which had first been considerably slowed down by large daily amounts of chronic stimulation (40 Hz, 50 per cent of total time, 4 weeks). During this experiment, the twitch contraction time of the ankle dorsiflexors was measured repeatedly using electrical stimulation and an external measuring device (ankle-twitch CT) (for method, see Eerbeek and Kernell (1991)). The plot shows ankle-twitch CT (means ± SE) versus time during the recovery period following the 40 Hz chronic stimulation. During the period shown in the graph, four of the cats received no extra stimulation (solid lines), and four other animals received peroneal nerve stimulation with 100 Hz bursts for 0.5 per cent of total time (interrupted lines). This fast-rate treatment did not promote the speeding up of the ankle dorsiflexors (Reproduced with permission, from Kernell and Eerbeek 1991.)

11.3.4. **Contralateral effects of chronic stimulation**

Studies of peripheral motor axon sprouting have shown the existence of unexpected crossed effects, apparently somehow transferred via the spinal cord from the MNs on one side to homologous cells on the other side (see Chapter 10, section 10.5), and contralateral cytochemical muscle effects have also been observed in cross-reinnervation experiments (Reichmann et al. 1983). In experiments with heavy patterns of chronic stimulation, unexpected kinds of contralateral effects have been seen with regard to contractile muscle properties (cats with deafferentation and spinal cord transection on the stimulated side); the non-stimulated contralateral muscles (peroneus longus) often become less capable of maintaining a steady force during 1 s high-rate bursts (100 Hz test stimulation) (Eerbeek *et al.* 1984, Fig. 5B), possibly because of a failure of neuromuscular transmission. From other points of view these contralateral muscles seemed normal; this included their maximum tetanic force, twitch speed, and fatigue resistance as tested with 40 Hz bursts. In the absence of chronic stimulation, both the ipsilateral and contralateral muscles of these animals had normal properties (see section 11.2.2). On the chronically stimulated side, forces were well maintained during 100 Hz stimulation. These intriguing contralateral effects were not seen with chronic stimulation programmes covering about 5.5 per cent or less of total time (Kernell *et al.* 1987b).

11.3.5. Sequence of muscle changes following the end of training or chronic stimulation (detraining)

The timing of the various muscle changes taking place during and after training is of practical as well as theoretical interest. Such timing studies are more easily performed using chronic stimulation than voluntary training programmes. Various aspects of the timing of changes during chronic stimulation have already been commented on in preceding sections (for further details, see reviews by Pette and Staron 2000; Pette 2002). Interestingly, the timing of detraining is not a simple mirror image of the rates at which various changes are acquired. Brown *et al.* (1989) treated fast-twitch rabbit muscles for 6 weeks with slow-rate chronic stimulation, which made them slower, more fatigue resistant, and weaker than normal controls. In the subsequent recovery period, maximum tetanic force and the time course and potentiation of the isometric twitch returned to normal in about 3–4 weeks, and this was also true for the increased percentage of slow type I fibres. However, the stimulation-evoked enhancements in fatigue resistance, capillary density, and oxidative enzyme activity declined over a longer period of time, and normal properties had only returned about 12 weeks after the end of the chronic stimulation. At an ultrastructural level, several of the changes did not recover to normal values until about 9–12 weeks after cessation of stimulation (Eisenberg *et al.* 1984). Several of the observations of Brown *et al.* (1989) were confirmed in experiments on a fast-twitch hindlimb muscle of the cat (peroneus longus) which had been subjected to large daily amounts of chronic stimulation for 4 weeks (Kernell and Eerbeek 1991). After 4 weeks of recovery, the stimulation-evoked changes in maximum force (weakening) and twitch time course (prolongation) had disappeared (Fig. 11.4B), fatigue resistance was decreasing but still remained greater than normal, and the enhanced twitch–tetanus ratio and EMG endurance (Fig. 11.2) had not yet started to recover from their post-stimulation levels. Thus, particularly for endurance-associated properties, there seems to be an interesting hysteresis in the training–detraining time course, which is potentially of a useful nature; endurance is apparently more quickly gained than lost.

The effects of detraining following voluntary exercise programmes also indicate that many of the training-induced properties revert to non-trained values relatively slowly.

In humans, a decline in capillary density may be seen within 3–4 weeks, and the percentage of oxidative fibres may decrease in endurance athletes and increase in strength-trained athletes within 8 weeks of stopping training (reviewed by Mujika and Padilla 2001). In horses, prolonged training programmes induced changes that were still present after 6 weeks of inactivity (e.g. increased fibre area, capillarization, mitochondrial volume, and treadmill run time) (Tyler *et al.* 1998), whereas in another study most of the exercise-induced alterations reverted after 3 months of detraining (e.g. increases of type IIa and type I MHC and oxidative enzymes, and decrease in anaerobic enzymes (Serrano *et al.* 2000).

11.3.6. Muscle use versus other factors in muscle plasticity

11.3.6.1. Motor nerves have activity-independent effects on muscle

It is a common clinical observation that muscles become more atrophic after denervation than after mere inactivity. Electrical activation counteracts some of the atrophy caused by denervation, but the effects are incomplete. For instance, chronic high-frequency stimulation, starting several months after denervation of rat hindlimb muscles, increased the mean maximum tetanic tension by a factor of 37 in the soleus and by a factor of 8 in the extensor digitorum longus (EDL). These values represented 40 per cent and 12 per cent, respectively, of the increases obtained by reinnervation after comparable periods of time (Hennig and Lomo 1987; cf. Westgaard 1975). Correspondingly, fast hindlimb muscles of the rat had lost more than 75 per cent of their original mass 2 weeks after denervation, whereas 2 weeks of almost complete lack of activation of innervated muscles caused an atrophy of only 40 per cent (inactivity caused by spinal cord isolation) (Hyatt *et al.* 2003). Part of the atrophy caused by denervation is counteracted by sciatic nerve extract injected into the muscle (rat) or even given systemically (intraperitoneally, mouse). The active factor is apparently a glycoprotein with a molecular weight of about 100 000; its exact nature still awaits clarification (Davis *et al.* 1985, 1988).

11.3.6.2. Activity-dependent effects may take place independently of innervation

Motoneuronal activity might conceivably exert effects on muscle properties, via the activity-dependent release of various biochemical inducing factors at the nerve terminal and/or by activating the muscle and causing it to contract. The latter type of MN effects is clearly very important, because most known effects of chronic stimulation on contractile muscle properties can also be obtained by direct activation of denervated muscle fibres (Lomo *et al.* 1974; Henriksson *et al.* 1982; Eken and Gundersen 1988; Gorza *et al.* 1988; Gundersen *et al.* 1988; Westgaard and Lomo 1988; Ausoni *et al.* 1990; Windisch *et al.* 1998; in organ culture, Barton-Davis *et al.* 1996; reviewed by Gardiner 2001), and this is also true for muscle membrane properties that are altered as a result of denervation and loss of activity (e.g. AChR distribution, Lomo and Rosenthal 1972; passive electrical properties, Westgaard 1975).

11.3.6.3. Individual muscles and muscle fibres may have different 'adaptive ranges'

Individual muscle fibres may differ from each other with regard to their use-related adaptability. This is most easily demonstrated by comparing the fibres of different muscles and animal species after the same kind of long-term treatment. For instance, in reponse to chronic stimulation, the activity of metabolic enzymes changes much less in mice than in rats, guinea pigs, and rabbits (Simoneau and Pette 1988), and a fast-to-slow transition of muscle fibres is more readily produced in rabbits than in rats (Kwong and Vrbova 1981; Kirschbaum *et al.* 1989); in rats, this process takes about 4 months (Windisch *et al.* 1998). When applying different patterns of direct chronic stimulation to the denervated slow soleus and the fast EDL muscles of the rat, the 'adaptive range' of induceable twitch-time course values was much wider for soleus than for EDL (Eken and Gundersen 1988; Westgaard and Lomo 1988). In the cat, 8 weeks of high daily amounts of chronic stimulation made the peroneus longus twitch as slow as that for slow units in the normal peroneus longus muscle, but not as slow as that for normal soleus units (Eerbeek *et al.* 1984). As was noted above (section 11.3.3.4), absence of activity does not make all fibres equal in myosin composition (e.g. Talmadge *et al.* 1999). After reinnervation the MNs may clearly change the myosin-type for many of their new muscle fibres (Chapter 10, section 10.4.3.2), but some individual muscle fibres are apparently resistant to change (Unguez *et al.* 1993; 1995). Thus many of the malleable properties of muscle fibres are somehow 'preset' with regard to the range within which they may be adjusted by activity. The nature of these presetting factors is still uncertain; possibly they include factors associated with non-neural differentiation mechanisms in early development (cf. Condon *et al.* 1990). Activity is clearly not the only factor determining how muscle fibres will differ from each other in their properties (Miller and Stockdale 1987).

11.3.6.4. Different muscle properties may, to some extent, be modified independently of each other

Particular patterns of activity may, to some extent, have different combined effects on muscle properties (Westgaard and Lomo 1988; Sutherland *et al.* 2003). One of several possible examples is illustrated in Table 11.2, where the effects on properties of the cat peroneus longus muscles are compared for three different patterns of chronic stimulation (Kernell *et al.* 1987a,b). All three patterns had the same effect of mild slowing on the time course of the isometric twitch (TwCT). Endurance was improved by the two patterns that were delivered during 5 per cent or more of total time (S1, S1F2). Force was decreased by the 5 per cent pattern given at the slow rate of 10 Hz (S1), but not by the two other patterns (S1F2, F2). Thus, each of these three stimulation patterns had a different profile of muscle effects. This implies that, whatever signals trigger the biochemical changes caused by long-term muscle activation, one such signal is not enough (see next section); several different triggering signals appear to be required.

Table 11.2 Differential effects of patterns of chronic stimulation on muscle properties

Group[a]	Stimulus[b] (% time)	Stimulus[c] (Hz)	L/R force	Fatigue index[d]	TwCT (ms)	Int50 (ms)
S1	5	10	69 ± 15* (6)	79 ± 7* (6)	29 ± 4* (6)	37 ± 8* (6)
S1F2	5 + 0.5	10 + 100	107 ± 21 (6)	80 ± 6* (6)	30 ± 3* (6)	35 ± 5* (6)
F2	0.5	100	113 ± 33 (6)	58 ± 6 (5)	29 ± 3* (6)	35 ± 2* (5)
Control	–	–	99 ± 13 (5)	56 ± 6 (4)	23 ± 2 (9)	28 ± 3 (9)

Data from experiments with different patterns of chronic stimulation delivered to a fast hindlimb muscle (peroneus longus) in the cat. Duration of stimulation 4–8 weeks (both durations had similar results for all displayed parameters). Results displayed as mean ± SD (*n*). Control values taken from normal untreated cats(fatigue index, TwCT, and Int50) and from unstimulated experimental animals (L/R force).

Abbreviations: L/R force, ratio (%) of experimental to control side for maximum tetanic force; TwCT, twitch contraction time (i.e. time to peak); Int50, stimulation interval needed for 50% of maximum tetanic force.

* Statistical significance of difference versus control value (*t*-test), $P < 0.05$.

[a] Experimental groups of animals, each treated in a different way.

[b] Daily amount of chronic stimulation as a percentage of total time.

[c] Pulse rate of chronic stimulation bursts.

[d] Burke test , reciprocal ratio (%) of maximum contraction during the test to that occuring 2 min later during the same test.

Data from Kernell *et al.* 1987a,b.

11.3.6.5. Biochemical factors

A detailed discussion of the nature of the biochemical signalling cascades involved in muscle plasticity (reviewed by Fluck and Hoppeler 2003) falls outside the scope of this physiological monograph. The candidates for triggering some of these cascades include sarcoplasmic Ca^{2+} ions (Sréter *et al.* 1987; Everts *et al.* 1993; Carroll *et al.* 1999; Freyssenet *et al.* 1999; Meissner *et al.* 2000), the ratio ratio ATP/ADP_{free} (Conjard *et al.* 1998; Pette 2002), and the concentrations of phosphocreatine (PCr), which decreases during activity, and inorganic phosphate (P_i), which increases during activity. Regulating factors involved in myosin transformation processes include, for instance, calcineurin (Chin *et al.* 1998; Serrano *et al.* 2001), and with regard to the regulation of muscle bulk an important role is played by muscle regulatory factors (MRFs) such as Myf-5, MyoD1, MRF4, and myogenin (Adams *et al.* 1999; Hyatt *et al.* 2003; for further comments and references, see Gardiner 2001). Membrane stretch sensors, such as the the the integrins (transmembrane glycoproteins), are believed to play a role in the long-term effects of muscle stretch and high-resistance force training (reviewed by Carson and Wei 2000; Mayer 2003). The number of intramuscular nuclei may be important for an appropriate quantitative response; functional overload produces no muscle hypertrophy if the mobilization of new nuclei from satellite cells is prevented with X-irradiation (Adams *et al.* 2002).

11.3.6.6. Hormonal effects

Several different hormones have effects on muscle bulk and maximum force (reviewed by Sheffield-Moore and Urban 2004). The most famous examples are undoubtedly testosterone and its synthetic derivatives, the androgenic anabolic steroids (AASs) (reviewed by Hartgens and Kuipers 2004). Such substances are widely used as (non-permitted) doping agents in sports activities (Juhn 2003), despite several serious side-effects of various kinds. In human subjects, AASs have been observed to produce gains of up to about 5–20 per cent of the initial strength and increments of 2–5 kg in lean body mass. The increase in muscle mass has been attributed to both muscle hypertrophy and the formation of new muscle fibres, and a key role seems to be played by proliferating satellite cells which are incorporated into muscle fibres undergoing hypertrophy. In addition to testosterone and its analogues, several other hormones, including growth hormone, insulin, and insulin-like growth factor I (IGF-I), also have complex anabolic effects on skeletal muscle. On the other hand, glucocorticoids have direct catabolic effects and induce protein loss and muscle wasting (Kelly *et al.* 1986; Sheffield-Moore and Urban 2004).

Thyroid hormone directly affects both the myosin composition and the metabolic enzyme profile of muscles, and also plays an important role in the development and maturation of the neuromuscular system. With regard to the MHC composition of muscles in adult animals, hyperthyroidism causes slow to fast conversions, and hypothyroidism has the opposite effect (reviewed by Pette and Staron 2000; Baldwin and Haddad 2001). With regard to metabolic systems, thyroid hormone may cause an increase in both oxidative and glycolytic enzyme activity (Sickles *et al.* 1987), converting both SO and FG fibres to FOG fibres (Nicol and Bruce 1981).

There are also hormone effects from muscles on the rest of the body; skeletal muscles themselves (probably the muscle fibres) apparently have important endocrine functions (reviewed by Pedersen *et al.* 2003). Contracting muscles have long been thought to release 'exercise' or 'work' factors that have general anti-inflammatory effects and beneficial regulating influences on the cardiovascular and other supporting systems. It has been proposed that such effects might be mediated by the cytokine interleukin 6 (IL-6) which is produced in large quantities by exercising muscle and secreted into circulating blood.

11.4. Plasticity of motoneurone properties

11.4.1. Endurance parameters

Differentially expressed properties of MNs which might relate to variations in neuronal endurance include the following.

(a) The 'fatigue-resistance' of neuromuscular transmission, i.e. the extent to which ACh release declines during maintained repetitive activation at different rates (Chapter 4, section 4.4.4, Fig. 4.3). In this context the postsynaptic response properties during maintained repetitive activation also have to be taken into account.

(b) The activity of metabolic enzymes in the MN soma (e.g. SDH) (Fig. 5.5C), which might possibly be of importance for the maintenance of neuronal functions during long-lasting periods of increased discharge.

(c) The characteristics of the late phase of spike-frequency adaptation, which is normally less conspicuous for MNs of slow and fatigue-resistant units, possibly simply because these cells fire at relatively slow rates (Fig. 6.3).

The effects of altered use on parameters (a) and (b) are discussed further below. The extent to which the late spike-frequency adaptation might also be specifically influenced by altered MN use is potentially interesting but still unknown.

11.4.1.1. Neuromuscular transmission

There is generally a systematic difference between the 'synaptic endurance' of NMJs of fast and slow units; during repetitive activation, the quantal content decreases less rapidly for slow (fatigue-resistant) NMJs than for those of faster units (Fig. 4.3) (Reid *et al.* 1999). Such type-associated differences might largely depend on the amounts and patterns of daily activity generated by the respective MNs. Reid *et al.* (2003) delivered different patterns of chronic stimulation to inactive nerves (proximal TTX block) of fast and slow hindlimb muscles in the rat ('fast' pattern of brief 150 Hz bursts, 'slow' pattern of longer 20 Hz trains; fast nerve to extensor digitorum longus, slow nerve to soleus). After 3–4 weeks of treatment with a 'fast' pattern, the slow nerve showed a fast-type decline of EPP quantal content, and treatment with a 'slow' pattern produced the opposite type of change for the fast nerve (Fig. 4.3). The TTX block alone did not change the run-down behaviour of the slow nerve EPPs.

In fast as well as slow NMJs, the 'safety factor' for neuromuscular transmission (Chapter 4, section 4.4.2) appears to be improved by voluntary training. Thus voluntary endurance exercise causes an increased quantal content of EPPs (mouse fast muscle, Dorlochter *et al.* 1991; rat soleus, Desaulniers *et al.* 2001), and there is also a decreased run-down during repetitive activation (i.e. an increased 'synaptic endurance') (Desaulniers *et al.* 2001). The quantal content of EPPs is also increased in hindlimb antigravity muscles that are overloaded after removal of synergists (Argaw *et al.* 2004). Furthermore, in NMJs of both fast and slow hindlimb muscles, endurance training gives rise to increased quantities of ACh receptors (Desaulniers *et al.* 1998) and an increased size of fast and slow presynaptic nerve terminals (Andonian and Fahim 1988). Paradoxically, inactivity may also cause an increase in size of the presynaptic nerve terminals of fast muscle fibres (rat diaphragm, NMJs of type II fibres) (Prakash *et al.* 1995).

11.4.1.2. Metabolic enzymes of motoneurones

In normal MN populations, a negative correlation is typically found between soma size and the activity of the oxidative enzyme SDH (see Chapter 5, section 5.3.1, Fig. 5.5C). It seems likely that differences in oxidative capacity between MNs have something to do with the total metabolic cost of their activities. However, it is still uncertain in which ways the functions of a MN would be at risk if the oxidative capacity were too low.

Chronic stimulation patterns which cause marked effects on the size and SDH activity of muscle fibres may have no effects on these parameters in the corresponding MNs (Donselaar *et al.* 1986). Similarly, no MN–SDH effects were found as a result of hindlimb extensor overload (Chalmers *et al.* 1991; Roy *et al.* 1999a), spinal transection or isolation (Chalmers *et al.* 1992), hindlimb suspension (Ishihara *et al.* 1997c), artificially increased force of gravity (rats in centrifuge) (Roy *et al.* 2001), voluntary exercise, or TTX block of motor nerves (Suzuki *et al.* 1991; Seburn *et al.* 1994). The only activity-related condition known so far which consistently tends to influence somatic SDH activity is microgravity; moderately sized hindlimb MNs of rats exhibited a decreased SDH activity after a 2 week space flight but no changes were observed in MNs of muscles with no weight-bearing functions, i.e. presumed perineal MNs (Ishihara *et al.* 2000).

Although voluntary motor exercise performed on Earth seems to have no consistent effect on somatic SDH activity, such contractions have been reported to cause an increase in other oxidative enzyme activities in rat MN cell bodies (malate dehydrogenase, Gerchman *et al.* 1975; citrate synthase in soleus MNs, Nakano *et al.* 1997). Furthermore, it should be remembered that somatic SDH activity can be influenced by other means than exercise; it is decreased after axotomy (Chalmers *et al.* 1992).

As was described above (section 11.3.6.6), thyroid hormone has an influence on the oxidative metabolism and MHC composition of muscle. Slow muscle fibres and their MNs (but not fast fibres and their MNs) both show increased NADH-tetrazolium reductase activity after treatment with thyroid hormone (Sickles *et al.* 1987).

11.4.2. Recruitment parameters

The ease with which MNs may become recruited is obviously important for the voluntary production of contractile force. In this context, three different factors will be discussed:

- intrinsic properties of the MNs that determine how much synaptic excitatory current will be needed to fire them (**intrinsic excitability**)
- the strength of the synaptic effects which may be mobilized for discharging the MNs
- conduction velocities of motor axons will also be considered, for two different reasons:
  - (i) a change in axonal conduction velocity might reflect a general change in MN excitability-related membrane properties (Carp *et al.* 2003)
  - (ii) conduction velocities of motor axons are used for categorizing MNs in studies of recruitment behaviour (see Chapter 8, section 8.2).

11.4.2.1. Motoneurone intrinsic excitability

The activating current needed to discharge a MN depends on its resting membrane potential, voltage threshold, input resistance, and subthreshold voltage-gated ion channels. There is clinical evidence suggesting that changes in MN recruitment parameters take place after spinal cord transection (ST); in chronic cases, there is not only muscle paralysis but also an increased reflex excitability and the occurrence of spasms (transient involuntary contractions) (section 11.2.3). However, investigations in anaesthetized animal preparations have produced rather little evidence for commensurate changes in intrinsic MN excitability in the chronic stage following ST. Gustafsson *et al.* (1982) noted a reduction in the electrotonic length of the dendrites (length of equivalent cylinder) and calculated that the peak voltage produced by a given synaptic input might be somewhat increased (cat, 2–3 weeks after ST). Baker and Chandler (1987a) found no significant changes in resting membrane potential, input resistance, rheobase current, or axonal conduction velocity (cat, 4–6 months after ST). Hochman and McCrea (1994b) also found no change of input resistance, rheobase current, or resting membrane potential. However, these authors found evidence for an increased voltage threshold (see also Cope *et al.* 1986) and an increased incidence or magnitude of subthreshold rectification, and they concluded that their results suggested, paradoxically, 'that ankle extensor motoneurons are less excitable in the chronic spinal state'. Finally, Bennett *et al.* (2001b), studying tail MNs of rats, also found no effect of chronic ST on input resistance or rheobase current (however, see below for effects on plateau behaviour).

The effects of keeping the target muscles inactive were investigated in rats by Cormery *et al.* (2000) using a TTX block of tibial motor nerve fibres. After 4 weeks, an increased rheobase current and voltage were observed in some of the MNs, but these responses were restricted to presumptive S-type MNs, the cells with the longest AHP durations, i.e. the same MN fraction which also reacted to muscle inactivity with a shortening of AHPs (see below). Thus muscle inactivity seemed mainly to decrease the excitability of those MNs that would normally be the most active. Changes in the opposite direction were indeed produced by chronic activation of motor nerves (cat medial gastrocnemius) (Munson *et al.* 1997a), which caused MNs to become more excitable (increased input resistance, decreased rheobase current), keeping them matched to the slowing produced in the stimulated muscle. Thus, to a limited extent, these kinds of extreme experimental conditions have generated data suggesting that activity promotes MN excitability, i.e. a (weak) positive feedback. None of these changes in passive MN properties help very much to explain the increased reflex excitability after chronic ST.

Things become more subtle when considering the effects of voluntary activation. Beaumont and Gardiner (2002, 2003) studied the effects of running in rats, and the main changes were again restricted to S-type MNs (cells with long AHPs) which showed a parallel shift in the voltage threshold and resting membrane potential towards more negative values. Such parallel changes in these parameters might, for instance, help to counteract Na^+ current inactivation in repetitive firing. Provided that the equilibrium potential for K^+ ions had not changed (i.e. that this was not the reason for the more negative membrane potential), a negative shift of voltage threshold might cause an increase in the slope of the *f–I* relation, thus promoting rate gradation during motor activity (see Chapter 6, section 6.6.2). For a recent summary of research along these lines, see Gardiner *et al.* (2005).

Another interesting type of voluntary 'training' has been explored by Wolpaw and his colleagues (reviewed by Wolpaw and Tennissen 2001); in monkeys and rats the H-reflex response of limb muscles was up- or downregulated with operant conditioning techniques. The effects of this long-term conditioning training (e.g. lasting 30–40 days) also remain after section of the spinal cord, i.e. changes (also) take place at a spinal level. In H-reflex down-conditioned monkeys, the MNs concerned had an increased voltage threshold (Carp and Wolpaw 1994), i.e. intrinsic MN excitability changed such that it helped to explain the decreased H-reflex responses. Furthermore, in rats as well as primates, H-reflex down-conditioning was associated with a decreased axonal conduction velocity for the target MNs (Carp and Wolpaw 1994; Carp et al. 2001), possibly as a result of a threshold increase also in the axonal membranes (shift in voltage dependence of Na^+ current?).

11.4.2.2. Motoneurone plateau behaviour

In contrast with the rather moderate or slight effects of chronic ST on passive membrane properties, there are dramatic ST-associated changes in MN 'plateau behaviour', i.e. in membrane properties underlying the depolarization-evoked appearance of excitatory persistent inward currents (PICs) (see Chapter 6, section 6.7)). In a recent series of publications, Bennett and colleagues describe these effects when investigated for tail MNs of the rat (Bennett et al. 1999, 2001a, 2004; Li et al. 2004b). Following transection of the spinal cord at S2, tail MNs are inactive for about 2 weeks. After this 'acute' phase, there is a gradual increase in classical symptoms of spasticity with hyper-reflexia and easily evoked spasms. The hyper-reflexia includes the appearance of extremely long-lasting discharges in response to brief and slight electrical or natural stimulation. The properties of the tail MNs were investigated in vitro, using intracellular techniques (Bennett et al. 2001b; Li and Bennett 2003, 2004a). After chronic ST (i.e. 1–5 months), almost all the MNs showed PICs when depolarized with slowly rising currents. These PICs were sufficient to drive many of the MNs in plateau discharges, maintained without the addition of external excitation (cf. Chapter 6, section 6.7, Fig. 6.5A). The PICs consisted of two components: a nimodipine-sensitive Ca^{2+} current (Cav1.3 L-type) with a slow activation (250 ms), no inactivation during the plateau, and a slow deactivation (>300 ms) after return to resting membrane potential, and a TTX-sensitive Na^+ current with a rapid activation and deactivation and a slow inactivation during the plateau. The Ca^{2+} component was responsible for about half the total PIC initially and about two-thirds later on. The Na^+ PIC was activated already at subthreshold membrane potentials, and the Ca^{2+} PIC emerged just below spike threshold for some MNs and just above for others. In these experiments, the ST brought MNs into states which are typically promoted by monoaminergic inputs; at first sight, this seems paradoxical because one of the effects of ST is to isolate the MNs from these particular inputs from the brainstem. However, segmental synapses should be capable of similar effects because plateau behaviour may also be facilitated by glutaminergic and cholinergic metabotropic receptors (Alaburda et al. 2002; for further comments, see Heckman et al. 2005). It would be interesting to know whether an increased tendency for plateau firing might also appear after a long-term selective monoaminergic denervation of the MNs (cf. test up to about

4 weeks, Kiehn *et al.* 1996). Recent studies of human subjects with long-standing spinal cord lesions have revealed that their (partly) paralysed muscles indeed have MNs with 'plateau-like' behaviours (see section 11.2.3 above; Zijdewind and Thomas 2001, 2003).

As well as spinal cord damage, there are probably also other long-term influences which might have an effect on MN intrinsic excitability and plateau behaviour; this is an important field for further experimental work. Such properties of MNs might, for instance, be under partial hormonal control. In hindlimb MNs, certain plateau-like effects were more common in female cats which had received treatment with oestradiol for seven preceding days (Kirkwood *et al.* 2002).

11.4.3. Motoneurone synaptic drive

11.4.3.1. Effects of spinal transection on segmental reflex circuits

The spinal cord contains the circuitry for many types of basic motor behaviour, including simple acts of posture and locomotion. After ST, the isolated cord segments may be systematically trained for the coordination of hindlimb standing or treadmill walking. However, these fascinating aspects of neuronal plasticity are likely mainly to concern pre-motoneuronal interneurones of various types; hence, this falls outside the scope of the present book (reviewed by Edgerton *et al.* 2001). In this context it is of interest that non-potentiated EPSPs from various sources tend to become larger after ST (Baker and Chandler 1987b; Hochman and McCrea 1994a), perhaps because of sprouting after degeneration of synapses from descending pathways.

11.4.3.2. Use-related effects on properties of Ia EPSPs

Excitation from muscle spindle afferents will normally contribute to the synaptic drive of MNs in voluntary contractions (Chapter 9, section 9.6.3). One aspect of the monosynaptic Ia EPSPs that has proved very interesting in relation to plasticity concerns its modulation during high-rate repetitive activation (HR modulation) (Koerber and Mendell 1991). Normally, HR modulation is negative for MNs with large Ia EPSPs (e.g. in S MNs) and positive for MNs with small Ia EPSPs (e.g. FF MNs) (Fig. 7.4B,C). Following chronic stimulation of the nerve to a mixed cat hindlimb muscle, which converted all muscle units to slow-type properties, the Ia EPSPs had acquired the negative HR modulation of S-type MNs (Munson *et al.* 1997a; Mendell and Munson 1999). For MNs of the chronically activated nerve, this was also true for the effects of afferents of a synergistic nerve which had itself not been treated with the chronic stimulation. Thus this property of the Ia synapses appears to be regulated via the MN itself, as is also indicated by the fact that the same Ia afferent elicits EPSPs with different HR-modulation properties in different individual MNs (Koerber and Mendell 1991).

11.4.3.3. Maximal voluntary activation intensity

As was described in Chapter 8, section 8.4.3, it is surprisingly difficult to achieve a fully maximal activation of a muscle in a voluntary contraction (Fig. 8.6B). The extent to which this can be done varies with the muscle and task concerned and may be influenced by training; for further discussion, see Enoka (1997). During strength training, the increase in maximum voluntary force is often associated with an increase in the accompanying EMG (Hakkinen and Komi 1983; Hakkinen *et al.* 1998). Correspondingly, the maximum force often increases faster than the cross-sectional area of the muscle (e.g. Hakkinen *et al.* 1998), indicating that part of the voluntary force increase was caused by a higher degree of maximal MN activation. During the training of rapid dorsiflexion movements of the foot, direct measurements showed that the resulting increase in maximum force and speed was indeed associated with an increase in maximum discharge rate of the MNs, indicating an increased central drive (Van Cutsem *et al.* 1998). In this case, part of the increased MN rate was due to an increased incidence of 'doublets', i.e. unusually brief interspike intervals (<2–5 ms). MNs have a very high gain just after the abrupt onset of a stimulating current, prior to the process of initial spike-frequency adaptation (see Fig. 6.2B). Thus an increased incidence of initial 'doublets' might simply indicate that the rate of rise of the synaptic activation had increased. However, the extra 'doublets' seen by Van Cutsem *et al.* (1998) sometimes also appeared at later times in the discharge, which might reflect a change in MN characteristics (e.g. an increased delayed depolarization, occasionally causing the discharge of an 'extra' spike soon after the preceding one (cf. Fig. 6.1B)).

The central MN activation mechanisms may be improved by purely mental exercises performed without any concurrent contractions. Such 'imaginary' motor training delivered significant improvements in the maximal voluntary force of a hand muscle (Yue and Cole 1992) as well as for ankle plantar-flexors (Zijdewind *et al.* 2003). Correspondingly, negative effects on the maximal voluntary MN drive are also very evident for various kinds of disuse. Thus a marked decrease in maximal voluntary activation is seen after prolonged bed rest (Duchateau 1995; Berg *et al.* 1997; Koryak 1998, 1999) or joint immobilization (Duchateau and Hainaut 1987, 1990; Vandenborne *et al.* 1998).

11.4.4. **Neuronal speed and frequency gradation parameters**

As was noted above, the isometric and shortening speed of slow muscle fibres tend to become faster when the muscles are kept inactive. Therefore the maintenance of a normal 'speed-match' between inactive muscles and MNs would require a shortening of the AHP in the MNs (see Chapter 6, section 6.9.3.3, Fig. 6.8). Such a shortening has indeed been observed in the slowest MNs, both after ST (cat soleus MNs) (Czéh *et al.* 1978; Gallego *et al.* 1978; Cope *et al.* 1986) and after TTX block of the motor nerve, causing muscle paralysis (Czéh *et al.* 1978; rat slowest tibial MNs, Cormery *et al.* 2000). Fast MNs apparently do not change in this respect (Gustafsson *et al.* 1982; Munson *et al.* 1986). In the slow soleus MNs, the shortening of the AHP could be counteracted by chronic stimulation activating the muscle (Fig. 11.5A), and this stimulation was effective when applied distal, but not proximal, to a TTX block of the nerve (Czéh *et al.* 1978). An influence from the muscle was also indicated by the finding that, after ST, the shortening of the AHP for soleus MNs did not take place if muscle atrophy was prevented by immobilizing the paralysed muscle in a lengthened position (Gallego *et al.* 1979).

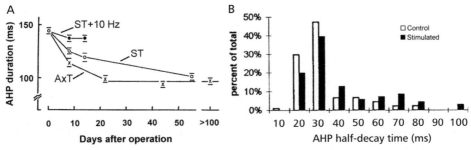

Figure 11.5 Effects of chronic stimulation on MN after-potentials. Experiments on cat spinal MNs, including intracellular measurements of the time course of after-hyperpolarization (AHP) following single spikes. (**A**) Decreased duration of AHP of soleus motoneurones after spinal cord transection (ST, open circles) or after section of the soleus nerve (axotomy) (AxT, crosses). The shortening of AHP following spinal cord transection was counteracted by additional daily stimulation of the sciatic nerve at 10 Hz (ST + 10 Hz, filled circles; means ± SE). (Reproduced with permission, from Czéh *et al.* 1978, labels added) (**B**) Histogram showing the distribution of AHP half-decay times (duration of AHP decline from peak to half-peak amplitude) for MNs of gastrocnemius medialis muscle. Open columns, controls; filled columns, animals treated for 8 weeks or more with chronic stimulation of the nerve to medial gastrocnemius (20 Hz covering 50 per cent of daily time). (Reproduced with permission, from Munson *et al.* 1997a.)

After chronic stimulation and intense endurance training, muscles might become slower. In this situation, there are also signs that MNs tend to change in a direction that would match their properties to the slowing muscle fibres; chronic stimulation which causes a slowing of isometric contractions also causes MNs to have more prolonged AHPs (Fig. 11.5B) (Munson *et al.* 1997a). However, as was the case for the effects of paralysis after spinal transection or motor nerve block (see above), the changes in AHP duration seemed often to concern slow-type MNs (S MNs) which became still slower. The original F-type MNs usually did not turn into S MNs. Thus the original S-type MNs seem particularly malleable, having a more extended 'adaptive range' than F MNs. This may be related to the fact that slow units and muscles, like those of the rat and cat soleus, have important anti-gravity postural functions which will alter markedly in relation to changes in animal weight (e.g. during growth); in these muscles, the development of normal adult properties depends strongly on normal usage patterns (see Chapter 12, section 12.11).

An interesting case of possibly increased activity of slow MNs concerns those units that remain innervated after a partial denervation of a muscle. Particularly during the initial period, the remaining units would be expected to have to compensate for the denervation by producing stronger unit contractions. Ultimately, however, much of the force loss would be compensated for by sprouting. Also in such cases, S-type MNs (and not the F-type cells) react by changing their AHP time course, although not always in the expected direction. Thus, for cat soleus at 3 weeks after a partial denervation, the remaining soleus

MNs acquired a faster AHP and, correspondingly but somewhat later, the twitches of their units also became faster (Huizar *et al.* 1977). On the other hand, for S-type units of cat gastrocnemius which remained 12 weeks after a partial denervation, the AHPs became slower and there was also a slowing of axonal conduction velocity (Havton *et al.* 2001). It is still unclear whether these findings differed because the MN properties were sampled at different times after the partial denervation. A prolongation of the AHP time course of MNs has also been seen after a lifelong overload of the medial gastrocnemius muscle in cats (synergists tenotomized in the first postnatal week) (Gollvik *et al.* 1986). In this case, the AHP prolongation took place for both S- and F-type MNs and, intriguingly, it did not appear to be associated with any signs of general muscle slowing.

11.4.5. MN morphology

Motoneuronal morphology may clearly be influenced in adult animals. However, owing to the relatively time-consuming nature of the measurements concerned, information about such types of plasticity is still very fragmentary.

11.4.5.1. Dendrites

Changes in the dimensions of the dendrites are particularly interesting because of the implications for the synaptic input to the MNs. Tenotomy of the slow soleus muscle led to a substantial muscle atrophy and an elimination of dendritic branches from soleus MNs (Gollvik *et al.* 1990). However, the opposite experiment, overload of the soleus by tenotomy of its synergists, did not affect the MN dendritic branching pattern (Gollvik *et al.* 1990). Furthermore, after transection of the spinal cord, the partially 'denervated' MNs below the lesion showed electrical signs of a possible dendrite retraction (shortened eletrotonic length) (Gustafsson *et al.* 1982); it might be interesting to confirm these suggestions using direct morphological measurements.

11.4.5.2. Soma

Changes in the size of the cell body might take place as a consequence of an altered intensity of synthetic processes within the MNs, by analogy with the swelling that takes place during the intense RNA and protein synthesis following axotomy (chromatolytic reaction) (Chapter 10, section 10.2.1). Mechanisms of this general nature might underlie the changes in soma dimensions after increased motor activity (increased soma size of rat soleus MNs) (Nakano *et al.* 1997) or in association with hypothyroidism (slight decrease in soma size of rat soleus MNs) (Bakels *et al.* 1998).

11.4.5.3. Axons

Changes in axon diameter and conduction velocity are of interest partly because these parameters are often used for categorization and comparisons across MN populations (cf. Chapter 8, section 8.2). There are few publications reporting systematic use-related changes in axonal properties (i.e. in the absence of lesions and regeneration). Andersson and Edström (1957) found smaller axons after a period of hyperactivity. On the other hand, Walsh *et al.* (1978) found an increased axonal conduction velocity for MNs that were presumably subjected to overuse (MNs of overloaded cat gastrocnemius muscle). However, an increased conduction velocity does not necessarily imply that axonal dimensions changed; differences in conduction velocity may also depend on differences in the spike-generating mechanisms of the axonal membrane (Carp *et al.* 2003).

11.4.6. Cytochemistry, axonal transport, and trophic signalling

Muscle fibres and MNs are clearly interdependent, and many aspects of the plasticity of MNs are likely to be (partially) caused by changes in various biochemical factors that are retrogradely transported from the muscle along the axon (cf. effects of axotomy, Chapter 10, section 10.2). Similarly, an altered use of the MNs might result in a change of inducing/controlling factors being transported from the MN to its muscle fibres. Only a few of these various factors are known; this is an important field for further investigation.

Many investigations concerning the biochemical interactions between MNs and their target cells concentrate on the role of neurotrophins, which are known to be important for MN survival during development (Chapter 12, section 12.6); Bartlett *et al.* (1998) have reviewed neurotrophin transport. The muscle content of NT-4 was found to be increased by muscle activation, and intramuscular injection of NT-4 was observed to promote sprouting of motor terminals (Funakoshi *et al.* 1995). It was suggested by these authors that NT-4 might mediate many of the activity-related interactions between MNs and their muscle fibres. No differences were found between fast and slow MNs with regard to their expression of mRNA for NT4 or its trkB receptor (Copray and Kernell 2000).

Gonzalez and Collins (1997) applied BDNF to the gastrocnemius muscle of adult rats, and 5 days later found that the MNs had acquired a lower current threshold and a smaller total capacitance (i.e. they presumably had a smaller size). Running exercises in rats resulted in an increase in BDNF in muscle (soleus) as well as in MNs (Gomez-Pinilla *et al.* 2001). However, running exercises have not been found to result in smaller MN sizes (see section 11.4.5). For information about effects of neurotrophins on axotomized MNs, see Chapter 10, section 10.2.6. In addition to their long-term actions, neurotrophins also have acute effects on the neuromuscular system. Thus it has been demonstrated that both NT-3 and BDNF exert strong effects of various kinds on synaptic transmission in the neonate spinal cord (reviewed by Mendell and Arvanian 2002).

In addition to the neurotrophins, there are of course many other important 'control substances' which are transported along motor axons. Gardiner and colleagues have found that exercise in rats causes an increased soma and axonal concentration of CGRP (Gharakhanlou *et al.* 1999), a general increase in the orthograde transport of proteins (Jasmin *et al.* 1988; Kang *et al.* 1995), an increase in the transport towards the muscle of SNAP-25 (important for synaptic functions) (Kang *et al.* 1995), and an increase in both ortho- and retrograde transport of AChE (Jasmin *et al.* 1987). Intriguingly, the transport enhancement of AChE did not appear to depend on the intensity of motor activity *per se*, because the effects were seen after chronic running exercise but not after swimming. Furthermore, the MN content of CGRP also becomes increased after block of neuromuscular activity, using alpha bungarotoxin or TTX (Sala *et al.* 1995).

There is a growing list of externally derived proteins with a life-saving effect on MNs during development, *in vitro*, and/or after axotomy (Henderson *et al.* 1998). The actions of these substances are not necessarily limited to the promotion of cell survival, but they might also exert long-term effects on various MN properties. These 'trophic' substances include:

- the neurotrophins proper (BDNF, NT-3, NT-4/5)

- members of the transforming growth factor beta family, for example glial cell-line-derived neurotrophic factor (GDNF) (Henderson *et al.* 1994; Munson and McMahon 1997), neurturin (NTN), persephin (PSP), and transforming growth factor β_3

- cytokines of the IL-6 family, for example ciliary neurotrophic factor (CNTF) (Oppenheim *et al.* 1991), leukaemia inhibiting factor (LIF), and cardiotrophin-1 (CT-1);

- members of the fibroblast growth factor (FGF) family (e.g. FGF-5)

- other growth and developmental factors, for example hepatocyte growth factor (HGF), insulin-like growth factor (IGF), growth-promoting activity (GPA), and choline acetyltransferase developmental factor (CDF) (McManaman *et al.* 1990).

The substances derive from various external sources, such as fibroblasts (FGF-5), skeletal muscle fibres (CDF), Schwann cells (CNTF), and central glial cells (GDNF).

11.5. Pathophysiological issue: motoneurone–muscle interactions in disease

There are clearly many kinds of mutual long-term interactions between MNs and their muscle fibres, and therefore it is relevant question to ask to what extent neuromuscular diseases are associated with disturbances in these interactions, either as a symptom or as a partial cause of malfunctions. There are a few intriguing observations suggesting that this is a promising field for further research. Thus, when using physiological methods for counting the numbers of units in various muscles, decreased unit numbers were found, as expected, in central MN diseases (e.g. ALS) but also, surprisingly, in various myogenic diseases (e.g. myotonic muscular dystrophy) (reviewed by McComas 1991). In investigations of MN firing properties in patients with Duchenne muscular dystrophy, evidence was found indicating that the MNs had more short-lasting AHPs than those of normal MNs (Piotrkiewicz *et al.* 1999), i.e. the properties of the MNs had changed in a supposedly 'pure' muscle disease.

Chapter 12

Genetic specification and lifespan development

12.1. General issues

It is of self-evident interest to find out how living organisms and their components come into being during embryonic development. In addition, from a clinical point of view, this knowledge is essential for understanding (and, it is hoped, in the future correcting) various kinds of inborn deficits and malfunctions. It is also often thought that the functions of an adult biological system might be more easily understood if one knows how it developed. For some adult functions this is clearly true. However, for other aspects this might be less evident because processes and regulating mechanisms that are important during early development might not be as dominant in later life; the period of embryonic and perinatal development is a highly specialized phase of life with its own complex sets of rules.

At a molecular level, there is a surprising degree of resemblance between the developmental processes of animals that are phylogenetically far apart. Understanding the rules of embryonic development of tissues and organs is one of the major challenges of modern molecular biology. A full review of the developmental biology of the neuromuscular system is not possible within the scope of this book. Instead, a limited number of separate 'highlights' will be commented on, concentrating on issues that seem important as a background for, and sometimes contrasting with, adult neuromuscular physiology. More complete surveys of neuromuscular development can be found in various reviews (Kelly 1983; Oppenheim 1991; McComas 1996; Jessell and Sanes 2000a,b).

The earliest stages of neuromuscular development in vertebrates have been particularly well studied in amphibia (Xenopus), birds (chick), and rodents (rat, mouse). As far as is known, similar general principles also apply to humans, albeit with different timescales. In rats and chicks the total gestation period is only about 21 days, i.e. less than 10 per cent of the human 38 weeks. Molecular aspects of development have been extensively studied in various invertebrates, including the fruitfly (*Drosophila melanogaster*). Some of the genetic mechanisms operating in *Drosophila* are also, with minor modifications, employed in many other species, including mammals (see sections 12.3 and 12.4).

Lifespan development includes not only the initial making of the system, but also its gradual 'unmaking' towards the end of life; a few final comments will be devoted to neuromuscular ageing processes. Mice start showing the signs of the deterioration normally accompanying old age after about 2 years, and rats after 2–3 years; hence these two short-lived species are often used in studies of ageing processes in the neuromuscular system.

12.2. **The classical initial stages of development**

Even before fertilization, the contents of the egg cell (e.g. its mRNA) is organized into an 'animal' and a 'vegetal' pole, roughly corresponding to the future caudal and cranial ends of the body. Fertilization of the egg by a sperm leads to the appearance of a 'grey crescent' on the opposite side of the egg due to further polarization of its contents. This 'grey crescent' portion will become the dorsal side of the embryo, including the nervous system.

Following fertilization there is an initial series of cell divisions, leading to the spherical structure of the blastula with a central fluid-filled blastocoele. The 'animal' portion of the blastula contains cells of the future ectoderm and the 'vegetal' portion contains the cells of the future endoderm. At the border between the 'animal' and 'vegetal' cells, induction factors from vegetal cells make borderline animal cells to differentiate into future mesoderm. In these early processes, various peptides are active as inducing factors, possibly including molecules which will also be important later, such as fibroblast growth factor (FGF) and transforming growth factor-β (TGF-β).

Expansion of the mesoderm causes invagination of the blastula to form the gastrula, which ultimately will have three principal cell layers: ectoderm (outside), endoderm (inside), and mesoderm (between the ectoderm and the endoderm). The dorsal mesoderm becomes organized into segmental tissue blocks, the **somites**. All skeletal muscles develop from the somites. Somitic mesoderm also gives rise to vertebrae, ribs, and deeper parts of the skin (dermis). Non-somite mesoderm gives rise to the notochord and also to the heart and blood vessels.

At the later neurula stage, the neural tube is formed on the dorsal side by invagination of ectoderm (Fig. 12.1A–C). The neural tube is surrounded by tissues which influence its further development via the secretion of inducing factors: laterally the mesoderm (future vertebrae) and ventrally the notochord. The neural tube gives rise to all central nerve and glia cells.

12.3. **Differentiation into motoneurones and interneurones**

During gastrulation, only the neural plate expresses **neural-cell adhesion factor** (N-CAM), and other neurone-specific molecules are also specifically expressed here at a stage before the formation of the neural tube. In vertebrates as well as, for instance, in *Drosophila*, early steps in neural development are regulated by **proneural** genes, which encode transcription factors of the **basic helix–loop–helix** (bHLH) type (reviewed by Bertrand *et al.* 2002). Cells of the neural tube will form the spinal cord and the brain. Part of the neural plate located outside the neural tube, the **neural crest**, will generate components of the peripheral nervous system (dorsal and autonomic ganglia, Schwann cells, etc.).

The neural tube begins as a single-layer epithelium surrounding a central cavity, the **ventricle**. Cells of this epithelium differentiate into neuroblasts, which then migrate to positions further from the ventricle. The first cells to migrate are the ventral ones, many

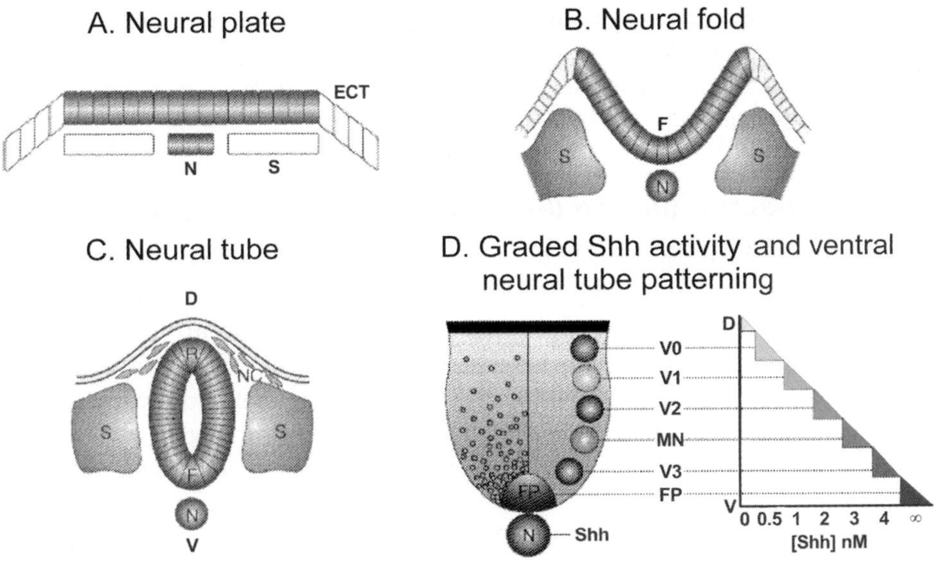

A. Neural plate

B. Neural fold

C. Neural tube

D. Graded Shh activity and ventral neural tube patterning

Figure 12.1 Early development of spinal cord and induction of MNs. (**A**)–(**C**) Schematic drawings showing stages during the development of the vertebrate (chick) spinal cord from the ectoderm (ECT) of the neural plate (**A**), which folds (**B**) to become the neural tube (**C**) with an underlying notochord (N), dorsal neural crest cells (NC), and laterally adjoining somitic mesoderm (S). (**D**) Schematic drawing of the ventral portion of the neural tube (left), including its lowermost portion, the floor plate (FP). Cells of the floor plate and notochord release sonic hedgehog protein (Shh), and the resulting Shh concentration gradient is symbolized by a gradient of vesicles (left). Depending on the Shh concentrations, neural progenitor cells at different loci within the neural tube will develop into different molecularly distinct classes of neurones, such as MNs and different types of ventral interneurones (V0, V1, V2, V3). *In vitro* observations have demonstrated that MNs, expressing Isl-1, will indeed emerge for Shh concentrations within a very limited range (right-hand graph). These experiments were performed with neural plate explants grown in different concentrations of recombinant amino-terminal fragment of Shh (Shh-N). (Modified with permission, from Jessell 2000.)

of which are destined to become motoneurones. Later on, more dorsal cells show the same proliferation and outward migration. Within the neural tube, the future fates of cells in the various regions are controlled by gradients of several inducing factors. Because of such gradients, the topographical position of neuroblasts within the neural tube is an important factor determining their future fates. This is clearly demonstrated by the effects of one of the major inducing substances, the **sonic hedgehog protein** (Shh) (reviewed by Jessell 2000; Briscoe and Ericson 2001).

Initially, Shh is released by cells of the notochord, and its concentration decreases from the ventral towards the dorsal regions of the neural tube. The highest concentrations are present for the most ventral cells in the tube which are soon induced to form the **floor plate**; these cells will then also start releasing Shh. *In vitro* experiments have confirmed that MNs are induced for a precise range of relatively high Shh concentrations, while other concentration ranges of Shh will instead induce various categories of spinal interneurones (Fig. 12.1D, MN versus V0, V1, V2, and V3) (Jessell 2000). In addition to Shh, (gradients of) other factors are also essential for inducing MNs, including FGF and retinoic acid (Novitch *et al.* 2003); retinoic acid is a derivative of vitamin A.

12.4. **Differentiation into different categories of motoneurones**

The genes that regulate the body layout are called **homeotic genes**. An important group of homeotic genes (regulating other genes) are the **homeobox genes** (Hox), which have as a common feature the code (homeobox) for a 60 amino acid sequence (homeodomain) which is part of the protein section that will bind to the DNA of the target gene. Homeobox genes of similar composition are used to control rostro-caudal body layout in, for instance, insects (*Drosophila*) and mammals (mice). The expression of the homeobox genes seems to be regulated by factors similar to those responsible for the initial induction of the mesoderm (e.g. activin A, activin B, FGF, TGF-β). An important feature of homeobox genes is that their effect seems to depend on the **homeobox gene combination** expressed in each target cell (cf. multi-digit numbers). Thus the target muscle destination and central connections for a given group of MNs might be 'labelled' and determined by their specific combination of switched-on homeobox genes. For a given group of developing MNs, this combination seems to be set by their three-dimensional position within a body-wide coordinate system of inducing factor gradients.

The differentiation of neuroblasts into a specified line or functional group of cells is caused by the induced expression of appropriate transcription factors, i.e. proteins that activate relevant (sets of) genes. During their Shh-induced development (and also often in the adult state), MNs are made to express several LIM homeodomain transcription factors including: *Isl-1, Isl-2, Lira-1* (*LHX1*), *Lira-3* (*LHX3*), and *Gsh-4* (*LHX4*). Subtypes of MNs, innervating different peripheral targets, express distinct combinatorial arrays of these genes (reviewed by Pfaff and Kintner 1998). For instance, Isl-1 and Isl-2 are initially present in all MNs, including visceral MNs (i.e. vegetative preganglionic neurones); however, Isl-2 is rapidly downregulated in the visceral MNs (Thaler *et al.* 2004). Homeodomain genes that are specifically expressed in developing MNs include *HB9* and *MNR2* (Thaler *et al.* 1999). As well as inducing the differentiation of MNs and various classes of spinal interneurones, Shh also regulates the expression of oligodendrocyte lineage genes (*Olig1* and *Olig2*), coding for transcription factors with bHLH domains. Expression of both Olig1 and Olig2 is essential for the differentiation of oligodendrocytes and, intriguingly, the expression of Olig2 is also essential for MN development (Bertrand *et al.* 2002; Lu *et al.* 2002).

Hoxc homeodomain proteins (transcription factors) apparently contribute to segmental rostro-caudal differences in MN central network identity and peripheral target destination. For instance, knockout of the Hoxc-8 gene leads to altered MN pool projections to distal forelimb muscles (Tiret *et al.* 1998). The expression of Hoxc-5 and Hoxc-6 is limited to MNs at rostral levels and Hoxc-8 and Hoxc-9 to those at more caudal sites, but the transition lines differ; for Hoxc-5 versus Hoxc-8 the transition occurs at a mid-brachial level, and for Hoxc-6 versus Hoxc-9 it occurs at the brachial–thoracic border. Rostro-caudal differences in motoneuronal Hoxc expression are probably induced by graded FGF signallling, increasing in concentration from rostral towards more caudal levels (Dasen *et al.* 2003). The known molecular definitions of MN identity have not yet reached a resolution corresponding to single muscle compartments and their MN pools, but this goal seems within reach; this complex research field is in a phase of rapid progress (see also section 12.13). Once a detailed molecular definition of MN identity has been reached, immuno-histochemical labelling techniques might replace the need for retrograde HRP labelling of MNs.

12.5. **Myotube generations and muscle fibre differentiation**

Muscle tissue is formed from the outer (lateral) portions of the somites (dermatomyotomes) under the influence of myogenic master regulatory genes, coding for the muscle regulatory factors (MRFs): Myo D, myogenin, myf-5, and myf-6 (Mrf 4), acting in cascade. Under the influence of activins A and/or B and other peptide growth factors, mesodermal cells of the somites multiply to form **myoblasts**. These are small cells with a single nucleus, containing little actin and almost no myosin. The membrane contains no functional ACh receptor molecules and the resting membrane potential is very low (-20 mV). The myoblasts will continue dividing until a sufficiently high concentration of proteins (inducing factors) is expressed by myogenic master regulatory genes (e.g. Myo D).

Above a critical inducing-factor concentration, myoblasts stop dividing and start to differentiate into muscle cells. Neighbouring myoblasts first form gap junctions with each other and then fuse to form **myotubes**, elongated cells with a single chain of many nuclei in a central position (i.e. not close to the membrane). In future limb muscles of rats, this process starts at around stage E14–15 (i.e. embryonic days 14–15). After a myotube has first been formed, new myoblasts will be added to it by fusion. However, there will be no mitosis of nuclei already inside the myotube. The myotubes will synthesize the thick (myosin) and thin (actin etc.) myofilaments, forming sarcomeres. Furthermore, there is an increase in mitochondria and development of the sarcoplasmic reticulum (SR) and associated structures such as the transverse tubular system (T system). Outside the muscle cells, the **basement membrane** comes into existence. Gradually the myotubes grow in size and become more mature in their properties. One of the last changes is that the nuclei leave their central position and become localized just under the cell membrane. The myotube has then become a mature muscle fibre.

Myotubes arise in two or more generations; each successive wave of myotubes emerges around those of the preceding generation, which are used as scaffolding for the fusing myoblasts. Myotubes become innervated very soon after their appearance; the outgrowth of MN axons takes place in parallel with the generation of myotubes and muscles. Compared with primary myotube generation, secondary (and tertiary) myotube formation appears to be more dependent on innervation for a normal completion. However, fibres of the first generation are also dependent on innervation for their ultimate survival, as is also true for adult muscle (critically reviewed by McLennan 1994).

Primary and secondary (and sometimes tertiary) myotubes/muscle fibres differ with regard to their future contractile specializations and adaptive range (reviewed by Hoh 1991). Furthermore, embryonic muscle fibres often contain mixtures of different iso-forms of myosin heavy chains (MHCs) including types that are not normally present in adults (e.g. 'embryonic' or foetal and 'neonatal' MHC) (cf. Table 3.4). In later life, many of the primary myotubes will keep their slow type I MHC (perhaps mainly those arising early on) (Narusawa et al. 1987), and some other primaries will later tend to become fast with varieties of type II MHC. Some of the secondary myotubes some will become slow (type I MHC) in later life, but many will turn out to be fast (type II MHC). The differen-tial development of the primary myotubes and their surrounding secondaries (primaries are often slow and secondaries are often fast) is important for the normal 'checkerboard' appearance of a muscle cross-section, with fibres of different types intermingled (cf. Fig. 3.10A,B).

In postnatal life, motor nerves can modify the phenotype of muscle fibres; for instance, they can switch some of them from fast to slow depending on how they are activated (cf. Chapter 10, section 10.4.3.2 and Chapter 11, section 11.3). This is important for adapting the neuromuscular properties to changing motor tasks. However, for each (set of) muscle fibre(s) this can only be done within a myogenically determined range (cf. Chapter 11, section 11.3.6.3). In contrast with the postnatal situation, neural influences on muscle properties are apparently not very important for the prenatal period of neuromus-cular differentiation. Also in the absence of innervation, myotubes and muscle fibres will differentiate into preferentially 'fast' or 'slow' varieties, and this includes major aspects of the typical fibre type regionalization (i.e. deep slow regions) (Condon et al. 1990; see also Miller and Stockdale 1987). The preferential occurrence of slow type I fibres in deep muscle regions might even be 'vestiges of the original muscle primordium', reflecting the locations of early primary myotubes (Narusawa et al. 1987). In prenatal development, MNs and muscles are not matched by mutual interactions causing a modification of 'speed'-associated properties, but rather by selective innervation (see section 12.8).

12.6. Outgrowth of motoneurone axons and programmed motoneurone death

Even before they have finished their lateral migration, newly differentiated MNs send out axons to innervate newly formed myotubes in the limb buds and elsewhere. Under the influence of various attracting and repelling axonal guidance factors, this occurs in a very precise manner. MNs from a certain site in the spinal cord always connect to the same future muscle(s) in the periphery. For a given group of MNs, the peripheral commitment can be altered by transplanting them to a new spinal location before their specification has become completed and their axons have started to grow out (e.g. zebra fish, Appel et al. 1995). However, later on, after their 'destination specification' has become consolidated, MNs will innervate the same peripheral targets even if their intraspinal positions have been altered (chick, partial cord reversal, Lance-Jones and Landmesser 1980; reviewed by Landmesser 2001). Several molecules are known which may serve to guide outgrowing central or peripheral axons, using attracting as well as repulsing effects (e.g. netrins, semaphorins, ephrins, etc.) (reviewed by Sanes and Jessell 2000). However, their role in muscle (re)innervation is still not well understood, and it also remains a tantalizing mystery why the precision of embryonic muscle innervation by 'their own' MNs is no longer available for peripheral nerve regeneration in adults (cf. Chapter 10, section 10.4.2).

Innervation of myotubes takes place even before the muscle masses of the limbs have become split up into separate muscles (initially only dorsal versus ventral portions of the muscle masses are formed). During this innervation process, the muscles split up and the pools of motoneurones also become separated, as seen in a cross-section, into several different groups of cell bodies (about six for each limb). During the initial muscle innervation, the motor axons are unmyelinated; the Schwann cells follow later, coming from the neural crest.

About half of the early MNs that send axons out towards the muscles will die (reviewed by Oppenheim 1991). This process of an initial surplus production of neurones and a subsequent 'programmed cell death' is widely spread within the CNS, occurring at different locations and in various animal species. The functional meaning of such a seemingly 'wasteful' arrangement might be that the initial surplus minimizes the risk that some target cells (i.e. muscle fibres in the case of MNs) would receive too little innervation. Furthermore, the process may be needed for sculpting the gross structure of the CNS during early development. In animals with mutations of cell death genes, the programmed cell death within the CNS may be reduced or eliminated (e.g. in the worm *Caenorhabditis elegans*, the fruit fly *Drosophila melanogaster*, the zebra fish *Danio rerio*, and the mouse *Mus musculus*). Such cases show a mixed variety of symptoms; in some cases gross anatomical malformations are seen, while in other instances animals seem to develop normally but with an excess of neurones and glia (reviewed by Buss and Oppenheim 2004).

The MNs that die in the programmed cell death do so by *apoptosis* (i.e. in a controlled fashion), and their lives are apparently quickly curtailed by a lack of sufficiently effective contacts with muscles. The surviving MNs appear to profit from essential factors that they have obtained via their axon terminals from innervated muscle fibres and/or other cells in their immediate surrounding. The nature of these factors is still unknown although there are several interesting candidates, including the neurotrophins and GDNF, which also effectively rescues MNs after axotomy (Oppenheim *et al.* 1995). A dependence on muscular trophic factors explains why the number of surviving MNs may be increased by increasing the total muscle mass (supernumerary limb) and decreased by removal of muscle (Oppenheim 1991). However, there is a puzzling relation between the MN survival rate and muscle activity. Very early in development, the MNs are already spontaneously active and may excite the muscle fibres synaptically (see below). If the muscle is kept inactive by blocking neuromuscular transmission during the period of expected cell death, MN survival is drastically improved. On the other hand, the extent of MN death is enhanced if the target muscle is made super-active using chronic electrical stimulation (Oppenheim and Nunez 1982). Does neuromuscular activity somehow cause a decrease in the local concentration of trophic factor(s) around the motor terminals?

12.7. **Formation of neuromuscular junctions**

Once motor axons have made contact with a muscle fibre, synaptic transmission may take place within 1–2 h (reviews of the complex process of neuromuscular junction development are given by Bennett (1983) and Sanes and Lichtman (1999)). There is an inductive action from muscle fibres onto the motor axon terminal, causing it to increase its ACh release. Furthermore, factors from the muscle fibre promote the adhesion between axon terminal and muscle. Factors of probable inductive importance in this context include N-CAM and cadherin. Furthermore, signals from the muscle cell cause an increase in intracellular Ca^{2+} concentration in the axonal growth cone, which promotes its differentiation into a presynaptic nerve ending.

There are many important interactions between the presynaptic nerve terminal and the muscle fibre during the formation of the neuromuscular synapse. Via the release of **agrin** (synthesized in the MN soma), the terminal promotes clustering and anchoring of AChRs in the subsynaptic membrane (an important step is phosphorylation of the β-subunit of the AChR). Via the release of **calcitonin gene related peptide** (CGRP) the nerve terminal causes an increased transcription of AChR genes in muscle nuclei close to the endplate. Finally, as a result of muscle fibre activity caused by the innervating MN, the AChR genes in other myonuclei along the fibre are downregulated, leading to a disappearance of AChRs at membrane sites outside the endplate (cf. opposite effects of denervation (Chapter 10, section 10.3.1.3)). However, these processes are not all induced by the nerve terminal alone; recent findings show that, also independently of motor innervation, AChR genes are expressed and AChR clusters form preferentially in the prospective synaptic region of muscle (Arber *et al.* 2002). One or several days after synaptic transmission has become established, AChE is inserted into the basement membrane. After the neuromuscular junction has become established, myonuclei start to accumulate in its neighbourhood. The axon terminal acquires more synaptic vesicles, and the axon ultimately becomes myelinated by actions of Schwann cells which have followed the axons outwards from the neural crest.

12.8. **From poly- to mononeuronal muscle fibre innervation**

In the adult, each twitch muscle fibre is innervated by a single MN. This does not correspond to the situation during early development; the initial muscle innervation is polyneuronal with terminals from several MNs participating in each neuromuscular junction complex (e.g. for 5–7 day old rats, the mean number of terminals per muscle fibre is about three for the extensor digitorum longus and five for the soleus muscle (Jansen and Fladby 1990). During an initial period after the polyneuronal innervation has become established, there is a gradual 'reshuffling' of the intramuscular MN connections such that the muscle units gradually become more homogeneous in their fast versus slow fibre composition (MHC typing) (Fladby and Jansen 1990; Jansen and Fladby 1990). Thus, although different MNs have widely overlapping muscle units at this stage, the units that overlap with each other are all dominated by fibres belonging to the same contractile type, either fast or slow (Thompson *et al.* 1984). This indicates that, during this initial period, MN and muscle fibre properties become matched by type-specific innervation rather than by re-specification processes such as those seen in adult reinnervation (cf. Chapter 10, section 10.4.3.2). In the extreme situation when a single MN is made to innervate a whole (small) heterogeneous muscle, the neonatal muscle retains its normal heterogeneous composition (Gates and Ridge 1992).

The initial polyneuronal innervation of skeletal muscle is removed in the perinatal period (in rats, during the first two postnatal weeks) (reviewed by Jansen and Fladby 1990); the programmed MN death takes place earlier and plays no role in this context. During the period of removal of polyneuronal innervation the rats also gradually develop their motor behaviour and, at around 2 weeks, become capable of standing and walking in an almost adult manner (Geisler *et al.* 1993; Westerga and Gramsbergen 1993). In human muscle, part of this process takes place in the early postnatal period; for example, the psoas muscle has a mononeuronal innervation after about week 12 (Gramsbergen *et al.* 1997).

The activity of MNs (and/or, secondarily, of the muscle fibres) is clearly of importance for the removal of polyneuronal innervation. The general removal process is inhibited by muscle paralysis and is accelerated by the extra activity produced by chronic electrical stimulation (reviewed by Jansen and Fladby 1990). At the level of single muscle fibres, some experiments showed that silent nerve endings would remain while others were withdrawn (TTX block of selected nerves) (Callaway *et al.* 1987); these effects may perhaps be analogous to the general inhibitory effect of paralysis on terminal removal. Other experiments indicated that, among the competing terminals of one junctional complex, the most active ones had a greater chance of remaining (e.g. chronic stimulation of selected nerves) (Ridge and Betz 1984), and this was also implied by the outcome of experiments with localized blocks of AChRs within single endplates (Balice-Gordon and Lichtman 1994). In the removal of polyneuronal innervation, the loss of AChRs normally precedes the loss of terminals, and the competition between active and inactive sites apparently takes place within the muscle fibre (for further details and discussions of possible mechanisms, see Nguyen and Lichtman 1996; Personius and Balice-Gordon 2000). Further analysis of these processes is potentially of great interest as a model for long-term synaptic plasticity elsewhere, including the CNS.

Although neuronal activity is important, in various ways, for the removal processes of polyneuronal muscle innervation, other factors also play a role. For instance, across a muscle there is often a topographical relation between the intraspinal location of a MN and the intramuscular location of its nerve endings (cf. Fig. 5.6). This relationship becomes further accentuated after the removal of polyneuronal innervation (Brown and Booth 1983; Bennett and Ho 1988), i.e. there are also topographical factors of importance for this process (tissue gradients of inducing compounds?).

12.9. **Early changes in motoneurone electrophysiology and muscle speed**

In rats, MNs first appear at around stage E14. At this early age, the cells are already capable of discharging action potentials (Alessandri-Haber *et al.* 1999). Some of them are also capable of repetitive impulse firing, but the range of discharge rates is then very low (*in vitro* studies). Because of the low initial channel density, the early membrane resistivity and membrane time constant tend to be very high and action potentials tend to be slow and prolonged. The lack of repetitive firing properties in many of the early cells might also be associated with low ion channel densities. During the pre- and perinatal period, the membrane density gradually increases for the various ion channels and the repetitive discharge properties improve (Fulton and Walton 1986; Nunez-Abades *et al.* 1993; Gao and Ziskind-Conhaim 1998; Martin-Caraballo and Greer 1999).

Among the first voltage-gated channel types to appear are the classical rapidly inactivating Na^+ channel and the delayed rectifier K^+ channel, i.e. the types of channel primarily needed for action potentials and the only channels typically present in axons (Alessandri-Haber *et al.* 1999). During pre- and perinatal development there are many qualitative alterations in channel composition, in terms of both increasing and decreasing expressions of various channel types. For instance, in mouse MNs, L-type Ca^{2+} channels appear only at around day P7 (seventh postnatal day) (Jiang *et al.* 1999), and in rats there is an early postnatal decrease in the expression of low-voltage activated Ca^{2+} channels and an increase in the density of I_h current (Berger *et al.* 1995).

The medium duration AHP is more prolonged in neonatal rats and cats than in adult animals. In rats, the AHP duration of genioglossal MNs shows some decrease during the first week (Nunez-Abades *et al.* 1993), whereas spinal rat MNs keep a relatively long AHP during the initial 12 days with no clear signs of a systematic decrease (Fulton and Walton 1986). On the other hand, fast rat hindlimb muscles increase rapidly in both twitch and shortening speed during this initial period (Close 1964), i.e. there then appears to be a dissociation between the speed development of these two neuromuscular components. In fast-mixed muscles of cats, there is a gradual shortening of twitch speed during the first few weeks (Buller *et al.* 1960a), and roughly simultaneously there is also a shortening of AHP duration for MNs of fast muscle units, which reaches a minimum at about 10 weeks (Hammarberg and Kellerth 1975a). At the age of 6 weeks or more, but not at 1 or 2 weeks, kittens show a correlation between the duration of AHP and twitch speed (Hammarberg and Kellerth 1975a), i.e. the 'speed' of muscles and MNs in the cat does not seem closely linked just after birth. The postnatal speeding-up of fast MNs and muscles might be two independently preprogrammed events.

12.10. **Postnatal motoneurone morphology**

At birth, spinal MNs of cats have a small cell body but the normal adult number of dendritic stems. During further development, the area of the soma will about double and that of the dendrites will become about five times larger. Furthermore, for triceps surae MNs, the soma reaches its adult dimensions at a time (P44–46) when the dendrites still have only half their adult membrane area (Ulfhake and Cullheim 1988; cf. Cameron *et al.* 1991 for phrenic MNs). These developmental processes take place with a different timing for different motor nuclei along the neuraxis (Cameron *et al.* 1989). However, little is known about how the growth of MN dendrites is regulated and guided. *In vitro* experiments have shown that, under tissue culture conditions, the extension of MN dendrites is inhibited by glutamine, the main excitatory transmitter of the spinal cord (Metzger *et al.* 1998).

The large postnatal expansion of the total dendritic area will enable the MNs to increase their total synaptic input. However, initially there is also a developmental loss of synapses. In newborn kittens, synapses are found on the initial segment of the axon; these synapses disappear during the initial weeks (Ronnevi and Conradi 1974), and this may also be true for many of the original synapses on the soma, perhaps as part of a general reorganization of MN synaptic input during development (Conradi and Ronnevi 1975).

In embryos, adjacent cells within a tissue are often joined by gap junctions, which are believed to be important for the transfer of molecular signals of importance for the developmental process (Guthrie and Gilula 1989). During the initial postnatal week coupled gap junctions are relatively common between the MNs of the tongue muscle genioglossus (rat), but they are seldom seen in animals older than 10 days (Mazza *et al.* 1992). Thus, for the coordination of early development within MN pools, direct molecular communication between the pool members might be of importance (for the role of gap junctions in synaptic transmission, see Chapter 5, section 5.2.3).

12.11. **Postnatal neuromuscular use and differentiation**

In rats and cats, the twitch speed tends to be similarly slow for future slow and fast muscles at birth. During the first few weeks they acquire separate isometric speeds, and this happens while both kinds of muscle are actually speeding up, the fast more than the slow (Buller *et al.* 1960a; Close 1964; Buller and Lewis 1965b). In rats, there is also a gradual increase in maximum shortening velocity for fast, but not slow, muscle (Close 1964). Rats and cats are incapable of normal locomotion for some time after birth (altricial animals). In the sheep, a precocial animal that can walk just after birth, the twitch speeds of fast and slow limb muscles are already clearly separated at birth, and this prenatal differentiation is not influenced by an *in utero* transection of the spinal cord (Walker and Luff 1995). The timing of these preprogrammed differentiating events is apparently adapted so that the motor machinery will be ready for behavioural use when needed.

Following the initial period of differential speeding up, there is a secondary slowing of twitch speed for the future slow muscle (Buller *et al.* 1960a; Close 1964). This slowing depends on use, and it does not appear in kittens after a spinal cord transection

(Buller *et al.* 1960a). In rats, the progressive postnatal slowing of the soleus, and a concomitant increase in the percentage of slow type I fibres, is correlated with the increase in body weight (Kugelberg 1976), i.e. the slowing seems to result from a natural kind of 'endurance training' of the body-supporting soleus muscle. The final adult fibre type composition of the various skeletal muscles is apparently partly dependent on how the muscles were (and are) used during postnatal periods of life, and partly on a considerable amount of genetic preprogramming (cf. Chapter 3, section 3.6.1).

The neuromuscular transmission also adapts to the increasingly 'tonic' tasks of weight-supporting slow muscles. Adult mammalian slow-twitch muscles have lower levels of spontaneous and evoked neurotransmitter release than terminals in fast-twitch muscles, which means that the slow terminals can continue functioning for longer times without becoming depleted in releasable ACh (see Chapter 4, section 4.4.4). In rats, the mature pattern of differences in fast versus slow release properties (e.g. in quantal content, spontaneous release frequency) gradually develops at times from the third postnatal week and later (Bewick *et al.* 2004), i.e. these changes may well be usage dependent (cf. consistent effects of chronic stimulation on such parameters (Reid *et al.* 2003)).

As the body grows, muscle fibres increase in girth and, sometimes, in numbers. The increase in numbers can occur as a result of fibre splitting; thinner fibres have the functional advantage of shorter intracellular diffusion distances. Muscle fibres must also continuously adapt their length to the changing geometry and size of the skeleton. This is done by mechanisms in the muscle fibres themselves. Without any innervation, even adult muscle fibres will respond to prolonged periods of stretch by adding new sarcomeres at their ends (Tabary *et al.* 1972; Goldspink *et al.* 1974). Correspondingly, a muscle held in a shortened position will shorten its muscle fibres by deleting sarcomeres.

12.12. **Neuromuscular ageing**

The age-associated deterioration of motor abilities has already started in early adult life, as is evident from the ages of professional football players and record holders in various power- and force-dependent types of sport. Our neuromuscular capability is at its peak in our twenties and early thirties, and for some muscles the number of muscle fibres begins declining already at the age of 25–35 years (human rectus abdominis) (Inokuchi *et al.* 1975). We start becoming generally weaker from the sixth decade of life (reviewed by Vandervoort 2002), and from then on the weakening progresses at a steady pace; the loss of maximum isometric force for muscles around the ankle joint is about 1–1.5 per cent per year. In human limb muscles, the weakening is more pronounced for the lower than for the upper extremities. The loss of force depends mainly on a loss of muscle tissue; old muscles have fewer and, to some extent, thinner muscle fibres (Vandervoort 2002). There is no consistent evidence indicating that old muscles have a lowered specific tension (rat, Larsson and Ansved 1995) or that old individuals have a lower capability for maximum voluntary muscle activation (human, Klass *et al.* 2005). The loss of muscle tissue is probably mainly caused by the death of MNs. In humans, physiological methods of counting the number of motor units in single muscles have shown a decline starting at the age of about 60 (Fig. 12.2A) (McComas 1991), and corresponding results have also been obtained in direct counts of human ventral horn cells (Tomlinson and Irving 1977). Similarly, in aged rats there is a decrease in the number of retrogradely labelled MNs (Fig. 12.2B) (Hashizume *et al.* 1988) and a decline in the number of ventral root fibres (Larsson and Ansved 1995) (see cited articles for further references). These measurements in rats also indicated that the MNs that die are among the largest (Fig. 12.2B; cf. mice, Hirofuji *et al.* 2000) and, correspondingly, fast-type muscle fibres in particular seem to be lost (Larsson and Ansved 1995). Histochemically, aged muscles show changes that seem to result from cycles of denervation and reinnervation: the fine patterns of fibre type distribution are altered, there are greater numbers of fibres with a mixed MHC composition, and the remaining muscle units are larger, having become increased by sprouting (Larsson and Ansved 1995). However, sprouting does not provide a full compensation for the effects of MN death in ageing muscles (cf. Fig. 10.3), i.e. some of the denervated muscle fibres are lost. The sprouting mechanisms are also impaired in the elderly and axonal regeneration is slower (Pestronk *et al.* 1980).

There are also other age-related muscle changes in addition to weakening. Thus isometric twitches of aged muscles are typically slower than those of younger ones, probably because of changes in intramuscular Ca^{2+} kinetics (Larsson and Ansved 1995). Measurements on human subjects have indicated that endurance is, if anything, improved

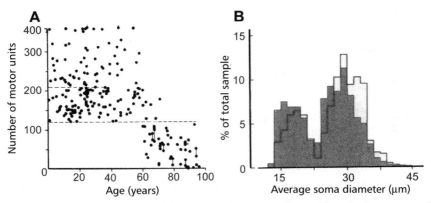

Figure 12.2 Loss of MNs on ageing. (**A**) Human subjects. Numbers of functioning motor units estimated by physiological methods in the foot muscle extensor digitorum brevis of 224 subjects, aged 6 months to 97 years. Bilateral values for the same subjects have been linked. The upper and lower horizontal lines indicate the mean and lower limit of values for healthy subjects below the age of 60 years (210 units and 120 units, respectively). (Reproduced with permission, from McComas 1991.) (**B**) Rat MNs of the gastrocnemius medialis muscle. Distribution of average soma sizes in middle-aged (10–13 months, bold lines, open bars) and very old (31 months, grey bars) rats. When combined with motoneuronal counts, these data suggest that the decrease in mean soma diameter was caused by a loss of predominantly large MNs in old age. (Reproduced with permission, from Hashizume *et al.* 1988.)

in the elderly. Moreover, aged neuromuscular systems are also susceptible to the beneficial effects of training (Vandervoort 2002).

About half the MN somata in aged rats have a reduced bouton coverage (Kullberg *et al.* 1998), and MNs of ageing mice showed a decreased oxidative enzyme activity in the soma (SDH, senescence-accelerated mice at 60 weeks) (Hirofuji *et al.* 2000). Compared with adult cats (1–3 years), aged animals (14–15 years) had an increased input resistance, a decreased rheobase, longer-lasting Ia EPSPs, and a lower axonal conduction velocity; no change was found in the duration of AHP (Chase *et al.* 1985; Morales *et al.* 1987). Thus ageing MNs also change their characteristics in various respects, and these alterations provide a possible starting point for the further unravelling of the ageing processes at the motoneuronal level. However, it is still difficult to predict what effects the various MN changes might have on neuromuscular input–output relations and on the motor behaviour of ageing animals. In addition to muscle weakening, most of the motor disabilities of ageing individuals are probably related to alterations in various motor command systems within the CNS, upstream from the MNs and outside the scope of this book.

12.13. **Applied issue: how to make motoneurones**

In section 12.3 it was briefly described how vertebrates make their own MNs from pluripotential cells using a few inducing molecules at precise concentrations (see also Fig. 12.1D). If this analysis includes all the essential steps for MN induction, it should be possible to repeat the whole procedure *in vitro*. This has been done using embryonic stem cells from mouse, which were first made to differentiate into spinal progenitor cells, and subsequently into MNs, by exposing them to various factors including retinoic acid and sonic hedgehog agonist (Wichterle *et al.* 2002). The stem-cell-derived MNs were able to populate the embryonic chick spinal cord, extend axons, and form synapses with target muscles. Furthermore, in physiological experiments (Miles *et al.* 2004), the cells were shown to display various electrophysiological properties essential for MNs, including a sensitivity to applied GABA, glycine, and glutamate, indications that they excited muscle fibres using ACh, and a capacity for delivering repetitive spike discharges when stimulated with steady currents. There still remains much to learn about, for instance, how to differentiate such MNs into cells with specific tasks (e.g. with regard to which muscle to innervate), how to make them acquire adult functional properties, and how to integrate them into the existing neuronal network of a living organism (e.g. an adult spinal cord). However, these and other parallel experiments (MacDonald *et al.* 2003) clearly mark the beginning of a new and fascinating chapter in applied and fundamental neuromuscular physiology. Perhaps replacement cells may one day become available for patients who have lost their own MNs.

Copyright acknowledgements

Permission from the following copyright holders to reproduce material that has previously been published elsewhere is gratefully acknowledged (for a detailed reference to each article, see citation in the relevant figure or table legend and bibliographic information in the reference list).

From *Acta Physiologica Scandinavica*, permission for Figures 6.2B, 6.8A, and 7.1.

From the *American Physiological Society*, permission for Figures 3.5A, 3.9B, 5.2B–D, 6.1C, 6.4, 6.9, 7.3, 7.6A, 7.6B, 8.1A, 8.4C, 9.3A, 9.3C, 9.3D, 11.1, 11.2, 11.4B, and 11.5B, and for material for Figures 3.4B–D and Table 6.1.

From *Archives Italiennes de Biologie*, permission for Figures 5.6, 8.2B, and 8.3B.

From Blackwell Publishing (*Journal of Anatomy*), permission for Figure 3.11.

From Blackwell Publishing (*Journal of Physiology*), permission for Figures 3.2, 3.3B, 3.8, 3.9A, 4.2A–D, 6.1A, 6.1D, 6.5B, 7.2A–D, 7.4A, 9.3B, 10.2, 11.3A, and 11.5A, and for material for Figure 3.5B. Furthermore, permission to reuse material from previous publications of the author in Figures 5.3A, 5.3B, 5.4C, 5.4D, 6.2A, 6.8B, 7.4D, 7.4E, 7.5D, 9.1B, and 11.3B–C.

From Elsevier, permission for Figures 3.1E, 3.3A, 3.3C, 3.3D, 4.1, 5.3C, 5.5A, 7.7, 8.2A, 8.4B, 8.7A, 10.3A, 10.3B and for material in Table 2.1 and Figure 3.4A. Furthermore, permission to reuse material from previous publications by the author in Figures 3.9D, 5.5B, 5.5D, 5.6 (insets), 6.1B, 6.6A, 6.7A, 7.5A–C, 8.1B, 8.1C, 9.2, 9.4C, and 10.1D.

From *Nature Reviews Genetics* (www.nature.com/reviews, Macmillan Magazines Ltd), permission for Fig.12.1.

From the Royal Society, permission for Figures 5.2A and 11.4A.

From S. Karger AG (Basel), permission for Figure 3.10D.

From Society for Neuroscience (*Journal of Neuroscience*), permission for Figure 4.3.

From Springer-Verlag, permission for Figures 2.1A, 3.1A–D, 3.6B, 3.7, 3.9C, 6.3A, 6.3B, 6.5A, 6.5C, 6.5D, 6.8C, 6.8D, 8.3A, 8.4A, 9.4A, and 9.4B.

From Wiley–Liss Inc. (a subsidiary of John Wiley & Sons Inc.), permission for Figures 5.1A, 5.1B, 5.1C, 5.4A, 5.4B, and 12.2B (originally published in *Journal of Comparative Neurology*), Figures 7.4B and 7.4C (originally published in *Journal of Neurobiology*), and for Figures 3.6A, 8.6, 10.1A–C, and 12.2A (originally published in *Muscle & Nerve*).

References

Aasheim G, **Fink BR**, and **Middaugh M** (1974). Inhibition of rapid axoplasmic transport by procaine hydrochloride. *Anesthesiology*, **41**, 549–53.

Adams GR, **Haddad F**, and **Baldwin KM** (1999). Time course of changes in markers of myogenesis in overloaded rat skeletal muscles. *Journal of Applied Physiology*, **87**, 1705–12.

Adams GR, **Caiozzo VJ**, **Haddad F**, and **Baldwin KM** (2002). Cellular and molecular responses to increased skeletal muscle loading after irradiation. *American Journal of Physiology*, **283**, C1182–95.

Adrian ED (1932). *The Mechanism of Nervous Action*. Oxford University Press, London.

Adrian ED and **Bronk DW** (1929). The discharge of impulses in motor nerve fibres. II: The frequency of discharge in reflex and voluntary contractions. *Journal of Physiology*, **67**, 119–51.

Akagi Y (1978). The localization of the motor neurons innervating the extraocular muscles in the oculomotor nuclei of the cat and rabbit, using horseradish peroxidase. *Journal of Comparative Neurology*, **181**, 745–61.

Alaburda A, **Perrier JF**, and **Hounsgaard J** (2002). Mechanisms causing plateau potentials in spinal motoneurones. *Advances in Experimental Medicine and Biology*, **508**, 219–26.

Alaimo MA, **Smith JL**, **Roy RR**, and **Edgerton VR** (1984). EMG activity of slow and fast ankle extensors following spinal cord transection. *Journal of Applied Physiology*, **56**, 1608–13.

al-Amood WS and **Lewis DM** (1987). The role of frequency in the effects of long-term intermittent stimulation of denervated slow-twitch muscle in the rat. *Journal of Physiology*, **392**, 377–95.

al-Amood WS and **Lewis DM** (1989). A comparison of the effects of denervation on the mechanical properties of rat and guinea-pig skeletal muscle. *Journal of Physiology*, **414**, 1–16.

al-Amood WS, **Buller AJ** and **Pope R** (1973). Long-term stimulation of cat fast-twitch skeletal muscle. *Nature*, **244**, 225–7.

al-Amood WS, **Lewis DM**, and **Schmalbruch H** (1991). Effects of chronic electrical stimulation on contractile properties of long-term denervated rat skeletal muscle. *Journal of Physiology*, **441**, 243–56.

Alberts B, **Johnson A**, **Lewis J**, **Raff M**, **Roberts K**, and **Walter P** (2002). *Molecular Biology of the Cell*. Garland Science, New York.

Albuquerque EX, **Schuh FT**, and **Kauffman FC** (1971). Early membrane depolarization of the fast mammalian muscle after denervation. *Pflügers Archiv*, **328**, 36–50.

Aldskogius H and **Thomander L** (1986). Selective reinnervation of somatotopically appropriate muscles after facial nerve transection and regeneration in the neonatal rat. *Brain Research*, **375**, 126–34.

Alessandri-Haber N, **Paillart C**, **Arsac C**, **Gola M**, **Couraud F**, and **Crest M** (1999). Specific distribution of sodium channels in axons of rat embryo spinal motoneurones. *Journal of Physiology*, **518**, 203–14.

Alexianu ME, **Ho BK**, **Mohamed AH**, **La Bella V**, **Smith RG**, and **Appel SH** (1994). The role of calcium-binding proteins in selective motoneuron vulnerability in amyotrophic lateral sclerosis. *Annals of Neurology*, **36**, 846–58.

Alford EK, **Roy RR**, **Hodgson JA**, and **Edgerton VR** (1987). Electromyography of rat soleus, medial gastrocnemius, and tibialis anterior during hind limb suspension. *Experimental Neurology*, **96**, 635–49.

Allum JH, **Dietz V**, and **Freund HJ** (1978). Neuronal mechanisms underlying physiological tremor. *Journal of Neurophysiology*, **41**, 557–71.

Al-Majed AA, Neumann CM, Brushart TM, and Gordon T (2000). Brief electrical stimulation promotes the speed and accuracy of motor axonal regeneration. *Journal of Neuroscience*, **20**, 2602–8.

Almenar-Queralt A and Goldstein LS (2001). Linkers, packages and pathways: new concepts in axonal transport. *Current Opinion in Neurobiology*, **11**, 550–7.

Alvarez FJ, Dewey DE, McMillin P, and Fyffe RE (1999). Distribution of cholinergic contacts on Renshaw cells in the rat spinal cord: a light microscopic study. *Journal of Physiology*, **515**, 787–97.

Alway SE, Winchester PK, Davis ME and Gonyea WJ (1989). Regionalized adaptations and muscle fiber proliferation in stretch-induced enlargement. *Journal of Applied Physiology*, **66**, 771–81.

Andersen P and Langmoen IA (1980). Intracellular studies on transmitter effects on neurones in isolated brain slices. *Quarterly Review of Biophysics*, **13**, 1–18.

Andersson Y and Edstrom JE (1957). Motor hyperactivity resulting in diameter decrease of peripheral nerves. *Acta Physiologica Scandinavica*, **39**, 240–5.

Andonian MH and Fahim MA (1988). Endurance exercise alters the morphology of fast- and slow-twitch rat neuromuscular junctions. *International Journal of Sports Medicine*, **9**, 218–23.

Andrews BJ (1992). Reducing 'FES' muscle fatigue. In A Pedotti and M Ferrarin (eds), *Restoration of Walking for Paraplegics. Recent Advancements and Trends*, pp. 197–202. IOS Press, Amsterdam.

Appel B, Korzh V, Glasgow E, *et al.* (1995). Motoneuron fate specification revealed by patterned LIM homeobox gene expression in embryonic zebrafish. *Development*, **121**, 4117–25.

Arancio O, Buffelli M, Cangiano A, and Pasino E (1992). Nerve stump effects in muscle are independent of synaptic connections and are temporally correlated with nerve degeneration phenomena. *Neuroscience Letters*, **146**, 1–4.

Arber S, Burden SJ, and Harris AJ (2002). Patterning of skeletal muscle. *Current Opinion in Neurobiology*, **12**, 100–3.

Argaw A, Desaulniers P, and Gardiner PF (2004). Enhanced neuromuscular transmission efficacy in overloaded rat plantaris muscle. *Muscle & Nerve*, **29**, 97–103.

Ariano MA, Armstrong RB, and Edgerton VR (1973). Hindlimb muscle fiber populations of five mammals. *Journal of Histochemistry and Cytochemistry*, **21**, 51–5.

Armstrong RB (1980). Properties and distributions of the fiber types in the locomotory muscles of mammals. In K Schmidt-Nielsen, L Bolis and CR Taylor (eds), *Comparative Physiology: Primitive Mammals*, pp. 243–54. Cambridge University Press, Cambridge.

Asmussen G and Gaunitz U (1981a). Changes in mechanical properties of the inferior oblique muscle of the rabbit after denervation. *Pflügers Archiv*, **392**, 198–205.

Asmussen G and Gaunitz U (1981b). Mechanical properties of the isolated inferior oblique muscle of the rabbit. *Pflügers Archiv*, **392**, 183–90.

Asmussen G, Beckers-Bleukx G, and Marechal G (1994). The force–velocity relation of the rabbit inferior oblique muscle; influence of temperature. *Pflügers Archiv*, **426**, 542–7.

Attwell D and Iadecola C (2002). The neural basis of functional brain imaging signals. *Trends in Neurosciences*, **25**, 621–5.

Augustine JR, Deschamps EG, and Ferguson JG Jr (1981). Functional organization of the oculomotor nucleus in the baboon. *American Journal of Anatomy*, **161**, 393–403.

Ausoni S, Gorza L, Schiaffino S, Gundersen K, and Lomo T (1990). Expression of myosin heavy chain isoforms in stimulated fast and slow rat muscles. *Journal of Neuroscience*, **10**, 153–60.

Axelsson J and Thesleff S (1959). A study of supersensitivity in denervated mammalian skeletal muscle. *Journal of Physiology*, **147**, 178–93.

Bagust J, Lewis DM, and Luck JC (1974). Post-tetanic effects in motor units of fast and slow twitch muscle of the cat. *Journal of Physiology*, **237**, 115–21.

Bagust J, Lewis DM, and **Westerman RA** (1981). Motor units in cross-reinnervated fast and slow twitch muscle of the cat. *Journal of Physiology*, **313**, 223–35.

Bakels R and **Kernell D** (1993a). Average but not continuous speed match between motoneurons and muscle units of rat tibialis anterior. *Journal of Neurophysiology*, **70**, 1300–6.

Bakels R and **Kernell D** (1993b). Matching between motoneurone and muscle unit properties in rat medial gastrocnemius. *Journal of Physiology*, **463**, 307–24.

Bakels R and **Kernell D** (1994). Threshold-spacing in motoneurone pools of rat and cat: possible relevance for manner of force gradation. *Experimental Brain Research*, **102**, 69–74.

Bakels R, Nijenhuis M, **Mast L**, and **Kernell D** (1998). Hypothyroidism in the rat results in decreased soleus motoneurone soma size. *Neuroscience Letters*, **254**, 149–52.

Baker LL and **Chandler SH** (1987a). Characterization of hindlimb motoneuron membrane properties in acute and chronic spinal cats. *Brain Research*, **420**, 333–9.

Baker LL and **Chandler SH** (1987b). Characterization of postsynaptic potentials evoked by sural nerve stimulation in hindlimb motoneurons from acute and chronic spinal cats. *Brain Research*, **420**, 340–50.

Baldissera F and **Gustafsson B** (1971). Supraspinal control of the discharge evoked by constant current in the alpha-motoneurones. *Brain Research*, **25**, 642–4.

Baldissera F and **Gustafsson B** (1974). Firing behaviour of a neurone model based on the after-hyperpolarization conductance time course and algebraical summation. Adaptation and steady state firing. *Acta Physiologica Scandinavica*, **92**, 27–47.

Baldissera F and **Parmiggiani F** (1975). Relevance of motoneuronal firing adaptation to tension development in the motor unit. *Brain Research*, **91**, 315–20.

Baldissera F, **Gustafsson B** and **Parmiggiani F** (1978). Saturating summation of the after-hyperpolarization conductance in spinal motoneurones: a mechanism for 'secondary range' repetitive firing. *Brain Research*, **146**, 69–82.

Baldissera F, **Hultborn H** and **Illert M** (1981). Integration in spinal neuronal systems. In VB Brooks (ed.), *Handbook of Physiology*, Section 1, Volume II, pp. 509–95. American Physiological Society, Bethesda, MD.

Baldissera F, **Campadelli P**, and **Piccinelli L** (1987). The dynamic response of cat gastrocnemius motor units investigated by ramp-current injection into their motoneurones. *Journal of Physiology*, **387**, 317–30.

Baldwin KM and **Haddad F** (2001). Effects of different activity and inactivity paradigms on myosin heavy chain gene expression in striated muscle. *Journal of Applied Physiology*, **90**, 345–57.

Balice-Gordon RJ and **Lichtman JW** (1994). Long-term synapse loss induced by focal blockade of postsynaptic receptors. *Nature*, **372**, 519–24.

Balice-Gordon RJ and **Thompson WJ** (1988). The organization and development of compartmentalized innervation in rat extensor digitorum longus muscle. *Journal of Physiology*, **398**, 211–31.

Barany M (1967). ATPase activity of myosin correlated with speed of muscle shortening. *Journal of General Physiology*, **50** (Suppl), 197–218.

Barmack NH, **Bell CC**, and **Rence BG** (1971). Tension and rate of tension development during isometric responses of extraocular muscle. *Journal of Neurophysiology*, **34**, 1072–9.

Barnard EA, **Dolly JO**, **Porter CW**, and **Albuquerque EX** (1975). The acetylcholine receptor and the ionic conductance modulation system of skeletal muscle. *Experimental Neurology*, **48**, 1–28.

Barrett EF, **Barrett JN**, and **Crill WE** (1980). Voltage-sensitive outward currents in cat motoneurones. *Journal of Physiology*, **304**, 251–76.

Barrett JN and Crill WE (1974). Specific membrane properties of cat motoneurones. *Journal of Physiology*, **239**, 301–24.

Barrett JN and Crill WE (1980). Voltage clamp of cat motoneurone somata: properties of the fast inward current. *Journal of Physiology*, **304**, 231–49.

Bartlett SE, Reynolds AJ, and Hendry IA (1998). Retrograde axonal transport of neurotrophins: differences between neuronal populations and implications for motor neuron disease. *Immunology and Cell Biology*, **76**, 419–23.

Barton-Davis ER, LaFramboise WA, and Kushmerick MJ (1996). Activity-dependent induction of slow myosin gene expression in isolated fast-twitch mouse muscle. *American Journal of Physiology*, **271**, C1409–14.

Basmajian JV (1963). Control and training of individual motor units. *Science*, **141**, 440–1.

Baumann H, Jaggi M, Soland F, Howald H, and Schaub MC (1987). Exercise training induces transitions of myosin isoform subunits within histochemically typed human muscle fibres. *Pflügers Archiv*, **409**, 349–60.

Bawa P and Calancie B (1983). Repetitive doublets in human flexor carpi radialis muscle. *Journal of Physiology*, **339**, 123–32.

Bawa P, Binder MD, Ruenzel P, and Henneman E (1984). Recruitment order of motoneurons in stretch reflexes is highly correlated with their axonal conduction velocity. *Journal of Neurophysiology*, **52**, 410–20.

Bayliss DA, Sirois JE, and Talley EM (2003). The TASK family: two-pore domain background K^+ channels. *Molecular Interventions*, **3**, 205–19.

Beaumont E and Gardiner P (2002). Effects of daily spontaneous running on the electrophysiological properties of hindlimb motoneurones in rats. *Journal of Physiology*, **540**, 129–38.

Beaumont E and Gardiner PF (2003). Endurance training alters the biophysical properties of hindlimb motoneurons in rats. *Muscle & Nerve*, **27**, 228–36.

Belanger AY and McComas AJ (1981). Extent of motor unit activation during effort. *Journal of Applied Physiology*, **51**, 1131–5.

Bellemare F and Bigland-Ritchie B (1987). Central components of diaphragmatic fatigue assessed by phrenic nerve stimulation. *Journal of Applied Physiology*, **62**, 1307–16.

Beltman JG, Sargeant AJ, Van Mechelen W, and De Haan A (2004). Voluntary activation level and muscle fiber recruitment of human quadriceps during lengthening contractions. *Journal of Applied Physiology*, **97**, 619–26.

Bennett DJ, Hultborn H, Fedirchuk B, and Gorassini M (1998a). Short-term plasticity in hindlimb motoneurons of decerebrate cats. *Journal of Neurophysiology*, **80**, 2038–45.

Bennett DJ, Hultborn H, Fedirchuk B, and Gorassini M (1998b). Synaptic activation of plateaus in hindlimb motoneurons of decerebrate cats. *Journal of Neurophysiology*, **80**, 2023–37.

Bennett DJ, Gorassini M, Fouad K, Sanelli L, Han Y, and Cheng J (1999). Spasticity in rats with sacral spinal cord injury. *Journal of Neurotrauma*, **16**, 69–84.

Bennett DJ, Li Y, Harvey PJ and Gorassini M (2001a). Evidence for plateau potentials in tail motoneurons of awake chronic spinal rats with spasticity. *Journal of Neurophysiology*, **86**, 1972–82.

Bennett DJ, Li Y and Siu M (2001b). Plateau potentials in sacrocaudal motoneurons of chronic spinal rats, recorded *in vivo*. *Journal of Neurophysiology*, **86**, 1955–71.

Bennett DJ, Sanelli L, Cooke CL, Harvey PJ and Gorassini MA (2004). Spastic long-lasting reflexes in the awake rat after sacral spinal cord injury. *Journal of Neurophysiology*, **91**, 2247–58.

Bennett MR (1983). Development of neuromuscular synapses. *Physiological Reviews*, **63**, 915–1048.

Bennett MR and Hacker PM (2002). The motor system in neuroscience: a history and analysis of conceptual developments. *Progress in Neurobiology*, **67**, 1–52.

Bennett MR and Ho S (1988). The formation of topographical maps in developing rat gastrocnemius muscle during synapse elimination. *Journal of Physiology*, **396**, 471–96.

Bennett MR and Lavidis NA (1984). Segmental motor projections to rat muscles during the loss of polyneuronal innervation. *Develomental Brain Research*, **13**, 1–7.

Bensimon G, Lacomblez L and Meininger V (1994). A controlled trial of riluzole in amyotrophic lateral sclerosis. ALS/Riluzole Study Group. *New England Journal of Medicine*, **330**, 585–91.

Berg DK and Hall ZW (1974). Fate of alpha-bungarotoxin bound to acetylcholine receptors of normal and denervated muscle. *Science*, **184**, 473–5.

Berg DK and Hall ZW (1975). Loss of alpha-bungarotoxin from junctional and extrajunctional acetylcholine receptors in rat diaphragm muscle *in vivo* and in organ culture. *Journal of Physiology*, **252**, 771–89.

Berg HE, Dudley GA, Haggmark T, Ohlsen H, and Tesch PA (1991). Effects of lower limb unloading on skeletal muscle mass and function in humans. *Journal of Applied Physiology*, **70**, 1882–5.

Berg HE, Larsson L, and Tesch PA (1997). Lower limb skeletal muscle function after 6 wk of bed rest. *Journal of Applied Physiology*, **82**, 182–8.

Berger AJ, Bayliss DA, and Viana F (1992). Modulation of neonatal rat hypoglossal motoneuron excitability by serotonin. *Neuroscience Letters*, **143**, 164–8.

Berger AJ, Bayliss DA, Bellingham MC, Umemiya M, and Viana F (1995). Postnatal development of hypoglossal motoneuron intrinsic properties. *Advances in Experimental Medicine and Biology*, **381**, 63–71.

Bergmans J (1970). *The Physiology of Single Human Nerve Fibres*. Vander, Louvain, Belgium.

Bernheim L, Hamann M, Liu JH, Fischer-Lougheed J, and Bader CR (1996). Role of nicotinic acetylcholine receptors at the vertebrate myotendinous junction: a hypothesis. *Neuromuscular Disorders*, **6**, 211–14.

Bernstein JJ and Guth L (1961). Nonselectivity in establishment of neuromuscular connections following nerve regeneration in the rat. *Experimental Neurology*, **4**, 262–75.

Bertrand N, Castro DS, and Guillemot F (2002). Proneural genes and the specification of neural cell types. *Nature Reviews Neuroscience*, **3**, 517–30.

Bessou P, Emonet-Denand F, and Laporte Y (1963). [Relation between the conduction rate of motor nerve fibers and the contraction time of their motor units.] *Comptes Rendus Hebdomadaires des Seances de l'Academie des Sciences*, **256**, 5625–7.

Bewick GS, Reid B, Jawaid S, Hatcher T, and Shanley L (2004). Postnatal emergence of mature release properties in terminals of rat fast- and slow-twitch muscles. *European Journal of Neuroscience*, **19**, 2967–76.

Bigland-Ritchie B and Woods JJ (1984). Changes in muscle contractile properties and neural control during human muscular fatigue. *Muscle & Nerve*, **7**, 691–9.

Bigland-Ritchie B, Jones DA, and Woods JJ (1979). Excitation frequency and muscle fatigue: electrical responses during human voluntary and stimulated contractions. *Experimental Neurology*, **64**, 414–27.

Bigland-Ritchie B, Kukulka CG, Lippold OC, and Woods JJ (1982). The absence of neuromuscular transmission failure in sustained maximal voluntary contractions. *Journal of Physiology*, **330**, 265–78.

Bigland-Ritchie B, Johansson R, Lippold OC, Smith S, and Woods JJ (1983a). Changes in motoneurone firing rates during sustained maximal voluntary contractions. *Journal of Physiology*, **340**, 335–46.

Bigland-Ritchie B, Johansson R, Lippold OC, and Woods JJ (1983b). Contractile speed and EMG changes during fatigue of sustained maximal voluntary contractions. *Journal of Neurophysiology*, **50**, 313–24.

Bigland-Ritchie BR, Dawson NJ, Johansson RS, and **Lippold OC** (1986). Reflex origin for the slowing of motoneurone firing rates in fatigue of human voluntary contractions. *Journal of Physiology*, **379**, 451–9.

Bigland-Ritchie B, Thomas CK, Rice CL, Howarth JV, and **Woods JJ** (1992a). Muscle temperature, contractile speed, and motoneuron firing rates during human voluntary contractions. *Journal of Applied Physiology*, **73**, 2457–61.

Bigland-Ritchie BR, Furbush FH, Gandevia SC, and **Thomas CK** (1992b). Voluntary discharge frequencies of human motoneurons at different muscle lengths. *Muscle & Nerve*, **15**, 130–7.

Bigland-Ritchie B, Zijdewind I, and **Thomas CK** (2000). Muscle fatigue induced by stimulation with and without doublets. *Muscle & Nerve*, **23**, 1348–55.

Billeter R, Heizmann CW, Howald H, and **Jenny E** (1981). Analysis of myosin light and heavy chain types in single human skeletal muscle fibers. *European Journal of Biochemistry*, **116**, 389–95.

Binder MC, Bawa P, Ruenzel P, and **Henneman E** (1983). Does orderly recruitment of motoneurons depend on the existence of different types of motor units? *Neuroscience Letters*, **36**, 55–8.

Binder MD (2002). Integration of synaptic and intrinsic dendritic currents in cat spinal motoneurons. *Brain Research Reviews*, **40**, 1–8.

Binder MD, Heckman CJ, and **Powers RK** (1996). The physiological control of motoneuron activity. In LB Rowell and JT Shepherd (eds), *Handbook of Physiology*, Section 12, pp. 3–53. American Physiological Society, Bethesda, MD.

Binder MD, Robinson FR, and **Powers RK** (1998). Distribution of effective synaptic currents in cat triceps surae motoneurons. VI: Contralateral pyramidal tract. *Journal of Neurophysiology*, **80**, 241–8.

Binder-Macleod SA (1992). Force–frequency relation in skeletal muscle. In DP Currier and RM Nelson (eds), *Dynamics of Human Biological Tissues*, pp. 97–113. F.A.Davis, Philadelphia, PA.

Binder-Macleod SA and **Barker CB** (1991). Use of a catchlike property of human skeletal muscle to reduce fatigue. *Muscle & Nerve*, **14**, 850–7.

Binder-Macleod SA and **Clamann HP** (1989). Force output of cat motor units stimulated with trains of linearly varying frequency. *Journal of Neurophysiology*, **61**, 208–17.

Binder-Macleod S and **Kesar T** (2005). Catchlike property of skeletal muscle: recent findings and clinical implications. *Muscle & Nerve*, **31**, 681–93.

Black J (1999). Claude Bernard on the action of curare. *British Medical Journal*, **319**, 622.

Blankenship JE (1968). Action of tetrodotoxin on spinal motoneurons of the cat. *Journal of Neurophysiology*, **31**, 186–94.

Blewett C and **Elder GC** (1993). Quantitative EMG analysis in soleus and plantaris during hindlimb suspension and recovery. *Journal of Applied Physiology*, **74**, 2057–66.

Blinkov SM and **Glezer II** (1968). *The Human Brain in Figures and Tables. A Quantitative Handbook.* Plenum Press, New York.

Blinzinger K and **Kreutzberg G** (1968). Displacement of synaptic terminals from regenerating motoneurons by microglial cells. *Zeitschrift für Zellforschung und Mikroskopische Anatomie*, **85**, 145–57.

Bodine SC, Roy RR, Eldred E, and **Edgerton VR** (1987). Maximal force as a function of anatomical features of motor units in the cat tibialis anterior. *Journal of Neurophysiology*, **57**, 1730–45.

Bodine-Fowler SC, Meyer S, Moskovitz A, Abrams R and **Botte MJ** (1997). Inaccurate projection of rat soleus motoneurons: a comparison of nerve repair techniques. *Muscle & Nerve*, **20**, 29–37.

Bonen A, McDermott JC, and **Hutber CA** (1989). Carbohydrate metabolism in skeletal muscle: an update of current concepts. *International Journal of Sports Medicine*, **10**, 385–401.

Bongiovanni LG and **Hagbarth KE** (1990). Tonic vibration reflexes elicited during fatigue from maximal voluntary contractions in man. *Journal of Physiology*, **423**, 1–14.

Botterman BR and Cope TC (1988). Motor-unit stimulation patterns during fatiguing contractions of constant tension. *Journal of Neurophysiology*, **60**, 1198–1214.

Botterman BR, Iwamoto GA, and Gonyea WJ (1986). Gradation of isometric tension by different activation rates in motor units of cat flexor carpi radialis muscle. *Journal of Neurophysiology*, **56**, 494–506.

Bottinelli R, Betto R, Schiaffino S, and Reggiani C (1994). Unloaded shortening velocity and myosin heavy chain and alkali light chain isoform composition in rat skeletal muscle fibres. *Journal of Physiology*, **478**, 341–9.

Boyd IA and Davey MR (1968). *Composition of Peripheral Nerves*. E & S Livingstone Ltd, Edinburgh.

Boyd JA and Martin AR (1956). The end-plate potential in mammalian muscle. *Journal of Physiology*, **132**, 74–91.

Bradley K and Somjen GG (1961). Accommodation in motoneurones of the rat and the cat. *Journal of Physiology*, **156**, 75–92.

Brannstrom T (1993). Quantitative synaptology of functionally different types of cat medial gastrocnemius alpha-motoneurons. *Journal of Comparative Neurology*, **330**, 439–54.

Brannstrom T and Kellerth JO (1998). Changes in synaptology of adult cat spinal alpha-motoneurons after axotomy. *Experimental Brain Research*, **118**, 1–13.

Brannstrom T, Havton L, and Kellerth JO (1992a). Changes in size and dendritic arborization patterns of adult cat spinal alpha-motoneurons following permanent axotomy. *Journal of Comparative Neurology*, **318**, 439–51.

Brannstrom T, Havton L, and Kellerth JO (1992b). Restorative effects of reinnervation on the size and dendritic arborization patterns of axotomized cat spinal alpha-motoneurons. *Journal of Comparative Neurology*, **318**, 452–61.

Bray JJ, Hawken MJ, Hubbard JI, Pockett S, and Wilson L (1976). The membrane potential of rat diaphragm muscle fibres and the effect of denervation. *Journal of Physiology*, **255**, 651–67.

Brenner HR, Witzemann V, and Sakmann B (1990). Imprinting of acetylcholine receptor messenger RNA accumulation in mammalian neuromuscular synapses. *Nature*, **344**, 544–7.

Briscoe J and Ericson J (2001). Specification of neuronal fates in the ventral neural tube. *Current Opinion in Neurobiology*, **11**, 43–9.

Brizzi L, Meunier C, Zytnicki D, *et al.* (2004). How shunting inhibition affects the discharge of lumbar motoneurones: a dynamic clamp study in anaesthetized cats. *Journal of Physiology*, **558**, 671–83.

Brock LG, Coombs JS, and Eccles JC (1952). The recording of potentials from motoneurones with an intracellular electrode. *Journal of Physiology*, **117**, 431–60.

Brodal A (1973). Self-observations and neuro-anatomical considerations after a stroke. *Brain*, **96**, 675–94.

Brody IA (1976). Regulation of isometric contraction in skeletal muscle. *Experimental Neurology*, **50**, 673–83.

Brooke MH and Kaiser KK (1970). Muscle fiber types: how many and what kind? *Archives of Neurology*, **23**, 369–79.

Brown AG and Fyffe RE (1981). Direct observations on the contacts made between Ia afferent fibres and alpha-motoneurones in the cat's lumbosacral spinal cord. *Journal of Physiology*, **313**, 121–40.

Brown GL and von Euler US (1938). The after effects of a tetanus on mammalian muscle. *Journal of Physiology*, **93**, 39–60.

Brown IE, Cheng EJ, and Loeb GE (1999). Measured and modeled properties of mammalian skeletal muscle. II. The effects of stimulus frequency on force–length and force–velocity relationships. *Journal of Muscle Research and Cell Motility*, **20**, 627–43.

Brown JM, Henriksson J, and Salmons S (1989). Restoration of fast muscle characteristics following cessation of chronic stimulation: physiological, histochemical and metabolic changes during slow-to-fast transformation. *Proceedings of the Royal Society of London, Series B*, **235**, 321–46.

Brown MC (1984). Sprouting of motor nerves in adult muscles: a recapitulation of ontogeny. *Trends in Neurosciences*, 7, 10–14.

Brown MC and Booth CM (1983). Postnatal development of the adult pattern of motor axon distribution in rat muscle. *Nature*, 304, 741–2.

Brownstone RM, Jordan LM, Kriellaars DJ, Noga BR and Shefchyk SJ (1992). On the regulation of repetitive firing in lumbar motoneurones during fictive locomotion in the cat. *Experimental Brain Research*, 90, 441–55.

Bruijn LI, Miller TM, and Cleveland DW (2004). Unraveling the mechanisms involved in motor neuron degeneration in ALS. *Annual Review of Neuroscience*, 27, 723–49.

Brushart TM (1988). Preferential reinnervation of motor nerves by regenerating motor axons. *Journal of Neuroscience*, 8, 1026–31.

Brushart TM (1993). Motor axons preferentially reinnervate motor pathways. *Journal of Neuroscience*, 13, 2730–8.

Brushart TM and Mesulam MM (1980). Alteration in connections between muscle and anterior horn motoneurons after peripheral nerve repair. *Science*, 208, 603–5.

Brushart TM, Hoffman PN, Royall RM, Murinson BB, Witzel C, and Gordon T (2002). Electrical stimulation promotes motoneuron regeneration without increasing its speed or conditioning the neuron. *Journal of Neuroscience*, 22, 6631–8.

Bruusgaard JC, Liestol K, Ekmark M, Kollstad K, and Gundersen K (2003). Number and spatial distribution of nuclei in the muscle fibres of normal mice studied *in vivo. Journal of Physiology*, 551, 467–78.

Buchthal F and Schmalbruch H (1980). Motor unit of mammalian muscle. *Physiological Reviews*, 60, 90–142.

Buck CR, Seburn KL, and Cope TC (2000). Neurotrophin expression by spinal motoneurons in adult and developing rats. *Journal of Comparative Neurology*, 416, 309–18.

Buller AJ and Lewis DM (1965a). Further observations on mammalian cross-innervated skeletal muscle. *Journal of Physiology*, 178, 343–58.

Buller AJ and Lewis DM (1965b). Further observations on the differentiation of skeletal muscles in the kitten hind limb. *Journal of Physiology*, 176, 355–70.

Buller AJ and Lewis DM (1965c). The rate of tension development in isometric tetanic contractions of mammalian fast and slow skeletal muscle. *Journal of Physiology*, 176, 337–54.

Buller AJ, Eccles JC and Eccles RM (1960a). Differentiation of fast and slow muscles in the cat hind limb. *Journal of Physiology*, 150, 399–416.

Buller AJ, Eccles JC and Eccles RM (1960b). Interactions between motoneurones and muscles in respect of the characteristic speeds of their responses. *Journal of Physiology*, 150, 417–39.

Buller AJ, Kean CJ and Ranatunga KW (1987). Transformation of contraction speed in muscle following cross-reinnervation; dependence on muscle size. *Journal of Muscle Research and Cell Motility*, 8, 504–16.

Bunge MB, Clark MB, Dean AC, Eldridge CF and Bunge RP (1990). Schwann cell function depends upon axonal signals and basal lamina components. *Annals of the New York Academy of Science*, 580, 281–7.

Burke RE (1967a). Composite nature of the monosynaptic excitatory postsynaptic potential. *Journal of Neurophysiology*, 30, 1114–37.

Burke RE (1967b). Motor unit types of cat triceps surae muscle. *Journal of Physiology*, 193, 141–60.

Burke RE (1968a). Firing patterns of gastrocnemius motor units in the decerebrate cat. *Journal of Physiology*, 196, 631–54.

Burke RE (1968b). Group Ia synaptic input to fast and slow twitch motor units of cat triceps surae. *Journal of Physiology*, **196**, 605–30.

Burke RE (1981). Motor units: anatomy, physiology and functional organization. In VB Brooks (ed.), *Handbook of Physiology*, Section 1, Volume II, pp. 345–422. American Physiological Society, Bethesda, MD.

Burke RE (2000). Comparison of alternative designs for reducing complex neurons to equivalent cables. *Journal of Computational Neuroscience*, **9**, 31–47.

Burke RE (2004). Spinal cord: ventral horn. In GM Shepherd (ed.), *The Synaptic Organization of the Brain*, pp. 79–123. Oxford University Press, Oxford.

Burke RE and Glenn LL (1996). Horseradish peroxidase study of the spatial and electrotonic distribution of group Ia synapses on type-identified ankle extensor motoneurons in the cat. *Journal of Comparative Neurology*, **372**, 465–85.

Burke RE and Nelson PG (1971). Accommodation to current ramps in motoneurons of fast and slow twitch motor units. *International Journal of Neuroscience*, **1**, 347–56.

Burke RE and Rudomin P (1977). Spinal neurons and synapses. In ER Kandel (ed.), *Handbook of Physiology*, Section 1, Volume I, pp. 877–944. American Physiological Society, Bethesda, MD.

Burke RE and Rymer WZ (1976). Relative strength of synaptic input from short-latency pathways to motor units of defined type in cat medial gastrocnemius. *Journal of Neurophysiology*, **39**, 447–58.

Burke RE and ten Bruggencate G (1971). Electrotonic characteristics of alpha motoneurones of varying size. *Journal of Physiology*, **212**, 120.

Burke RE, Jankowska E, and ten Bruggencate G (1970). A comparison of peripheral and rubrospinal synaptic input to slow and fast twitch motor units of triceps surae. *Journal of Physiology*, **207**, 709–32.

Burke RE, Fedina L, and Lundberg A (1971a). Spatial synaptic distribution of recurrent and group Ia inhibitory systems in cat spinal motoneurones. *Journal of Physiology*, **214**, 305–26.

Burke RE, Levine DN, and Zajac FE 3rd (1971b). Mammalian motor units: physiological-histochemical correlation in three types in cat gastrocnemius. *Science*, **174**, 709–12.

Burke RE, Levine DN, Tsairis P, and Zajac FE 3rd (1973). Physiological types and histochemical profiles in motor units of the cat gastrocnemius. *Journal of Physiology*, **234**, 723–48.

Burke RE, Levine DN, Salcman M, and Tsairis P (1974). Motor units in cat soleus muscle: physiological, histochemical and morphological characteristics. *Journal of Physiology*, **238**, 503–14.

Burke RE, Rudomin P and Zajac FE 3rd (1976). The effect of activation history on tension production by individual muscle units. *Brain Research*, **109**, 515–29.

Burke RE, Strick PL, Kanda K, Kim CC, and Walmsley B (1977). Anatomy of medial gastrocnemius and soleus motor nuclei in cat spinal cord. *Journal of Neurophysiology*, **40**, 667–80.

Burke RE, Dum RP, Fleshman JW, *et al.* (1982). A HRP study of the relation between cell size and motor unit type in cat ankle extensor motoneurons. *Journal of Comparative Neurology*, **209**, 17–28.

Buss RR and Oppenheim RW (2004). Role of programmed cell death in normal neuronal development and function. *Anatomical Science International*, **79**, 191–7.

Caldero J, Casanovas A, Sorribas A and Esquerda JE (1992). Calcitonin gene-related peptide in rat spinal cord motoneurons: subcellular distribution and changes induced by axotomy. *Neuroscience*, **48**, 449–61.

Callaway EM, Soha JM, and Van Essen DC (1987). Competition favouring inactive over active motor neurons during synapse elimination. *Nature*, **328**, 422–6.

Calvin WH (1975). Generation of spike trains in CNS neurons. *Brain Research*, **84**, 1–22.

Cameron WE, Fang H, Brozanski BS, and Guthrie RD (1989). The postnatal growth of motoneurons at three levels of the cat neuraxis. *Neuroscience Letters*, **104**, 274–80.

Cameron WE, He F, Kalipatnapu P, Jodkowski JS, and Guthrie RD (1991). Morphometric analysis of phrenic motoneurons in the cat during postnatal development. *Journal of Comparative Neurology*, **314**, 763–76.

Campa JF and Engel WK (1970a). Histochemical classification of anterior horn neurons. *Neurology*, **20**, 386.

Campa JF and Engel WK (1970b). Histochemistry of motor neurons and interneurons in the cat lumbar spinal cord. *Neurology*, **20**, 559–68.

Campa JF and Engel WK (1973). Histochemistry of motoneurons innervating slow and fast motor units. In JE Desmedt (ed.), *New Developments in Electromyography and Clinical Neurophysiology*, pp. 178–85. Karger, Basel.

Campbell KB, Razumova MV, Kirkpatrick RD, and Slinker BK (2001). Myofilament kinetics in isometric twitch dynamics. *Annals of Biomedical Engineering*, **29**, 384–405.

Carp JS and Wolpaw JR (1994). Motoneuron plasticity underlying operantly conditioned decrease in primate H-reflex. *Journal of Neurophysiology*, **72**, 431–42.

Carp JS, Powers RK, and Rymer WZ (1991). Alterations in motoneuron properties induced by acute dorsal spinal hemisection in the decerebrate cat. *Experimental Brain Research*, **83**, 539–48.

Carp JS, Herchenroder PA, Chen XY, and Wolpaw JR (1999). Sag during unfused tetanic contractions in rat triceps surae motor units. *Journal of Neurophysiology*, **81**, 2647–61.

Carp JS, Chen XY, Sheikh H, and Wolpaw JR (2001). Operant conditioning of rat H-reflex affects motoneuron axonal conduction velocity. *Experimental Brain Research*, **136**, 269–73.

Carp JS, Tennissen AM, and Wolpaw JR (2003). Conduction velocity is inversely related to action potential threshold in rat motoneuron axons. *Experimental Brain Research*, **150**, 497–505.

Carroll S, Nicotera P, and Pette D (1999). Calcium transients in single fibers of low-frequency stimulated fast-twitch muscle of rat. *American Journal of Physiology*, **277**, C1122–9.

Carson JA and Wei L (2000). Integrin signaling's potential for mediating gene expression in hypertrophying skeletal muscle. *Journal of Applied Physiology*, **88**, 337–43.

Castro MJ, Apple DFJr, Staron RS, Campos GE, and Dudley GA (1999). Influence of complete spinal cord injury on skeletal muscle within 6 mo of injury. *Journal of Applied Physiology*, **86**, 350–8.

Chalmers GR and Edgerton VR (1989). Single motoneuron succinate dehydrogenase activity. *Journal of Histochemistry and Cytochemistry*, **37**, 1107–14.

Chalmers GR, Roy RR, and Edgerton VR (1991). Motoneuron and muscle fiber succinate dehydrogenase activity in control and overloaded plantaris. *Journal of Applied Physiology*, **71**, 1589–92.

Chalmers GR, Roy RR, and Edgerton VR (1992). Adaptability of the oxidative capacity of motoneurons. *Brain Research*, **570**, 1–10.

Chamberlain S and Lewis DM (1989). Contractile characteristics and innervation ratio of rat soleus motor units. *Journal of Physiology*, **412**, 1–21.

Chan AK, Edgerton VR, Goslow GE Jr, Kurata H, Rasmussen SA, and Spector SA (1982). Histochemical and physiological properties of cat motor units after self-and cross-reinnervation. *Journal of Physiology*, **332**, 343–61.

Chanaud CM, Pratt CA, and Loeb GE (1991). Functionally complex muscles of the cat hindlimb. V. The roles of histochemical fiber-type regionalization and mechanical heterogeneity in differential muscle activation. *Experimental Brain Research*, **85**, 300–13.

Chang Q, Pereda A, Pinter MJ, and Balice-Gordon RJ (2000). Nerve injury induces gap junctional coupling among axotomized adult motor neurons. *Journal of Neuroscience*, **20**, 674–84.

Chase MH, Morales FR, Boxer PA and Fung SJ (1985). Aging of motoneurons and synaptic processes in the cat. *Experimental Neurology*, **90**, 471–8.

Chaudhuri A and Behan PO (2004). Fatigue in neurological disorders. *Lancet*, **363**, 978–88.

Chen XY and Wolpaw JR (1994). Triceps surae motoneuron morphology in the rat: a quantitative light microscopic study. *Journal of Comparative Neurology*, **343**, 143–57.

Chin ER, Olson EN, Richardson JA *et al.* (1998). A calcineurin-dependent transcriptional pathway controls skeletal muscle fiber type. *Genes & Development*, **12**, 2499–509.

Chiu SY, Ritchie JM, Rogart RB, and Stagg D (1979). A quantitative description of membrane currents in rabbit myelinated nerve. *Journal of Physiology*, **292**, 149–66.

Christou EA, Jakobi JM, Critchlow A, Fleshner M, and Enoka RM (2004). The 1- to 2-Hz oscillations in muscle force are exacerbated by stress, especially in older adults. *Journal of Applied Physiology*, **97**, 225–35.

Clamann HP and Henneman E (1976). Electrical measurement of axon diameter and its use in relating motoneuron size to critical firing level. *Journal of Neurophysiology*, **39**, 844–51.

Clamann HP and Kukulka CG (1977). The relation between size of motoneurons and their position in the cat spinal cord. *Journal of Morphology*, **153**, 461–6.

Clamann HP and Robinson AJ (1985). A comparison of electromyographic and mechanical fatigue properties in motor units of the cat hindlimb. *Brain Research*, **327**, 203–19.

Clamann HP and Schelhorn TB (1988). Nonlinear force addition of newly recruited motor units in the cat hindlimb. *Muscle & Nerve*, **11**, 1079–89.

Clamann HP, Henneman E, Luscher HR, and Mathis J (1985). Structural and topographical influences on functional connectivity in spinal monosynaptic reflex arcs in the cat. *Journal of Physiology*, **358**, 483–507.

Clausen T (2003). Na$^+$–K$^+$ pump regulation and skeletal muscle contractility. *Physiological Reviews*, **83**, 1269–1324.

Clements JD and Redman SJ (1989). Cable properties of cat spinal motoneurones measured by combining voltage clamp, current clamp and intracellular staining. *Journal of Physiology*, **409**, 63–87.

Cleveland S, Kuschmierz A, and Ross HG (1981). Static input-output relations in the spinal recurrent inhibitory pathway. *Biological Cybernetics*, **40**, 223–31.

Close R (1964). Dynamic properties of fast and slow skeletal muscles of the rat during development. *Journal of Physiology*, **173**, 74–95.

Close R (1965). The relation between intrinsic speed of shortening and duration of the active state of muscle. *Journal of Physiology*, **180**, 542–59.

Close R (1969). Dynamic properties of fast and slow skeletal muscles of the rat after nerve cross-union. *Journal of Physiology*, **204**, 331–46.

Clough JFM, Kernell D, and Phillips CG (1968a). Conduction velocity in proximal and distal portions of forelimb axons in the baboon. *Journal of Physiology*, **198**, 167–78.

Clough JFM, Kernell D, and Phillips CG (1968b). The distribution of monosynaptic excitation from the pyramidal tract and from primary spindle afferents to motoneurones of the baboon's hand and forearm. *Journal of Physiology*, **198**, 145–66.

Cohen MJ (1987). The shape of nerve cells. In G Adelman (ed.), *Encyclopedia of Neuroscience*, pp. 1088–9. Birkhäuser, Boston, MA.

Collins DF, Burke D, and Gandevia SC (2002). Sustained contractions produced by plateau-like behaviour in human motoneurones. *Journal of Physiology*, **538**, 289–301.

Condon K, Silberstein L, Blau HM, and Thompson WJ (1990). Differentiation of fiber types in aneural musculature of the prenatal rat hindlimb. *Developmental Biology*, **138**, 275–95.

Conjard A, Peuker H, and Pette D (1998). Energy state and myosin heavy chain isoforms in single fibres of normal and transforming rabbit muscles. *Pflügers Archiv*, **436**, 962–9.

Conradi S and Ronnevi LO (1975). Spontaneous elimination of synapses on cat spinal motoneurons after birth: do half of the synapses on the cell bodies disappear? *Brain Research*, **92**, 505–10.

Conradi S and Skoglund S (1969). Observations on the ultrastruture and distribution of neuronal and glial elements on the motoneuron surface in the lumbosacral spinal cord of the cat during postnatal development. *Acta Physiologica Scandinavica Supplementum*, **333**, 5–52.

Conradi S, Kellerth JO, Berthold CH, and Hammarberg C (1979). Electron microscopic studies of serially sectioned cat spinal alpha-motoneurons. IV: Motoneurons innervating slow-twitch (type S) units of the soleus muscle. *Journal of Comparative Neurology*, **184**, 769–82.

Conway BA, Hultborn H, Kiehn O, and Mintz I (1988). Plateau potentials in alpha-motoneurones induced by intravenous injection of L-dopa and clonidine in the spinal cat. *Journal of Physiology*, **405**, 369–84.

Coombs JS, Eccles JC, and Fatt P (1955). The electrical properties of the motoneurone membrane. *Journal of Physiology*, **130**, 291–325.

Cooper S and Eccles JC (1930). The isometric responses of mammalian muscles. *Journal of Physiology*, **69**, 377–85.

Cooper S and Sherrington CS (1940). Gower's tract and spinal border cells. *Brain*, **63**, 123–34.

Cope T and Pinter M (1995). The size principle: still working after all these years. *News in Physiological Sciences*, **10**, 280–6.

Cope TC, Bodine SC, Fournier M, and Edgerton VR (1986). Soleus motor units in chronic spinal transected cats: physiological and morphological alterations. *Journal of Neurophysiology*, **55**, 1202–20.

Copray JC and Brouwer N (1994). Selective expression of neurotrophin-3 messenger RNA in muscle spindles of the rat. *Neuroscience*, **63**, 1125–35.

Copray JC, Liem RS, and Kernell D (1996). Calreticulin expression in spinal motoneurons of the rat. *Journal of Chemical Neuroanatomy*, **11**, 57–65.

Copray JC, Jaarsma D, Kust BM, *et al.* (2003). Expression of the low affinity neurotrophin receptor p75 in spinal motoneurons in a transgenic mouse model for amyotrophic lateral sclerosis. *Neuroscience*, **116**, 685–94.

Copray S and Kernell D (2000). Neurotrophins and trk-receptors in adult rat spinal motoneurons: differences related to cell size but not to 'slow/fast' specialization. *Neuroscience Letters*, **289**, 217–20.

Cormery B, Marini JF, and Gardiner PF (2000). Changes in electrophysiological properties of tibial motoneurones in the rat following 4 weeks of tetrodotoxin-induced paralysis. *Neuroscience Letters*, **287**, 21–4.

Cragg BG (1970). What is the signal for chromatolysis? *Brain Research*, **23**, 1–21.

Cramer KS and Van-Essen DC (1995). Lack of topography in the spinal cord projection to the rabbit soleus muscle. *Journal of Comparative Neurology*, **351**, 404–14.

Creed RS, Denny-Brown D, Eccles JC, Liddell EGT, and Sherrington CS (1932). *Reflex Activity of the Spinal Cord*. Oxford University Press, London.

Crill WE (1996). Persistent sodium current in mammalian central neurons. *Annual Review of Physiology*, **58**, 349–62.

Crill WE (1999). Functional implications of dendritic voltage-dependent conductances. *Journal de Physiologie*, **93**, 17–21.

Crill WE and Kennedy TT (1967). Inferior olive of the cat: intracellular recording. *Science*, **157**, 716–18.

Crone C, Hultborn H, Kiehn O, Mazieres L, and Wigstrom H (1988). Maintained changes in motoneuronal excitability by short-lasting synaptic inputs in the decerebrate cat. *Journal of Physiology*, **405**, 321–43.

Crow MT and Kushmerick MJ (1982). Chemical energetics of slow- and fast-twitch muscles of the mouse. *Journal of General Physiology*, **79**, 147–66.

Cull-Candy SG, Miledi R, and Uchitel OD (1982). Properties of junctional and extrajunctional acetylcholine-receptor channels in organ cultured human muscle fibres. *Journal of Physiology*, **333**, 251–67.

Cullheim S (1978). Relations between cell body size, axon diameter and axon conduction velocity of cat sciatic alpha-motoneurons stained with horseradish peroxidase. *Neuroscience Letters*, **8**, 17–20.

Cullheim S and Kellerth JO (1978a). A morphological study of the axons and recurrent axon collaterals of cat alpha-motoneurones supplying different functional types of muscle unit. *Journal of Physiology*, **281**, 301–13.

Cullheim S and Kellerth JO (1978b). A morphological study of the axons and recurrent axon collaterals of cat alpha-motoneurones supplying different hind-limb muscles. *Journal of Physiology*, **281**, 285–99.

Cullheim S and Kellerth JO (1978c). A morphological study of the axons and recurrent axon collaterals of cat sciatic alpha-motoneurons after intracellular staining with horseradish peroxidase. *Journal of Comparative Neurology*, **178**, 537–57.

Cullheim S and Kellerth JO (1981). Two kinds of recurrent inhibition of cat spinal alpha-motoneurones as differentiated pharmacologically. *Journal of Physiology*, **312**, 209–24.

Cullheim S, Kellerth JO, and Conradi S (1977). Evidence for direct synaptic interconnections between cat spinal alpha-motoneurons via the recurrent axon collaterals: a morphological study using intracellular injection of horseradish peroxidase. *Brain Research*, **132**, 1–10.

Cullheim S, Lipsenthal L, and Burke RE (1984). Direct monosynaptic contacts between type-identified alpha-motoneurons in the cat. *Brain Research*, **308**, 196–9.

Cullheim S, Fleshman JW, Glenn LL, and Burke RE (1987a). Membrane area and dendritic structure in type-identified triceps surae alpha motoneurons. *Journal of Comparative Neurology*, **255**, 68–81.

Cullheim S, Fleshman JW, Glenn LL, and Burke RE (1987b). Three-dimensional architecture of dendritic trees in type-identified alpha-motoneurons. *Journal of Comparative Neurology*, **255**, 82–96.

Curtis DR and Eccles JC (1960). Synaptic action during and after repetitive stimulation. *Journal of Physiology*, **150**, 374–98.

Cushing S, Bui T, and Rose PK (2005). Effect of nonlinear summation of synaptic currents on the input–output properties of spinal motoneurons. *Journal of Neurophysiology*, **94**, 3465–78.

Czéh G, Gallego R, Kudo N, and Kuno M (1978). Evidence for the maintenance of motoneurone properties by muscle activity. *Journal of Physiology*, **281**, 239–52.

Dasen JS, Liu JP, and Jessell TM (2003). Motor neuron columnar fate imposed by sequential phases of Hox-c activity. *Nature*, **425**, 926–33.

Davis HL, Heinicke EA, Cook RA, and Kiernan JA (1985). Partial purification from mammalian peripheral nerve of a trophic factor that ameliorates atrophy of denervated muscle. *Experimental Neurology*, **89**, 159–71.

Davis HL, Bressler BH, and Jasch LG (1988). Myotrophic effects on denervated fast-twitch muscles of mice: correlation of physiologic, biochemical, and morphologic findings. *Experimental Neurology*, **99**, 474–89.

de Haan A, Jones DA, and Sargeant AJ (1989). Changes in velocity of shortening, power output and relaxation rate during fatigue of rat medial gastrocnemius muscle. *Pflügers Archiv*, **413**, 422–8.

de Jongh HR and Kernell D (1982). Limits of usefulness of electrophysiological methods for estimating dendritic length in neurones. *Journal of Neuroscience Methods*, **6**, 129–38.

De Luca CJ and Erim Z (1994). Common drive of motor units in regulation of muscle force. *Trends in Neurosciences*, **17**, 299–305.

De Luca CJ, LeFever RS, McCue MP, and Xenakis AP (1982). Behaviour of human motor units in different muscles during linearly varying contractions. *Journal of Physiology*, **329**, 113–28.

De Ruiter CJ and De Haan A (2000). Temperature effect on the force/velocity relationship of the fresh and fatigued human adductor pollicis muscle. *Pflügers Archiv*, **440**, 163–70.

De Ruiter CJ, De Haan A, and Sargeant AJ (1995). Physiological characteristics of two extreme muscle compartments in gastrocnemius medialis of the anaesthetized rat. *Acta Physiologica Scandinavica*, **153**, 313–24.

de Ruiter CJ, Jones DA, Sargeant AJ, and de Haan A (1999). Temperature effect on the rates of isometric force development and relaxation in the fresh and fatigued human adductor pollicis muscle. *Experimental Physiology*, **84**, 1137–50.

Debold EP, Dave H, and Fitts RH (2004). Fiber type and temperature dependence of inorganic phosphate: implications for fatigue. *American Journal of Physiology*, **287**, C673–81.

Degens H, Turek Z, Hoofd LJ, Van't Hof MA, and Binkhorst RA (1992). The relationship between capillarisation and fibre types during compensatory hypertrophy of the plantaris muscle in the rat. *Journal of Anatomy*, **180**, 455–63.

Delgado-Lezama R, Perrier JF, Nedergaard S, Svirskis G, and Hounsgaard J (1997). Metabotropic synaptic regulation of intrinsic response properties of turtle spinal motoneurones. *Journal of Physiology*, **504**, 97–102.

Delp MD and Duan C (1996). Composition and size of type I, IIA, IID/X, and IIB fibers and citrate synthase activity of rat muscle. *Journal of Applied Physiology*, **80**, 261–70.

Denny-Brown D (1929). On the nature of postural reflexes. *Proceedings of the Royal Society of London, Series B*, **104**, 252–301.

DeSantis M, Berger PK, Laskowski MB, and Norton AS (1992). Regeneration by skeletomotor axons in neonatal rats is topographically selective at an early stage of reinnervation. *Experimental Neurology*, **116**, 229–39.

Desaulniers P, Lavoie PA, and Gardiner PF (1998). Endurance training increases acetylcholine receptor quantity at neuromuscular junctions of adult rat skeletal muscle. *Neuroreport*, **9**, 3549–52.

Desaulniers P, Lavoie PA, and Gardiner PF (2001). Habitual exercise enhances neuromuscular transmission efficacy of rat soleus muscle in situ. *Journal of Applied Physiology*, **90**, 1041–8.

Desmedt JE and Godaux E (1977). Ballistic contractions in man: characteristic recruitment pattern of single motor units of the tibialis anterior muscle. *Journal of Physiology*, **264**, 673–93.

Desmedt JE and Godaux E (1981). Spinal motoneuron recruitment in man: rank deordering with direction but not with speed of voluntary movement. *Science*, **214**, 933–6.

Destombes J, Horcholle-Bossavit G, Thiesson D, and Jami L (1992). Alpha and gamma motoneurons in the peroneal nuclei of the cat spinal cord: an ultrastructural study. *Journal of Comparative Neurology*, **317**, 79–90.

Deuschl G, Raethjen J, Lindemann M, and Krack P (2001). The pathophysiology of tremor. *Muscle & Nerve*, **24**, 716–35.

Devanandan MS, Eccles RM, and Westerman RA (1965). Single motor units of mammalian muscle. *Journal of Physiology*, **178**, 359–67.

Devasahayam SR and Sandercock TG (1992). Velocity of shortening of single motor units from rat soleus. *Journal of Neurophysiology*, **67**, 1133–45.

Dienel GA (2004). Lactate muscles its way into consciousness: fueling brain activation. *American Journal of Physiology*, **287**, R519–21.

Dietz V, Bischofberger E, Wita C, and Freund HJ (1976). Correlation between the discharges of two simultaneously recorded motor units and physiological tremor. *Electroencephalography and Clinical Neurophysiology*, **40**, 97–105.

Dimitrijevic MR, McKay WB, Sarjanovic I, Sherwood AM, Svirtlih L, and Vrbova G (1992). Co-activation of ipsi- and contralateral muscle groups during contraction of ankle dorsiflexors. *Journal of the Neurological Sciences*, **109**, 49–55.

Doble A (1996). The pharmacology and mechanism of action of riluzole. *Neurology*, **47**, S233–41.

Dodge FA and Cooley JW (1973). Action potential of motoneuron. *IBM Journal of Research and Development*, **17**, 219–29.

Donselaar Y, Kernell D, Eerbeek O, and Verhey BA (1985). Somatotopic relations between spinal motoneurones and muscle fibres of the cat's musculus peroneus longus. *Brain Research*, **335**, 81–8.

Donselaar Y, Kernell D, and Eerbeek O (1986). Soma size and oxidative enzyme activity in normal and chronically stimulated motoneurones of the cat's spinal cord. *Brain Research*, **385**, 22–9.

Donselaar Y, Eerbeek O, Kernell D, and Verhey BA (1987). Fibre sizes and histochemical staining characteristics in normal and chronically stimulated fast muscle of cat. *Journal of Physiology*, **382**, 237–54.

Dorlochter M, Irintchev A, Brinkers M, and Wernig A (1991). Effects of enhanced activity on synaptic transmission in mouse extensor digitorum longus muscle. *Journal of Physiology*, **436**, 283–92.

Duchateau J (1995). Bed rest induces neural and contractile adaptations in triceps surae. *Medicine and Science in Sports and Exercise*, **27**, 1581–9.

Duchateau J and Hainaut K (1987). Electrical and mechanical changes in immobilized human muscle. *Journal of Applied Physiology*, **62**, 2168–73.

Duchateau J and Hainaut K (1990). Effects of immobilization on contractile properties, recruitment and firing rates of human motor units. *Journal of Physiology*, **422**, 55–65.

Dum RP and Kennedy TT (1980a). Physiological and histochemical characteristics of motor units in cat tibialis anterior and extensor digitorum longus muscles. *Journal of Neurophysiology*, **43**, 1615–30.

Dum RP and Kennedy TT (1980b). Synaptic organization of defined motor-unit types in cat tibialis anterior. *Journal of Neurophysiology*, **43**, 1631–44.

Dum RP, O'Donovan MJ, Toop J, and Burke RE (1985a). Cross-reinnervated motor units in cat muscle. I: Flexor digitorum longus muscle units reinnervated by soleus motoneurons. *Journal of Neurophysiology*, **54**, 818–36.

Dum RP, O'Donovan MJ, Toop J, Tsairis P, Pinter MJ, and Burke RE (1985b). Cross-reinnervated motor units in cat muscle. II: Soleus muscle reinnervated by flexor digitorum longus motoneurons. *Journal of Neurophysiology*, **54**, 837–51.

Dunlop J, Beal McIlvain H, She Y, and Howland DS (2003). Impaired spinal cord glutamate transport capacity and reduced sensitivity to riluzole in a transgenic superoxide dismutase mutant rat model of amyotrophic lateral sclerosis. *Journal of Neuroscience*, **23**, 1688–96.

Durand D (1984). The somatic shunt cable model for neurons. *Biophysical Journal*, **46**, 645–53.

Dziegielewska KM, Evans CA, and Saunders NR (1980). Rapid effect of nerve injury upon axonal transport of phospholipids. *Journal of Physiology*, **304**, 83–98.

Eccles JC (1957). *The Physiology of Nerve Cells*. Johns Hopkins University Press, Baltimore, MD.

Eccles JC (1964). *The Physiology of Synapses*. Springer, Berlin.

Eccles JC and Hoff HE (1932). The rhythmic discharge of motoneurones. *Proceedings of the Royal Society of London, Series B*, **110**, 483–514.

Eccles JC and Sherrington CS (1930). Numbers and contraction-values of individual motor-units examined in some muscles of the limb. *Proceedings of the Royal Society of London, Series B*, **106**, 326–57.

Eccles JC, Fatt P, and Koketsu K (1954). Cholinergic and inhibitory synapses in a pathway from motor-axon collaterals to motoneurones. *Journal of Physiology*, **126**, 524–62.

Eccles JC, Eccles RM, and Lundberg A (1957). The convergence of monosynaptic excitatory afferents on to many different species of alpha motoneurones. *Journal of Physiology*, **137**, 22–50.

Eccles JC, Eccles RM, and Lundberg A (1958a). The action potentials of the alpha motoneurones supplying fast and slow muscles. *Journal of Physiology*, **142**, 275–91.

Eccles JC, Libet B, and Young RR (1958b). The behaviour of chromatolysed motoneurones studied by intracellular recording. *Journal of Physiology*, **143**, 11–40.

Eccles JC, Eccles RM, Iggo A, and Ito M (1961). Distribution of recurrent inhibition among motoneurones. *Journal of Physiology*, **159**, 479–99.

Edgerton VR, Goslow GE Jr, Rasmussen SA, and Spector SA (1980). Is resistance of a muscle to fatigue controlled by its motoneurones? *Nature*, **285**, 589–90.

Edgerton VR, Leon RD, Harkema SJ, *et al.* (2001). Retraining the injured spinal cord. *Journal of Physiology*, **533**, 15–22.

Edin BB and Vallbo AB (1990). Muscle afferent responses to isometric contractions and relaxations in humans. *Journal of Neurophysiology*, **63**, 1307–13.

Edman KA (1979). The velocity of unloaded shortening and its relation to sarcomere length and isometric force in vertebrate muscle fibres. *Journal of Physiology*, **291**, 143–59.

Edman KA, Reggiani C, Schiaffino S, and te Kronnie G (1988). Maximum velocity of shortening related to myosin isoform composition in frog skeletal muscle fibres. *Journal of Physiology*, **395**, 679–94.

Edström L and Kugelberg E (1968). Histochemical composition, distribution of fibres and fatiguability of single motor units. Anterior tibial muscle of the rat. *Journal of Neurology, Neurosurgery and Psychiatry*, **31**, 424–33.

Edwards RH, Hill DK, Jones DA, and Merton PA (1977). Fatigue of long duration in human skeletal muscle after exercise. *Journal of Physiology*, **272**, 769–78.

Eerbeek O and Kernell D (1991). External recording of twitch time course in cat ankle muscles. *Muscle & Nerve*, **14**, 422–8.

Eerbeek O, Kernell D, and Verhey BA (1984). Effects of fast and slow patterns of tonic long-term stimulation on contractile properties of fast muscle in the cat. *Journal of Physiology*, **352**, 73–90.

Eisenberg BR and Salmons S (1981). The reorganization of subcellular structure in muscle undergoing fast-to-slow type transformation. A stereological study. *Cell and Tissue Research*, **220**, 449–71.

Eisenberg BR, Brown JM, and Salmons S (1984). Restoration of fast muscle characteristics following cessation of chronic stimulation. The ultrastructure of slow-to-fast transformation. *Cell and Tissue Research*, **238**, 221–30.

Eken T (1998). Spontaneous electromyographic activity in adult rat soleus muscle. *Journal of Neurophysiology*, **80**, 365–76.

Eken T and Gundersen K (1988). Electrical stimulation resembling normal motor-unit activity: effects on denervated fast and slow rat muscles. *Journal of Physiology*, **402**, 651–69.

Emonet-Denand F, Laporte Y, and Proske U (1971). Contraction of muscle fibers in two adjacent muscles innervated by branches of the same motor axon. *Journal of Neurophysiology*, **34**, 132–8.

Emonet-Denand F, Filippi GM, Laporte Y, and Petit J (1987). [Summation of maximal tetanic tensions developed by slow or fast motor units of the peroneus longus muscle in the cat.] *Comptes Rendus de l'Academie des Sciences, Serie III, Sciences de la Vie*, **305**, 417–22.

Emonet-Denand F, Hunt CC, Petit J, and Pollin B (1988). Proportion of fatigue-resistant motor units in hindlimb muscles of cat and their relation to axonal conduction velocity. *Journal of Physiology*, **400**, 135–58.

Emonet-Denand F, Laporte Y, and Proske U (1990). Summation of tension in motor units of the soleus muscle of the cat. *Neuroscience Letters*, **116**, 112–17.

English AW (1984). An electromyographic analysis of compartments in cat lateral gastrocnemius muscle during unrestrained locomotion. *Journal of Neurophysiology*, **52**, 114–25.

English AW and Letbetter WD (1982). A histochemical analysis of identified compartments of cat lateral gastrocnemius muscle. *Anatomical Record*, **204**, 123–30.

Enoka RM (1997). Neural adaptations with chronic physical activity. *Journal of Biomechanics*, **30**, 447–55.

Enoka RM and Fuglevand AJ (2001). Motor unit physiology: some unresolved issues. *Muscle & Nerve*, **24**, 4–17.

Enoka RM, Rankin LL, Joyner MJ, and Stuart DG (1988). Fatigue-related changes in neuromuscular excitability of rat hindlimb muscles. *Muscle & Nerve*, **11**, 1123–32.

Erlanger J and Gasser HS (1937). *Electrical Signs of Nervous Activity*. University of Pennsylvania Press, Philadelphia, PA.

Eusebi F, Farini D, Grassi F, Monaco L, and Ruzzier F (1988). Effects of calcitonin gene-related peptide on synaptic acetylcholine receptor-channels in rat muscle fibres. *Proceedings of the Royal Society of London, Series B*, **234**, 333–42.

Everts ME, Lomo T and Clausen T (1993). Changes in K$^+$, Na$^+$ and calcium contents during *in vivo* stimulation of rat skeletal muscle. *Acta Physiologica Scandinavica*, **147**, 357–68.

Evinger C, Graf WM, and Baker R (1987). Extra- and intracellular HRP analysis of the organization of extraocular motoneurons and internuclear neurons in the guinea pig and rabbit. *Journal of Comparative Neurology*, **262**, 429–45.

Eyzaguirre C and Kuffler SW (1955). Processes of excitation in the dendrites and in the soma of single isolated sensory nerve cells of the lobster and crayfish. *Journal of General Physiology*, **39**, 87–119.

Falk G and Fatt P (1964). Linear electrical properties of striated muscle fibers observed with intracellular electrodes. *Proceedings of the Royal Society of London, Series B*, **160**, 69–123.

Farmer SF, Halliday DM, Conway BA, Stephens JA, and Rosenberg JR (1997). A review of recent applications of cross-correlation methodologies to human motor unit recording. *Journal of Neuroscience Methods*, **74**, 175–87.

Fedirchuk B and Dai Y (2004). Monoamines increase the excitability of spinal neurones in the neonatal rat by hyperpolarizing the threshold for action potential production. *Journal of Physiology*, **557**, 355–61.

Filippi GM and Troiani D (1994). Relations among motor unit types, generated forces and muscle length in single motor units of anaesthetized cat peroneus longus muscle. *Experimental Brain Research*, **101**, 406–14.

Finol HJ, Lewis DM, and Owens R (1981). The effects of denervation on contractile properties or rat skeletal muscle. *Journal of Physiology*, **319**, 81–92.

Fitts RH, McDonald KS, and Schluter JM (1991). The determinants of skeletal muscle force and power: their adaptability with changes in activity pattern. *Journal of Biomechanics*, **24** (Suppl 1), 111–22.

Fitzpatrick R, Burke D, and Gandevia SC (1996). Loop gain of reflexes controlling human standing measured with the use of postural and vestibular disturbances. *Journal of Neurophysiology*, **76**, 3994–4008.

Fladby T and Jansen JK (1990). Development of homogeneous fast and slow motor units in the neonatal mouse soleus muscle. *Development*, **109**, 723–32.

Fleshman JW, Munson JB, Sypert GW, and Friedman WA (1981). Rheobase, input resistance, and motor-unit type in medial gastrocnemius motoneurons in the cat. *Journal of Neurophysiology*, **46**, 1326–38.

Flood P (2005). The importance of myorelaxants in anesthesia. *Current Opinion in Pharmacology*, **5**, 322–7.

Fluck M and Hoppeler H (2003). Molecular basis of skeletal muscle plasticity—from gene to form and function. *Reviews of Physiology, Biochemistry and Pharmacology*, **146**, 159–216.

Foehring RC and Munson JB (1990). Motoneuron and muscle-unit properties after long-term direct innervation of soleus muscle by medial gastrocnemius nerve in cat. *Journal of Neurophysiology*, **64**, 847–61.

Foehring RC, Sypert GW, and Munson JB (1986). Properties of self-reinnervated motor units of medial gastrocnemius of cat. II: Axotomized motoneurons and time course of recovery. *Journal of Neurophysiology*, **55**, 947–65.

Foehring RC, Sypert GW, and Munson JB (1987a). Motor-unit properties following cross-reinnervation of cat lateral gastrocnemius and soleus muscles with medial gastrocnemius nerve. I: Influence of motoneurons on muscle. *Journal of Neurophysiology*, **57**, 1210–26.

Foehring RC, Sypert GW, and Munson JB (1987b). Motor-unit properties following cross-reinnervation of cat lateral gastrocnemius and soleus muscles with medial gastrocnemius nerve. II: Influence of muscle on motoneurons. *Journal of Neurophysiology*, **57**, 1227–45.

Fohr UG, Weber BR, Muntener M, *et al.* (1993). Human alpha and beta parvalbumins. Structure and tissue-specific expression. *European Journal of Biochemistry*, **215**, 719–27.

Fontaine B, Klarsfeld A, Hokfelt T, and Changeux JP (1986). Calcitonin gene-related peptide, a peptide present in spinal cord motoneurons, increases the number of acetylcholine receptors in primary cultures of chick embryo myotubes. *Neuroscience Letters*, **71**, 59–65.

Fournier M, Roy RR, Perham H, Simard CP and Edgerton VR (1983). Is limb immobilization a model of muscle disuse? *Experimental Neurology*, **80**, 147–56.

Fournier M, Alula M, and Sieck GC (1991). Neuromuscular transmission failure during postnatal development. *Neuroscience Letters*, **125**, 34–6.

Frankenhaeuser B and Huxley AF (1964). The action potential in the myelinated nerve fibre of *Xenopus laevis* as computed on the basis of voltage clamp data. *Journal of Physiology*, **171**, 302–15.

Freund HJ (1983). Motor unit and muscle activity in voluntary motor control. *Physiological Reviews*, **63**, 387–436.

Freund HJ, Budingen HJ, and Dietz V (1975). Activity of single motor units from human forearm muscles during voluntary isometric contractions. *Journal of Neurophysiology*, **38**, 933–46.

Freyssenet D, Di Carlo M, and Hood DA (1999). Calcium-dependent regulation of cytochrome c gene expression in skeletal muscle cells. Identification of a protein kinase C-dependent pathway. *Journal of Biological Chemistry*, **274**, 9305–11.

Friederich JA and Brand RA (1990). Muscle fiber architecture in the human lower limb. *Journal of Biomechanics*, **23**, 91–5.

Friedman WA, Sypert GW, Munson JB, and Fleshman JW (1981). Recurrent inhibition in type-identified motoneurons. *Journal of Neurophysiology*, **46**, 1349–59.

Fuglevand AJ (1995). The role of the sarcolemma action potential in fatigue. *Advances in Experimental Medicine and Biology*, **384**, 101–8.

Fuglevand AJ and Johns RK (2004). Saturation of motor unit firing rate. In CJ Heckman and R Enoka (eds), *Active Dendrites in Motor Neurons* (available online at: http://www.colorado.edu/intphys/news/Summaries.html)

Fuglevand AJ and Keen DA (2003). Re-evaluation of muscle wisdom in the human adductor pollicis using physiological rates of stimulation. *Journal of Physiology*, **549**, 865–75.

Fuglevand AJ and Segal SS (1997). Simulation of motor unit recruitment and microvascular unit perfusion: spatial considerations. *Journal of Applied Physiology*, **83**, 1223–34.

Fuglevand AJ, Winter DA, and Patla AE (1993). Models of recruitment and rate coding organization in motor-unit pools. *Journal of Neurophysiology*, **70**, 2470–88.

Fuglevand AJ, Bilodeau M, and Enoka RM (1995). Short-term immobilization has a minimal effect on the strength and fatigability of a human hand muscle. *Journal of Applied Physiology*, **78**, 847–55.

Fuglevand AJ, Macefield VG, and Bigland-Ritchie B (1999). Force-frequency and fatigue properties of motor units in muscles that control digits of the human hand. *Journal of Neurophysiology*, **81**, 1718–29.

Fulton BP and Walton K (1986). Electrophysiological properties of neonatal rat motoneurones studied *in vivo*. *Journal of Physiology*, **370**, 651–78.

Funakoshi H, Belluardo N, Arenas E, *et al.* (1995). Muscle-derived neurotrophin-4 as an activity-dependent trophic signal for adult motor neurons. *Science*, **268**, 1495–9.

Furutani R, Izawa T, and Sugita S (2004). Distribution of facial motoneurons innervating the common facial muscles of the rabbit and rat. *Okajimas Folia Anatomica Japan*, **81**, 101–8.

Fyffe RE (1991). Spatial distribution of recurrent inhibitory synapses on spinal motoneurons in the cat. *Journal of Neurophysiology*, **65**, 1134–49.

Gage PW and Eisenberg RS (1969). Capacitance of the surface and transverse tubular membrane of frog sartorius muscle fibers. *Journal of General Physiology*, **53**, 265–78.

Gallego R, Huizar P, Kudo N, and Kuno M (1978). Disparity of motoneurone and muscle differentiation following spinal transection in the kitten. *Journal of Physiology*, **281**, 253–65.

Gallego R, Kuno M, Nunez R, and Snider WD (1979). Dependence of motoneurone properties on the length of immobilized muscle. *Journal of Physiology*, **291**, 179–89.

Gandevia SC (2001). Spinal and supraspinal factors in human muscle fatigue. *Physiological Reviews*, **81**, 1725–89.

Gao BX and Ziskind-Conhaim L (1998). Development of ionic currents underlying changes in action potential waveforms in rat spinal motoneurons. *Journal of Neurophysiology*, **80**, 3047–61.

Gardiner PF (1993). Physiological properties of motoneurons innervating different muscle unit types in rat gastrocnemius. *Journal of Neurophysiology*, **69**, 1160–70.

Gardiner PF (2001). *Neuromuscular Aspects of Physical Activity*. Human Kinetics, Champaign, IL.

Gardiner P, Michel R, Browman C, and Noble E (1986). Increased EMG of rat plantaris during locomotion following surgical removal of its synergists. *Brain Research*, **380**, 114–21.

Gardiner P, Beaumont E and Cormery B (2005). Motoneurones 'learn' and 'forget' physical activity. *Canadian Journal of Applied Physiology*, **30**, 352–70.

Garland SJ and Griffin L (1999). Motor unit double discharges: statistical anomaly or functional entity? *Canadian Journal of Applied Physiology*, **24**, 113–30.

Garland SJ, Enoka RM, Serrano LP, and Robinson GA (1994). Behavior of motor units in human biceps brachii during a submaximal fatiguing contraction. *Journal of Applied Physiology*, **76**, 2411–9.

Garnett R and Stephens JA (1981). Changes in the recruitment threshold of motor units produced by cutaneous stimulation in man. *Journal of Physiology*, **311**, 463–73.

Garnett RA, O'Donovan MJ, Stephens JA, and Taylor A (1979). Motor unit organization of human medial gastrocnemius. *Journal of Physiology*, **287**, 33–43.

Garry DJ, Ordway GA, Lorenz JN, et al. (1998). Mice without myoglobin. *Nature*, **395**, 905–8.

Gasser HS and Erlanger J (1929). The role of fiber size in the establishment of a nerve block by pressure or cocaine. *American Journal of Physiology*, **88**, 581–91.

Gates HJ and Ridge RM (1992). The importance of competition between motoneurones in developing rat muscle; effects of partial denervation at birth. *Journal of Physiology*, **445**, 457–72.

Gauthier GF and Hobbs AW (1982). Effects of denervation on the distribution of myosin isozymes in skeletal muscle fibers. *Experimental Neurology*, **76**, 331–46.

Gauthier A, Davenne D, Martin A, Cometti G, and Van Hoecke J (1996). Diurnal rhythm of the muscular performance of elbow flexors during isometric contractions. *Chronobiology International*, **13**, 135–46.

Geisler HC, Westerga J, and Gramsbergen A (1993). Development of posture in the rat. *Acta Neurobiologiae Experimentalis (Warsaw)*, **53**, 517–23.

Gelfan S and Tarlov IM (1963). Altered neuron population in L7 segment of dogs with experimental hind-limb rigidity. *American Journal of Physiology*, **205**, 606–16.

Gerchman LB, Edgerton VR, and Carrow RE (1975). Effects of physical training on the histochemistry and morphology of ventral motor neurons. *Experimental Neurology*, **49**, 790–801.

Gerding R, Robbins N, and Antosiak J (1977). Efficiency of reinnervation of neonatal rat muscle of original and foreign nerves. *Developmental Biology*, **61**, 177–83.

Gertler RA and Robbins N (1978). Differences in neuromuscular transmission in red and white muscles. *Brain Research*, **142**, 160–4.

Gharakhanlou R, Chadan S, and Gardiner P (1999). Increased activity in the form of endurance training increases calcitonin gene-related peptide content in lumbar motoneuron cell bodies and in sciatic nerve in the rat. *Neuroscience*, **89**, 1229–39.

Giddings CJ and Gonyea WJ (1992). Morphological observations supporting muscle fiber hyperplasia following weight-lifting exercise in cats. *Anatomical Record*, **233**, 178–95.

Gillespie MJ and Stein RB (1983). The relationship between axon diameter, myelin thickness and conduction velocity during atrophy of mammalian peripheral nerves. *Brain Research*, **259**, 41–56.

Gillespie MJ, Gordon T, and Murphy PR (1986). Reinnervation of the lateral gastrocnemius and soleus muscles in the rat by their common nerve. *Journal of Physiology*, **372**, 485–500.

Glenn LL, Samojla BG, and Whitney JF (1987). Electrotonic parameters of cat spinal alpha-motoneurons evaluated with an equivalent cylinder model that incorporates non-uniform membrane resistivity. *Brain Research*, **435**, 398–402.

Glicksman MA (1980). Localization of motoneurons controlling the extraocular muscles of the rat. *Brain Research*, **188**, 53–62.

Gogan P, Gueritaud JP, Horcholle-Bossavit G, and Tyc-Dumont S (1974). Electronic coupling between motoneurones in the abducens nucleus of the cat. *Experimental Brain Research*, **21**, 139–54.

Gogan P, Gueritaud JP, Horcholle-Bossavit G, and Tyc-Dumont S (1977). Direct excitatory interactions between spinal motoneurones of the cat. *Journal of Physiology*, **272**, 755–67.

Goldspink G (1999). Changes in muscle mass and phenotype and the expression of autocrine and systemic growth factors by muscle in response to stretch and overload. *Journal of Anatomy*, **194**, 323–34.

Goldspink G, Tabary C, Tabary JC, Tardieu C, and Tardieu G (1974). Effect of denervation on the adaptation of sarcomere number and muscle extensibility to the functional length of the muscle. *Journal of Physiology*, **236**, 733–42.

Gollnick PD, Timson BF, Moore RL, and Riedy M (1981). Muscular enlargement and number of fibers in skeletal muscles of rats. *Journal of Applied Physiology*, **50**, 936–43.

Gollvik L, Kellerth JO, and Ulfhake B (1986). The effects of tenotomy and overload on the postnatal development of medial gastrocnemius motor units in the cat. *Acta Physiologica Scandinavica*, **128**, 485–94.

Gollvik L, Ornung G, Kellerth JO, and Ulfhake B (1990). Anatomy of soleus alpha-motoneurone dendrites in normal cats and in cats subjected to chronic postnatal tenotomy or overload of the soleus muscle. *Experimental Brain Research*, **80**, 34–43.

Gomez-Pinilla F, Ying Z, Opazo P, Roy RR, and Edgerton VR (2001). Differential regulation by exercise of BDNF and NT-3 in rat spinal cord and skeletal muscle. *European Journal of Neuroscience*, **13**, 1078–84.

Gomez Segade LA and Labandeira Garcia JL (1983). Location and quantitative analysis of the motoneurons innervating the extraocular muscles of the guinea-pig, using horseradish peroxidase (HRP) and double or triple labelling with fluorescent substances. *Journal für Hirnforschung*, **24**, 613–26.

Gonyea WJ and Ericson GC (1976). An experimental model for the study of exercise-induced skeletal muscle hypertrophy. *Journal of Applied Physiology*, **40**, 630–3.

Gonzalez M and Collins WF, 3rd (1997). Modulation of motoneuron excitability by brain-derived neurotrophic factor. *Journal of Neurophysiology*, **77**, 502–6.

Gonzalez-Serratos H (1975). Graded activation of myofibrils and the effect of diameter on tension development during contractures in isolated skeletal muscle fibres. *Journal of Physiology*, **253**, 321–39.

Gorassini M, Eken T, Bennett DJ, Kiehn O, and Hultborn H (2000). Activity of hindlimb motor units during locomotion in the conscious rat. *Journal of Neurophysiology*, **83**, 2002–11.

Gorassini M, Yang JF, Siu M, and Bennett DJ (2002). Intrinsic activation of human motoneurons: reduction of motor unit recruitment thresholds by repeated contractions. *Journal of Neurophysiology*, **87**, 1859–66.

Gordon AM, Huxley AF, and Julian FJ (1966). The variation in isometric tension with sarcomere length in vertebrate muscle fibres. *Journal of Physiology*, **184**, 170–92.

Gordon AM, Homsher E, and Regnier M (2000). Regulation of contraction in striated muscle. *Physiological Reviews*, **80**, 853–924.

Gordon G and Phillips CG (1953). Slow and rapid components in a flexor muscle. *Quarterly Journal of Experimental Physiology*, **38**, 35–45.

Gordon T and **Stein RB** (1982a). Reorganization of motor-unit properties in reinnervated muscles of the cat. *Journal of Neurophysiology*, **48**, 1175–90.

Gordon T and **Stein RB** (1982b). Time course and extent of recovery in reinnervated motor units of cat triceps surae muscles. *Journal of Physiology*, **323**, 307–23.

Gordon T, **Stein RB**, and **Thomas CK** (1986a). Innervation and function of hind-limb muscles in the cat after cross-union of the tibial and peroneal nerves. *Journal of Physiology*, **374**, 429–41.

Gordon T, **Stein RB** and **Thomas CK** (1986b). Organization of motor units following cross-reinnervation of antagonistic muscles in the cat hind limb. *Journal of Physiology*, **374**, 443–56.

Gordon T, **Thomas CK, Stein RB**, and **Erdebil S** (1988). Comparison of physiological and histochemical properties of motor units after cross-reinnervation of antagonistic muscles in the cat hindlimb. *Journal of Neurophysiology*, **60**, 365–78.

Gordon DC, **Loeb GE**, and **Richmond FJ** (1991a). Distribution of motoneurons supplying cat sartorius and tensor fasciae latae, demonstrated by retrograde multiple-labelling methods. *Journal of Comparative Neurology*, **304**, 357–72.

Gordon T, **Gillespie J, Orozco R**, and **Davis L** (1991b). Axotomy-induced changes in rabbit hindlimb nerves and the effects of chronic electrical stimulation. *Journal of Neuroscience*, **11**, 2157–69.

Gordon T, **Yang JF, Ayer K, Stein RB**, and **Tyreman N** (1993). Recovery potential of muscle after partial denervation: a comparison between rats and humans. *Brain Research Bulletin*, **30**, 477–82.

Gordon T, **Tyreman N, Rafuse VF**, and **Munson JB** (1997). Fast-to-slow conversion following chronic low-frequency activation of medial gastrocnemius muscle in cats. I. Muscle and motor unit properties. *Journal of Neurophysiology*, **77**, 2585–604.

Gordon T, **Sulaiman O**, and **Boyd JG** (2003). Experimental strategies to promote functional recovery after peripheral nerve injuries. *Journal of the Peripheral Nervous System*, **8**, 236–50.

Gordon T, **Thomas CK, Munson JB**, and **Stein RB** (2004). The resilience of the size principle in the organization of motor unit properties in normal and reinnervated adult skeletal muscles. *Canadian Journal of Physiology and Pharmacology*, **82**, 645–61.

Gorman RB, **McDonagh JC, Hornby TG, Reinking RM**, and **Stuart DG** (2005). Measurement and nature of firing rate adaptation in turtle spinal neurons. *Journal of Comparative Physiology A*, **191**, 583–603.

Gorza L (1990). Identification of a novel type 2 fiber population in mammalian skeletal muscle by combined use of histochemical myosin ATPase and anti-myosin monoclonal antibodies. *Journal of Histochemistry and Cytochemistry*, **38**, 257–65.

Gorza L, **Gundersen K, Lomo T, Schiaffino S**, and **Westgaard RH** (1988). Slow-to-fast transformation of denervated soleus muscles by chronic high-frequency stimulation in the rat. *Journal of Physiology*, **402**, 627–49.

Gossen ER, **Ivanova TD**, and **Garland SJ** (2003). The time course of the motoneurone after-hyperpolarization is related to motor unit twitch speed in human skeletal muscle. *Journal of Physiology*, **552**, 657–64.

Graham SC, **Roy RR, Navarro C**, *et al.* (1992). Enzyme and size profiles in chronically inactive cat soleus muscle fibers. *Muscle & Nerve*, **15**, 27–36.

Grampp W, **Harris JB**, and **Thesleff S** (1972). Inhibition of denervation changes in skeletal muscle by blockers of protein synthesis. *Journal of Physiology*, **221**, 743–54.

Gramsbergen A, **Ijkema-Paassen J, Westerga J**, and **Geisler HC** (1996). Dendrite bundles in motoneuronal pools of trunk and extremity muscles in the rat. *Experimental Neurology*, **137**, 34–42.

Gramsbergen A, **Ijkema-Paassen J, Nikkels PG**, and **Hadders-Algra M** (1997). Regression of polyneural innervation in the human psoas muscle. *Early Human Development*, 49, 49–61.

Granit R (1975). The functional role of the muscle spindles–facts and hypotheses. *Brain*, **98**, 531–56.

Granit R and Renkin B (1961). Net depolarization and discharge rate of motoneurones, as measured by recurrent inhibition. *Journal of Physiology*, **158**, 461–75.

Granit R, Henatsch HD, and Steg G (1956). Tonic and phasic ventral horn cells differentiated by post-tetanic potentiation in cat extensors. *Acta Physiologica Scandinavica*, **37**, 114–26.

Granit R, Phillips CG, Skoglund S, and Steg G (1957). Differentiation of tonic from phasic alpha ventral horn cells by stretch, pinna and crossed extensor reflexes. *Journal of Neurophysiology*, **20**, 470–81.

Granit R, Kernell D, and Shortess GK (1963a). The behaviour of mammalian motoneurones during long-lasting orthodromic, antidromic and trans-membrane stimulation. *Journal of Physiology*, **169**, 743–54.

Granit R, Kernell D, and Shortess GK (1963b). Quantitative aspects of repetitive firing of mammalian motoneurones, caused by injected currents. *Journal of Physiology*, **168**, 911–31.

Granit R, Kernell D, and Smith RS (1963c). Delayed depolarization and the repetitive response to intracellular stimulation of mammalian motoneurones. *Journal of Physiology*, **168**, 890–910.

Granit R, Kernell D, and Lamarre Y (1966a). Algebraical summation in synaptic activation of motoneurones firing within the 'primary range' to injected currents. *Journal of Physiology*, **187**, 379–99.

Granit R, Kernell D, and Lamarre Y (1966b). Synaptic stimulation superimposed on motoneurones firing in the 'secondary range' to injected current. *Journal of Physiology*, **187**, 401–15.

Grantyn R and Grantyn A (1978). Morphological and electrophysiological properties of cat abducens motoneurons. *Experimental Brain Research*, **31**, 249–74.

Green HJ, Ball-Burnett M, Chin ER, Dux L, and Pette D (1992). Time-dependent increases in Na^+,K^+-ATPase content of low-frequency-stimulated rabbit muscle. *FEBS Letters*, **310**, 129–31.

Grimby L, Hannerz J, and Hedman B (1979). Contraction time and voluntary discharge properties of individual short toe extensor motor units in man. *Journal of Physiology*, **289**, 191–201.

Grimby L, Hannerz J, and Hedman B (1981). The fatigue and voluntary discharge properties of single motor units in man. *Journal of Physiology*, **316**, 545–54.

Grotmol S, Totland GK, and Kryvi H (1988). A general, computer-based method for study of the spatial distribution of muscle fiber types in skeletal muscle. *Anatomy and Embryology*, **177**, 421–6.

Grotmol S, Totland GK, Kryvi H, Breistol A, Essen-Gustavsson B, and Lindholm A (2002). Spatial distribution of fiber types within skeletal muscle fascicles from Standardbred horses. *Anatomical Record*, **268**, 131–6.

Grow WA, Kendall-Wassmuth E, Grober MS, Ulibarri C, and Laskowski MB (1996). Muscle fiber type correlates with innervation topography in the rat serratus anterior muscle.*Muscle & Nerve*, **19**, 605–13.

Gruber H and Zenker W (1978). Acetylcholinesterase activity in motor nerve fibres in correlation to muscle fibre types in rat. *Brain Research*, **141**, 325–34.

Guertin PA and Hounsgaard J (1998). Chemical and electrical stimulation induce rhythmic motor activity in an *in vivo* preparation of the spinal cord from adult turtles. *Neuroscience Letters*, **245**, 5–8.

Gundersen K, Leberer E, Lomo T, Pette D, and Staron RS (1988). Fibre types, calcium-sequestering proteins and metabolic enzymes in denervated and chronically stimulated muscles of the rat. *Journal of Physiology*, **398**, 177–89.

Gurahian SM and Goldberg SJ (1987). Fatigue of lateral rectus and retractor bulbi motor units in cat. *Brain Research*, **415**, 281–92.

Gurney ME, Cutting FB, Zhai P, *et al.* (1996). Benefit of vitamin E, riluzole, and gabapentin in a transgenic model of familial amyotrophic lateral sclerosis. *Annals of Neurology*, **39**, 147–57.

Gustafsson B (1979). Changes in motoneurone electrical properties following axotomy. *Journal of Physiology*, **293**, 197–215.

Gustafsson B and Pinter MJ (1984a). Effects of axotomy on the distribution of passive electrical properties of cat motoneurones. *Journal of Physiology*, **356**, 433–42.

Gustafsson B and Pinter MJ (1984b). An investigation of threshold properties among cat spinal alpha-motoneurones. *Journal of Physiology*, **357**, 453–83.

Gustafsson B and Pinter MJ (1984c). Relations among passive electrical properties of lumbar alpha-motoneurones of the cat. *Journal of Physiology*, **356**, 401–31.

Gustafsson B and Pinter MJ (1985a). Factors determining the variation of the afterhyperpolarization duration in cat lumbar alpha-motoneurones. *Brain Research*, **326**, 392–5.

Gustafsson B and Pinter MJ (1985b). On factors determining orderly recruitment of motor units: a role for intrinsic properties. *Trends in Neurosciences*, **8**, 431–3.

Gustafsson B, Katz R and Malmsten J (1982). Effects of chronic partial deafferentiation on the electrical properties of lumbar alpha-motoneurones in the cat. *Brain Research*, **246**, 23–33.

Guth L and Samaha FJ (1970). Procedure for the histochemical demonstration of actomyosin ATPase. *Experimental Neurology*, **28**, 365–7.

Guth L, Kemerer VF, Samaras TA, Warnick JE, and Albuquerque EX (1981). The roles of disuse and loss of neurotrophic function in denervation atrophy of skeletal muscle. *Experimental Neurology*, **73**, 20–36.

Guthrie SC and Gilula NB (1989). Gap junctional communication and development. *Trends in Neurosciences*, **12**, 12–16.

Gydikov A and Kosarov D (1974). Some features of different motor units in human biceps brachii. *Pflügers Archiv*, **347**, 75–88.

Hagbarth KE and Macefield VG (1995). The fusimotor system. Its role in fatigue. *Advances in Experimental Medicine and Biology*, **384**, 259–70.

Hakkinen K and Komi PV (1983). Electromyographic changes during strength training and detraining. *Medicine and Science in Sports and Exercise*, **15**, 455–60.

Hakkinen K, Newton RU, Gordon SE, et al. (1998). Changes in muscle morphology, electromyographic activity, and force production characteristics during progressive strength training in young and older men. *Journal of Gerontology A*, **53**, B415–23.

Hamm TM, Sasaki S, Stuart DG, Windhorst U, and Yuan CS (1987). Distribution of single-axon recurrent inhibitory post-synaptic potentials in a single spinal motor nucleus in the cat. *Journal of Physiology*, **388**, 653–64.

Hammarberg C and Kellerth JO (1975a). The postnatal development of some twitch and fatigue properties of single motor units in the ankle muscles of the kitten. *Acta Physiologica Scandinavica*, **95**, 243–57.

Hammarberg C and Kellerth JO (1975b). Studies of some twitch and fatigue properties of different motor unit types in the ankle muscles of the adult cat. *Acta Physiologica Scandinavica*, **95**, 231–42.

Harada Y and Takahashi T (1983). The calcium component of the action potential in spinal motoneurones of the rat. *Journal of Physiology*, **335**, 89–100.

Hardman VJ and Brown MC (1987). Accuracy of reinnervation of rat internal intercostal muscles by their own segmental nerves. *Journal of Neuroscience*, **7**, 1031–6.

Harris AJ, Duxson MJ, Butler JE, Hodges PW, Taylor JL, and Gandevia SC (2005). Muscle fiber and motor unit behavior in the longest human skeletal muscle. *Journal of Neuroscience*, **25**, 8528–33.

Harris JB and Thesleff S (1972). Nerve stump length and membrane changes in denervated skeletal muscle. *Nature New Biology*, **236**, 60–1.

Harrison PJ, Hultborn H, Jankowska E, Katz R, Storai B, and Zytnicki D (1984). Labelling of interneurones by retrograde transsynaptic transport of horseradish peroxidase from motoneurones in rats and cats. *Neuroscience Letters*, **45**, 15–9.

Hartgens F and Kuipers H (2004). Effects of androgenic-anabolic steroids in athletes. *Sports Medicine*, **34**, 513–54.

Hashizume K, and Kanda K, and Burke RE (1988). Medial gastrocnemius motor nucleus in the rat: age-related changes in the number and size of motoneurons. *Journal of Comparative Neurology*, **269**, 425–30.

Hatcher DD and Luff AR (1988). Contractile properties of cat skeletal muscle after repetitive stimulation. *Journal of Applied Physiology*, **64**, 502–10.

Hather BM, Tesch PA, Buchanan P and Dudley GA (1991). Influence of eccentric actions on skeletal muscle adaptations to resistance training. *Acta Physiologica Scandinavica*, **143**, 177–85.

Havton L and Kellerth JO (1987). Regeneration by supernumerary axons with synaptic terminals in spinal motoneurons of cats. *Nature*, **325**, 711–14.

Havton L and Kellerth JO (1990). Elimination of intramedullary axon collaterals of cat spinal alpha-motoneurons following peripheral nerve injury. *Experimental Brain Research*, **79**, 65–74.

Havton LA and Kellerth JO (2001). Transformation of synaptic vesicle phenotype in the intramedullary axonal arbors of cat spinal motoneurons following peripheral nerve injury. *Experimental Brain Research*, **139**, 297–302.

Havton LA, Hotson JR and Kellerth JO (2001). Partial peripheral motor nerve lesions induce changes in the conduction properties of remaining intact motoneurons. *Muscle & Nerve*, **24**, 662–6.

Heckman CJ (1994). Computer simulations of the effects of different synaptic input systems on the steady-state input-output structure of the motoneuron pool. *Journal of Neurophysiology*, **71**, 1727–39.

Heckman CJ and Binder MD (1988). Analysis of effective synaptic currents generated by homonymous Ia afferent fibers in motoneurons of the cat. *Journal of Neurophysiology*, **60**, 1946–66.

Heckman CJ and Binder MD (1991a). Analysis of Ia-inhibitory synaptic input to cat spinal motoneurons evoked by vibration of antagonist muscles. *Journal of Neurophysiology*, **66**, 1888–93.

Heckman CJ and Binder MD (1991b). Computer simulation of the steady-state input-output function of the cat medial gastrocnemius motoneuron pool. *Journal of Neurophysiology*, **65**, 952–67.

Heckman CJ and Binder MD (1993a). Computer simulations of motoneuron firing rate modulation. *Journal of Neurophysiology*, **69**, 1005–8.

Heckman CJ and Binder MD (1993b). Computer simulations of the effects of different synaptic input systems on motor unit recruitment. *Journal of Neurophysiology*, **70**, 1827–40.

Heckman CJ, Lee RH, and Brownstone RM (2003). Hyperexcitable dendrites in motoneurons and their neuromodulatory control during motor behavior. *Trends in Neurosciences*, **26**, 688–95.

Heckman CJ, Gorassini MA, and Bennett DJ (2005). Persistent inward currents in motoneuron dendrites: Implications for motor output. *Muscle & Nerve*, **31**, 135–56.

Hellsing G and Lindstrom L (1983). Rotation of synergistic activity during isometric jaw closing muscle contraction in man. *Acta Physiologica Scandinavica*, **118**, 203–7.

Hellstrom J, Oliveira AL, Meister B, and Cullheim S (2003). Large cholinergic nerve terminals on subsets of motoneurons and their relation to muscarinic receptor type 2. *Journal of Comparative Neurology*, **460**, 476–86.

Henatsch HD, Schulte FJ, and Busch G (1959). Wandelbarkeit des tonisch-phasischen Reaktionstyps einzelner Extensor-Motoneurone bei Variation ihrer Antriebe. *Pflügers Archiv*, **270**, 161–73.

Henderson CE, Phillips HS, Pollock RA, *et al.* (1994). GDNF: a potent survival factor for motoneurons present in peripheral nerve and muscle. *Science*, **266**, 1062–4.

Henderson CE, Yamamoto Y, Livet J, Arce V, Garces A, and deLapeyriere O (1998). Role of neurotrophic factors in motoneuron development. *Journal de Physiologie*, **92**, 279–81.

Henneman E (1957). Relation between size of neurons and their susceptibility to discharge. *Science*, **126**, 1345–7.

Henneman E and Mendell LM (1981). Functional organization of motoneuron pool and its inputs. In VB Brooks (ed.), *Handbook of Physiology*, Section 1, Volume II pp. 423–507. American Physiological Society, Bethesda, MD.

Henneman E, Somjen G, and Carpenter DO (1965). Functional significance of cell size in spinal motoneurons. *Journal of Neurophysiology*, **28**, 560–80.

Henneman E, Shahani BT, and Young RR (1976). Voluntary control of human motor units. In M Shahani (ed.), *The Motor System: Neurophysiology and Muscle Mechanisms*, pp. 73–8. Elsevier, Amsterdam.

Hennig R and Lomo T (1985). Firing patterns of motor units in normal rats. *Nature*, **314**, 164–6.

Hennig R and Lomo T (1987). Effects of chronic stimulation on the size and speed of long-term denervated and innervated rat fast and slow skeletal muscles. *Acta Physiologica Scandinavica*, **130**, 115–31.

Henriksson J, Galbo H, and Blomstrand E (1982). Role of the motor nerve in activity-induced enzymatic adaptation in skeletal muscle. *American Journal of Physiology*, **242**, C272–7.

Henriksson J, Chi MM, Hintz CS, *et al.* (1986). Chronic stimulation of mammalian muscle: changes in enzymes of six metabolic pathways. *American Journal of Physiology*, **251**, C614–32.

Hensbergen E and Kernell D (1992). Task-related differences in distribution of electromyographic activity within peroneus longus muscle of spontaneously moving cats. *Experimental Brain Research*, **89**, 682–5.

Hensbergen E and Kernell D (1997). Daily durations of spontaneous activity in cat's ankle muscles. *Experimental Brain Research*, **115**, 325–32.

Hensbergen E and Kernell D (1998). Circadian and individual variations in duration of spontaneous activity among ankle muscles of the cat. *Muscle & Nerve*, **21**, 345–51.

Heron MI and Richmond FJ (1993). In-series fiber architecture in long human muscles. *Journal of Morphology*, **216**, 35–45.

Herzog W, Kamal S, and Clarke HD (1992). Myofilament lengths of cat skeletal muscle: theoretical considerations and functional implications. *Journal of Biomechanics*, **25**, 945–8.

Hess A (1970). Vertebrate slow muscle fibers. *Physiological Reviews*, **50**, 40–62.

Heuser J (1976). Morphology and synaptic vesicle discharge and reformation at the frog neuromuscular junction. In S Thesleff (ed.), *Motor Innervation of Muscle*, pp. 51–115. Academic Press, London.

Heyer CB and Llinas R (1977). Control of rhythmic firing in normal and axotomized cat spinal motoneurons. *Journal of Neurophysiology*, **40**, 480–8.

Hicks A and McComas AJ (1989). Increased sodium pump activity following repetitive stimulation of rat soleus muscles. *Journal of Physiology*, **414**, 337–49.

Hill AV (1970). *First and Last Experiments in Muscle Mechanics*. Cambridge University Press, Cambridge.

Hille B (1967). The selective inhibition of delayed potassium currents in nerve by tetraethylammonium ion. *Journal of General Physiology*, **50**, 1287–1302.

Hille B (2001). *Ion Channels of Excitable Membranes*, Sinauer, Sunderland, MA.

Hirofuji C, Ishihara A, Roy RR, *et al.* (2000). SDH activity and cell size of tibialis anterior motoneurons and muscle fibers in SAMP6. *Neuroreport*, **11**, 823–8.

Hirokawa N and Takemura R (2005). Molecular motors and mechanisms of directional transport in neurons. *Nature Reviews Neuroscience*, **6**, 201–14.

Hnik P, Holas M, Krekule I, *et al.* (1976). Work-induced potassium changes in skeletal muscle and effluent venous blood assessed by liquid ion-exchanger microelectrodes. *Pflügers Archiv*, **362**, 85–94.

Hochman S and McCrea DA (1994a). Effects of chronic spinalization on ankle extensor motoneurons. I: Composite monosynaptic Ia EPSPs in four motoneuron pools. *Journal of Neurophysiology*, **71**, 1452–67.

Hochman S and McCrea DA (1994b). Effects of chronic spinalization on ankle extensor motoneurons. II: Motoneuron electrical properties. *Journal of Neurophysiology*, **71**, 1468–79.

Hochman S and Schmidt BJ (1998). Whole cell recordings of lumbar motoneurons during locomotor-like activity in the *in vivo* neonatal rat spinal cord. *Journal of Neurophysiology*, **79**, 743–52.

Hodes R (1949). Selective destruction of large motoneurons by poliomyelitis virus. I: Conduction velocity of motor nerve fibers of chronic poliomyelitis patients. *Journal of Neurophysiology*, **12**, 257–66.

Hodes R, Peacock SMJ, and Bodian D (1949). Selective destruction of large motoneurons by poliomyelitis virus; size of motoneurons in the spinal cord of rhesus monkeys. *Journal of Neuropathology and Experimental Neurology*, **4**, 400–10.

Hodgkin AL (1948). The local electric changes associated with repetitive action in a non-medullated nerve. *Journal of Physiology*, **107**, 165–81.

Hodgkin AL and Huxley AF (1952). A quantitative description of membrane current and its application to conduction and excitation in nerve. *Journal of Physiology*, **117**, 500–44.

Hodgson JA, Wichayanuparp S, Recktenwald MR, *et al.* (2001). Circadian force and EMG activity in hindlimb muscles of rhesus monkeys. *Journal of Neurophysiology*, **86**, 1430–44.

Hoffer JA, O'Donovan MJ, Pratt CA, and Loeb GE (1981). Discharge patterns of hindlimb motoneurons during normal cat locomotion. *Science*, **213**, 466–7.

Hoffer JA, Loeb GE, Sugano N, Marks WB, O'Donovan MJ, and Pratt CA (1987). Cat hindlimb motoneurons during locomotion. III: Functional segregation in sartorius. *Journal of Neurophysiology*, **57**, 554–62.

Hoffer JA, Stein RB, Haugland MK, *et al.* (1996). Neural signals for command control and feedback in functional neuromuscular stimulation: a review. *Journal of Rehabilitation Research and Development*, **33**, 145–57.

Hoffman PN and Lasek RJ (1980). Axonal transport of the cytoskeleton in regenerating motor neurons: constancy and change. *Brain Research*, **202**, 317–33.

Hogan EL, Dawson DM, and Romanul FC (1965). Enzymatic changes in denervated muscle. II: Biochemical studies. *Archives of Neurology*, **13**, 274–82.

Hoh JF (1975). Selective and non-selective reinnervation of fast-twitch and slow-twitch rat skeletal muscle. *Journal of Physiology*, **251**, 791–801.

Hoh JF (1991). Myogenic regulation of mammalian skeletal muscle fibres. *News in Physiological Sciences*, **6**, 1–6.

Hornberger TA Jr and Farrar RP (2004). Physiological hypertrophy of the FHL muscle following 8 weeks of progressive resistance exercise in the rat. *Canadian Journal of Applied Physiology*, **29**, 16–31.

Hornby TG, McDonagh JC, Reinking RM, and Stuart DG (2002a). Effects of excitatory modulation on intrinsic properties of turtle motoneurons. *Journal of Neurophysiology*, **88**, 86–97.

Hornby TG, McDonagh JC, Reinking RM, and Stuart DG (2002b). Electrophysiological properties of spinal motoneurons in the adult turtle. *Journal of Comparative Physiology A*, **188**, 397–408.

Hounsgaard J and Kiehn O (1989). Serotonin-induced bistability of turtle motoneurones caused by a nifedipine-sensitive calcium plateau potential. *Journal of Physiology*, **414**, 265–82.

Hounsgaard J, Hultborn H, Jespersen B, and Kiehn O (1984). Intrinsic membrane properties causing a bistable behaviour of alpha-motoneurones. *Experimental Brain Research*, **55**, 391–4.

Hounsgaard J, Hultborn H, and Kiehn O (1986). Transmitter-controlled properties of alpha-motoneurones causing long-lasting motor discharge to brief excitatory inputs. *Progress in Brain Research*, **64**, 39–49.

Hounsgaard J, Hultborn H, Jespersen B, and Kiehn O (1988a). Bistability of alpha-motoneurones in the decerebrate cat and in the acute spinal cat after intravenous 5-hydroxytryptophan. *Journal of Physiology*, **405**, 345–67.

Hounsgaard J, Kiehn O, and Mintz I (1988b). Response properties of motoneurones in a slice preparation of the turtle spinal cord. *Journal of Physiology*, **398**, 575–89.

Howald H (1982). Training-induced morphological and functional changes in skeletal muscle. *International Journal of Sports Medicine*, **3**, 1–12.

Howald H, Hoppeler H, Claassen H, Mathieu O, and Straub R (1985). Influences of endurance training on the ultrastructural composition of the different muscle fiber types in humans. *Pflügers Archiv*, **403**, 369–76.

Howell JN, Fuglevand AJ, Walsh ML, and **Bigland-Ritchie B** (1995). Motor unit activity during isometric and concentric–eccentric contractions of the human first dorsal interosseus muscle. *Journal of Neurophysiology*, **74**, 901–4.

Hoyle G (1983). *Muscles and their Neural Control*. John Wiley, New York.

Hsiao CF, **Trueblood PR, Levine MS**, and **Chandler SH** (1997). Multiple effects of serotonin on membrane properties of trigeminal motoneurons *in vivo*. *Journal of Neurophysiology*, **77**, 2910–24.

Hubbard JI, **Stenhouse D**, and **Eccles RM** (1967). Origin of synaptic noise. *Science*, **157**, 330–1.

Huizar P, **Kuno M, Kudo N**, and **Miyata Y** (1977). Reaction of intact spinal motoneurones to partial denervation of the muscle. *Journal of Physiology*, **265**, 175–91.

Hultborn H, **Jankowska E**, and **Lindstrom S** (1968). Inhibition in IA inhibitory pathway by impulses in recurrent motor axon collaterals. *Life Sciences*, **7**, 337–9.

Hultborn H, **Jankowska E, Lindstrom S**, and **Roberts W** (1971). Neuronal pathway of the recurrent facilitation of motoneurones. *Journal of Physiology*, **218**, 495–514.

Hultborn H, **Wigström H**, and **Wängberg B** (1975). Prolonged activation of soleus motoneurones following a conditioning train in soleus Ia afferents—a case for a reverberating loop? *Neuroscience Letters*, **1**, 147–52.

Hultborn H, **Lindstrom S**, and **Wigstrom H** (1979). On the function of recurrent inhibition in the spinal cord. *Experimental Brain Research*, **37**, 399–403.

Hultborn H, **Katz R**, and **Mackel R** (1988a). Distribution of recurrent inhibition within a motor nucleus. II: Amount of recurrent inhibition in motoneurones to fast and slow units. *Acta Physiologica Scandinavica*, **134**, 363–74.

Hultborn H, **Lipski J, Mackel R**, and **Wigstrom H** (1988b). Distribution of recurrent inhibition within a motor nucleus. I: Contribution from slow and fast motor units to the excitation of Renshaw cells. *Acta Physiologica Scandinavica*, **134**, 347–61.

Hultborn H, **Brownstone RB, Toth TI**, and **Gossard JP** (2004). Key mechanisms for setting the input-output gain across the motoneuron pool. *Progress in Brain Research*, **143**, 77–95.

Hultman E (1967). Physiological role of muscle glycogen in man, with special reference to exercise. *Circulation Research*, **21**, 99–112.

Hume RI, **Role LW**, and **Fischbach GD** (1983). Acetylcholine release from growth cones detected with patches of acetylcholine receptor-rich membranes. *Nature*, **305**, 632–4.

Hursh JB (1938). Conduction velocity and diameter of nerve fibers. *American Journal of Physiology*, **127**, 131–53.

Hyatt JP, **Roy RR, Baldwin KM**, and **Edgerton VR** (2003). Nerve activity-independent regulation of skeletal muscle atrophy: role of MyoD and myogenin in satellite cells and myonuclei. *American Journal of Physiology*, **285**, C1161–73.

Iansek R and **Redman SJ** (1973a). The amplitude, time course and charge of unitary excitatory post-synaptic potentials evoked in spinal motoneurone dendrites. *Journal of Physiology*, **234**, 665–88.

Iansek R and **Redman SJ** (1973b). An analysis of the cable properties of spinal motoneurones using a brief intracellular current pulse. *Journal of Physiology*, **234**, 613–36.

Iliya AR and **Dum RP** (1984). Somatotopic relations between the motor nucleus and its innervated muscle fibers in the cat tibialis anterior. *Experimental Neurology*, **86**, 272–92.

Illert M and **Kümmel H** (1999). Reflex pathways from large muscle spindle afferents and recurrent axon collaterals to motoneurones of wrist and digit muscles: a comparison in cats, monkeys and humans. *Experimental Brain Research*, **128**, 13–19.

Illert M, **Fritz N, Aschoff A**, and **Hollander H** (1982). Fluorescent compounds as retrograde tracers compared with horseradish peroxidase (HRP). II: A parametric study in the peripheral motor system of the cat. *Journal of Neuroscience Methods*, **6**, 199–218.

Ingjer F (1979). Capillary supply and mitochondrial content of different skeletal muscle fiber types in untrained and endurance-trained men. A histochemical and ultrastructural study. *European Journal of Applied Physiology*, **40**, 197–209.

Inokuchi S, Ishikawa H, Iwamoto S, and Kimura T (1975). Age-related changes in the histological composition of the rectus abdominis muscle of the adult human. *Human Biology*, **47**, 231–49.

Ishihara A, Roy RR, and Edgerton VR (1995). Succinate dehydrogenase activity and soma size of motoneurons innervating different portions of the rat tibialis anterior. *Neuroscience*, **68**, 813–22.

Ishihara A, Hayashi S, Roy RR, *et al.* (1997a). Mitochondrial density of ventral horn neurons in the rat spinal cord. *Acta Anatomica (Basel)*, **160**, 248–53.

Ishihara A, Hori A, Roy RR, *et al.* (1997b). Perineal muscles and their innervation: metabolic and functional significance of the motor unit. *Acta Anatomica (Basel)*, **159**, 156–66.

Ishihara A, Oishi Y, Roy RR, and Edgerton VR (1997c). Influence of two weeks of non-weight bearing on rat soleus motoneurons and muscle fibers. *Aviation, Space, and Environmental Medicine*, **68**, 421–5.

Ishihara A, Ohira Y, Roy RR, *et al.* (2000). Comparison of the response of motoneurons innervating perineal and hind limb muscles to spaceflight and recovery. *Muscle & Nerve*, **23**, 753–62.

Ito M and Kudo M (1994). Reinnervation by axon collaterals from single facial motoneurons to multiple muscle targets following axotomy in the adult guinea pig. *Acta Anatomica (Basel)*, **151**, 124–30.

Ito M and Oshima T (1962). Temporal summation of after-hyperpolarization following a motoneurone spike. *Nature*, **195**, 910–11.

Ito M and Oshima T (1965). Electrical behaviour of the motoneurone membrane during intracellularly applied current steps. *Journal of Physiology*, **180**, 607–35.

Ito M, Okoyama S, Furukawa M, Kitao Y, Moriizumi T, and Kudo M (1994). Non-selective reinnervation by regenerating facial motoneurons after peripheral nerve crush in the developing rat. *Kaibogaku Zasshi*, **69**, 168–74.

Jack JJB (1975). Physiology of peripheral nerve fibres in relation to their size. *British Journal of Anaesthesiology*, **47**, 173–82.

Jack JJ and Redman SJ (1971). An electrical description of the motoneurone, and its application to the analysis of synaptic potentials. *Journal of Physiology*, **215**, 321–52.

Jack JJ, Miller S, Porter R, and Redman SJ (1971). The time course of minimal excitory post-synaptic potentials evoked in spinal motoneurones by group Ia afferent fibres. *Journal of Physiology*, **215**, 353–80.

Jack JJB, Noble D, and Tsien RW (1975). *Electric Current Flow in Excitable Cells*. Clarendon Press, Oxford.

Jack JJ, Redman SJ, and Wong K (1981a). The components of synaptic potentials evoked in cat spinal motoneurones by impulses in single group Ia afferents. *Journal of Physiology*, **321**, 65–96.

Jack JJ, Redman SJ, and Wong K (1981b). Modifications to synaptic transmission at group Ia synapses on cat spinal motoneurones by 4-aminopyridine. *Journal of Physiology*, **321**, 111–26.

Jacobs BL and Fornal CA (1993). 5-HT and motor control: a hypothesis. *Trends in Neurosciences*, **16**, 346–52.

Jami L, Murthy KS, and Petit J (1982a). A quantitative study of skeletofusimotor innervation in the cat peroneus tertius muscle. *Journal of Physiology*, **325**, 125–44.

Jami L, Murthy KS, Petit J, and Zytnicki D (1982b). Distribution of physiological types of motor units in the cat peroneus tertius muscle. *Experimental Brain Research*, **48**, 177–84.

Jami L, Murthy KS, Petit J, and Zytnicki D (1983). After-effects of repetitive stimulation at low frequency on fast-contracting motor units of cat muscle. *Journal of Physiology*, **340**, 129–43.

Jankowska E and Roberts WJ (1972). Synaptic actions of single interneurones mediating reciprocal Ia inhibition of motoneurones. *Journal of Physiology*, **222**, 623–42.

Jankowska E and **Smith DO** (1973). Antidromic activation of Renshaw cells and their axonal projections. *Acta Physiologica Scandinavica*, **88**, 198–214.

Jansen JKS and **Fladby T** (1990). The perinatal reorganization of the innervation of skeletal muscle in mammals. *Progress in Neurobiology*, **34**, 39–90.

Jasmin BJ, **Lavoie PA**, and **Gardiner PF** (1987). Fast axonal transport of acetylcholinesterase in rat sciatic motoneurons is enhanced following prolonged daily running, but not following swimming. *Neuroscience Letters*, **78**, 156–60.

Jasmin BJ, **Lavoie PA**, and **Gardiner PF** (1988). Fast axonal transport of labeled proteins in motoneurons of exercise-trained rats. *American Journal of Physiology*, **255**, C731–6.

Jason LA, **Corradi K**, **Torres-Harding S**, **Taylor RR**, and **King C** (2005). Chronic fatigue syndrome: the need for subtypes. *Neuropsychological Reviews*, **15**, 29–58.

Jensen W, **Sinkjaer T**, and **Sepulveda F** (2002). Improving signal reliability for on-line joint angle estimation from nerve cuff recordings of muscle afferents. *IEEE Transactions on Neural Systems and Rehabilitation Engineering*, **10**, 133–9.

Jerregard H, **Nyberg T**, and **Hildebrand C** (2001). Sorting of regenerating rat sciatic nerve fibers with target-derived molecules. *Experimental Neurology*, **169**, 298–306.

Jessell TM (2000). Neuronal specification in the spinal cord: inductive signals and transcriptional codes. *Nature Reviews Genetics*, **1**, 20–9.

Jessell TM and **Sanes JR** (2000a). The generation and survival of nerve cells. In ER Kandel, JH Schwartz, and TM Jessell (eds), *Principles of Neural Science*, pp. 1041–62. McGraw-Hill, New York.

Jessell TM and **Sanes JR** (2000b). The induction and patterning of the nervouse system. In ER Kandel, JH Schwartz, and TM Jessell (eds), *Principles of Neural Science*, pp. 1019–40. McGraw-Hill, New York.

Jevsek M, **Mars T**, **Mis K**, and **Grubic Z** (2004). Origin of acetylcholinesterase in the neuromuscular junction formed in the *in vivo* innervated human muscle. *European Journal of Neuroscience*, **20**, 2865–71.

Jiang BA, **Roy RR**, **Navarro C**, **Nguyen Q**, **Pierotti D**, and **Edgerton VR** (1991). Enzymatic responses of cat medial gastrocnemius fibers to chronic inactivity. *Journal of Applied Physiology*, **70**, 231–9.

Jiang Z, **Rempel J**, **Li J**, **Sawchuk MA**, **Carlin KP**, and **Brownstone RM** (1999). Development of L-type calcium channels and a nifedipine-sensitive motor activity in the postnatal mouse spinal cord. *European Journal of Neuroscience*, **11**, 3481–7.

Jodkowski JS, **Viana F**, **Dick TE**, and **Berger AJ** (1988). Repetitive firing properties of phrenic motoneurons in the cat. *Journal of Neurophysiology*, **60**, 687–702.

Johnson JD, **Jiang Y**, and **Rall JA** (1999). Intracellular EDTA mimics parvalbumin in the promotion of skeletal muscle relaxation. *Biophysical Journal*, **76**, 1514–22.

Johnson KV, **Edwards SC**, **Van Tongeren C**, and **Bawa P** (2004). Properties of human motor units after prolonged activity at a constant firing rate. *Experimental Brain Research*, **154**, 479–87.

Johnson MA, **Polgar J**, **Weightman D**, and **Appleton D** (1973). Data on the distribution of fibre types in thirty-six human muscles: an autopsy study. *Journal of the Neurological Sciences*, **18**, 111–29.

Johnston IP and **Sears TA** (1989). Ultrastructure of axotomized alpha and gamma motoneurons in the cat thoracic spinal cord. *Neuropathology and Applied Neurobiology*, **15**, 149–63.

Jones DA (1996). High-and low-frequency fatigue revisited. *Acta Physiologica Scandinavica*, **156**, 265–70.

Jones D, **Round J**, **de Haan A**, and **Jones DA** (2004). *Skeletal Muscle—From Molecules to Movement*. Churchill Livingstone, London.

Jones LA (1995). The senses of effort and force during fatiguing contractions. *Advances in Experimental Medicine and Biology*, **384**, 305–13.

Jones LA and **Hunter IW** (1983). Effect of fatigue on force sensation. *Experimental Neurology*, **81**, 640–50.

Juhn M (2003). Popular sports supplements and ergogenic aids. *Sports Medicine*, **33**, 921–39.

Kallen RG, Sheng ZH, Yang J, Chen LQ, Rogart RB, and Barchi RL (1990). Primary structure and expression of a sodium channel characteristic of denervated and immature rat skeletal muscle. *Neuron*, **4**, 233–42.

Kamenskaya MA, Elmqvist D, and Thesleff S (1975). Guanidine and neuromuscular transmission. II: Effect on transmitter release in response to repetitive nerve stimulation. *Archives of Neurology*, **32**, 510–18.

Kanda K and Hashizume K (1992). Factors causing difference in force output among motor units in the rat medial gastrocnemius muscle. *Journal of Physiology*, **448**, 677–95.

Kanda K, Burke RE, and Walmsley B (1977). Differential control of fast and slow twitch motor units in the decerebrate cat. *Experimental Brain Research*, **29**, 57–74.

Kandel ER and Siegelbaum SA (2000a). Overview of synaptic transmission. In ER Kandel, JH Schwartz, and TM Jessell (eds), *Principles of Neural Science*, pp. 175–86. McGraw-Hill, New York.

Kandel ER and Siegelbaum SA (2000b). Signalling at the nerve–muscle synapse: directly gated transmission. In ER Kandel, JH Schwartz, and TM Jessell (eds), *Principles of Neural Science*, pp. 187–206. McGraw-Hill, New York.

Kandel ER and Siegelbaum SA (2000c). Synaptic integration. In ER Kandel, JH Schwartz, and TM Jessell (eds), *Principles of Neural Science*, pp. 207–28. McGraw-Hill, New York.

Kandel ER, Schwartz JH, and Jessell TM (eds) (2000). *Principles of Neural Science*. McGraw-Hill, New York.

Kandou TW and Kernell D (1989). Distribution of activity within the cat's peroneus longus muscle when activated in different ways via the central nervous system. *Brain Research*, **486**, 340–50.

Kang CM, Lavoie PA, and Gardiner PF (1995). Chronic exercise increases SNAP-25 abundance in fast-transported proteins of rat motoneurones. *Neuroreport*, **6**, 549–53.

Kashihara Y, Kuno M, and Miyata Y (1987). Cell death of axotomized motoneurones in neonatal rats, and its prevention by peripheral reinnervation. *Journal of Physiology*, **386**, 135–48.

Katz B (1950). Depolarization of sensory terminals and the initiation of impulses in the muscle spindle. *Journal of Physiology*, **3**, 261–82.

Kayser B (2003). Exercise starts and ends in the brain. *European Journal of Applied Physiology*, **90**, 411–9.

Kellerth JO, Berthold CH, and Conradi S (1979). Electron microscopic studies of serially sectioned cat spinal alpha-motoneurons. III: Motoneurons innervating fast-twitch (type FR) units of the gastrocnemius muscle. *Journal of Comparative Neurology*, **184**, 755–67.

Kelly AM (1983). Emergence of specialization in skeletal muscle. In LD Peachey and RH Adrian (eds), *Handbook of Physiology*, Section 10, pp. 507–37. American Physiological Society, Bethesda, MD.

Kelly FJ, McGrath JA, Goldspink DF, and Cullen MJ (1986). A morphological/biochemical study on the actions of corticosteroids on rat skeletal muscle. *Muscle & Nerve*, **9**, 1–10.

Kern DS, Semmler JG, and Enoka RM (2001). Long-term activity in upper- and lower-limb muscles of humans. *Journal of Applied Physiology*, **91**, 2224–32.

Kernell D (1964). The delayed depolarization in cat and rat motoneurones. *Progress in Brain Research*, **12**, 42–55.

Kernell D (1965a). The adaptation and the relation between discharge frequency and current strength of cat lumbosacral motoneurones stimulated by long-lasting injected currents. *Acta Physiologica Scandinavica*, **65**, 65–73.

Kernell D (1965b). High-frequency repetitive firing of cat lumbosacral motoneurones stimulated by long-lasting injected currents. *Acta Physiologica Scandinavica*, **65**, 74–86.

Kernell D (1965c). The limits of firing frequency in cat lumbosacral motoneurones possessing different time course of afterhyperpolarization. *Acta Physiologica Scandinavica*, **65**, 87–100.

Kernell D (1965d). Synaptic influence on the repetitive activity elicited in cat lumbosacral motoneurones by long-lasting injected currents. *Acta Physiologica Scandinavica*, **63**, 409–10.

Kernell D (1966a). Input resistance, electrical excitability, and size of ventral horn cells in cat spinal cord. *Science*, 152, 1637–40.

Kernell D (1966b). The repetitive discharge of motoneurones. In R Granit (ed.), *Muscular Afferents and Motor Control*, pp. 351–62. Almqvist & Wiksell, Stockholm.

Kernell D (1968). The repetitive impulse discharge of a simple neurone model compared to that of spinal motoneurones. *Brain Research*, **11**, 685–7.

Kernell D (1969). Synaptic conductance changes and the repetitive impulse discharge of spinal motoneurones. *Brain Research*, **15**, 291–4.

Kernell D (1971). Effects of synapses of dendrites and soma on the repetitive impulse firing of a compartmental neuron model. *Brain Research*, **35**, 551–5.

Kernell D (1972). The early phase of adaptation in repetitive impulse discharges of cat spinal motoneurones. *Brain Research*, **41**, 184–6.

Kernell D (1976). Recruitment, rate modulation and the tonic stretch reflex. *Progress in Brain Research*, **44**, 257–66.

Kernell D (1979). Rhythmic properties of motoneurones innervating muscle fibres of different speed in m. gastrocnemius medialis of the cat. *Brain Research*, **160**, 159–62.

Kernell D (1983). Functional properties of spinal motoneurons and gradation of muscle force. *Advances in Neurology*, **39**, 213–26.

Kernell D (1986). Organization and properties of spinal motoneurones and motor units. *Progress in Brain Research*, **64**, 21–30.

Kernell D (1992). Organized variability in the neuromuscular system: a survey of task-related adaptations. *Archives Italiennes de Biologie*, **130**, 19–66.

Kernell D (1995). Neuromuscular frequency-coding and fatigue. *Advances in Experimental Medicine and Biology*, **384**, 135–45.

Kernell D (1998). Muscle regionalization. *Canadian Journal of Applied Physiology*, **23**, 1–22.

Kernell D and Eerbeek O (1991). Recovery after intense chronic stimulation: a physiological study of cat's fast muscle. *Journal of Applied Physiology*, **70**, 1763–9.

Kernell D and Hultborn H (1990). Synaptic effects on recruitment gain: a mechanism of importance for the input-output relations of motoneurone pools? *Brain Research*, **507**, 176–9.

Kernell D and Lind A (1995). Systematic variations in metabolic properties within single-type muscle fibre populations. *Pflügers Archiv*, **430** (Suppl), R124.

Kernell D and Monster AW (1981). Threshold current for repetitive impulse firing in motoneurones innervating muscle fibres of different fatigue sensitivity in the cat. *Brain Research*, **229**, 193–6.

Kernell D and Monster AW (1982a). Motoneurone properties and motor fatigue. An intracellular study of gastrocnemius motoneurones of the cat. *Experimental Brain Research*, **46**, 197–204.

Kernell D and Monster AW (1982b). Time course and properties of late adaptation in spinal motoneurones of the cat. *Experimental Brain Research*, **46**, 191–6.

Kernell D and Sjoholm H (1973). Repetitive impulse firing: comparisons between neurone models based on 'voltage clamp equations' and spinal motoneurones. *Acta Physiologica Scandinavica*, **87**, 40–56.

Kernell D and Sjoholm H (1975). Recruitment and firing rate modulation of motor unit tension in a small muscle of the cat's foot. *Brain Research*, **98**, 57–72.

Kernell D and Zwaagstra B (1981). Input conductance axonal conduction velocity and cell size among hindlimb motoneurones of the cat. *Brain Research*, **204**, 311–26.

Kernell D and Zwaagstra B (1989a). Dendrites of cat's spinal motoneurones: relationship between stem diameter and predicted input conductance. *Journal of Physiology*, **413**, 255–69.

Kernell D and Zwaagstra B (1989b). Size and remoteness: two relatively independent parameters of dendrites, as studied for spinal motoneurones of the cat. *Journal of Physiology*, **413**, 233–54.

Kernell D, Ducati A, and Sjoholm H (1975). Properties of motor units in the first deep lumbrical muscle of the cat's foot. *Brain Research*, **98**, 37–55.

Kernell D, Eerbeek O, and Verhey BA (1983a). Motor unit categorization on basis of contractile properties: an experimental analysis of the composition of the cat's m. peroneus longus. *Experimental Brain Research*, **50**, 211–9.

Kernell D, Eerbeek O, and Verhey BA (1983b). Relation between isometric force and stimulus rate in cat's hindlimb motor units of different twitch contraction time. *Experimental Brain Research*, **50**, 220–7.

Kernell D, Verhey BA, and Eerbeek O (1985). Neuronal and muscle unit properties at different rostro-caudal levels of cat's motoneurone pool. *Brain Research*, **335**, 71–9.

Kernell D, Donselaar Y, and Eerbeek O (1987a). Effects of physiological amounts of high- and low-rate chronic stimulation on fast-twitch muscle of the cat hindlimb. II. Endurance-related properties. *Journal of Neurophysiology*, **58**, 614–27.

Kernell D, Eerbeek O, Verhey BA, and Donselaar Y (1987b). Effects of physiological amounts of high- and low-rate chronic stimulation on fast-twitch muscle of the cat hindlimb. I. Speed- and force-related properties. *Journal of Neurophysiology*, **58**, 598–613.

Kernell D, Lind A, van Diemen AB and De Haan A (1995). Relative degree of stimulation-evoked glycogen degradation in muscle fibres of different type in rat gastrocnemius. *Journal of Physiology*, **484**, 139–53.

Kernell D, Hensbergen E, Lind A, and Eerbeek O (1998). Relation between fibre composition and daily duration of spontaneous activity in ankle muscles of the cat. *Archives Italiennes de Biologie*, **136**, 191–203.

Kernell D, Bakels R, and Copray JC (1999). Discharge properties of motoneurones: how are they matched to the properties and use of their muscle units? *Journal de Physiologie*, **93**, 87–96.

Kiehn O, Erdal J, Eken T, and Bruhn T (1996). Selective depletion of spinal monoamines changes the rat soleus EMG from a tonic to a more phasic pattern. *Journal of Physiology*, **492**, 173–84.

Kiehn O, Kjaerulff O, Tresch MC, and Harris-Warrick RM (2000). Contributions of intrinsic motor neuron properties to the production of rhythmic motor output in the mammalian spinal cord. *Brain Research Bulletin*, **53**, 649–59.

Kirkwood PA, Lawton M, and Ford TW (2002). Plateau potentials in hindlimb motoneurones of female cats under anaesthesia. *Experimental Brain Research*, **146**, 399–403.

Kirschbaum BJ, Heilig A, Hartner KT, and Pette D (1989). Electrostimulation-induced fast-to-slow transitions of myosin light and heavy chains in rabbit fast-twitch muscle at the mRNA level. *FEBS Letters*, **243**, 123–6.

Klass M, Baudry S, and Duchateau J (2005). Aging does not affect voluntary activation of the ankle dorsiflexors during isometric, concentric, and eccentric contractions. *Journal of Applied Physiology*, **99**, 31–8.

Klaus W, Luellmann H, and Muscholl E (1960). [The effect of acetylcholine on potassium-42 loss from postnatal, denervated and reinnervated skeletal muscle.] *Experientia*, **16**, 498.

Klingman J, Chui H, Corgiat M, and Perry J (1988). Functional recovery. A major risk factor for the development of postpoliomyelitis muscular atrophy. *Archives of Neurology*, **45**, 645–7.

Klug GA, Leberer E, Leisner E, Simoneau JA, and Pette D (1988). Relationship between parvalbumin content and the speed of relaxation in chronically stimulated rabbit fast twitch muscle. *Pflügers Archiv*, **411**, 126–31.

Koerber HR and Mendell LM (1991). Modulation of synaptic transmission at Ia-afferent fiber connections on motoneurons during high-frequency stimulation: role of postsynaptic target. *Journal of Neurophysiology*, **65**, 590–7.

Komi PV, Viitasalo JH, Havu M, Thorstensson A, Sjodin B, and Karlsson J (1977). Skeletal muscle fibres and muscle enzyme activities in monozygous and dizygous twins of both sexes. *Acta Physiologica Scandinavica*, **100**, 385–92.

Koryak Y (1998). Electromyographic study of the contractile and electrical properties of the human triceps surae muscle in a simulated microgravity environment. *Journal of Physiology*, **510**, 287–95.

Koryak Y (1999). The effects of long-term simulated microgravity on neuromuscular performance in men and women. *European Journal of Applied Physiology*, **79**, 168–75.

Kouzaki M, Shinohara M, Masani K, Kanehisa H, and Fukunaga T (2002). Alternate muscle activity observed between knee extensor synergists during low-level sustained contractions. *Journal of Applied Physiology*, **93**, 675–84.

Kraemer WJ, Adams K, Cafarelli E, *et al.* (2002). American College of Sports Medicine position stand. Progression models in resistance training for healthy adults. *Medicine and Science in Sports and Exercise*, **34**, 364–80.

Krnjevic K and Mildedi R (1958). Failure of neuromuscular propagation in rats. *Journal of Physiology*, **140**, 440–61.

Krnjevic K, Puil E, and Werman R (1978). EGTA and motoneuronal afterpotentials. *Journal of Physiology*, **275**, 199–223.

Kroon GW, Naeije M, and Hansson TL (1986). Electromyographic power-spectrum changes during repeated fatiguing contractions of the human masseter muscle. *Archives of Oral Biology*, **31**, 603–8.

Kudina LP (1999). Analysis of firing behaviour of human motoneurones within 'subprimary range'. *Journal de Physiologie*, **93**, 115–23.

Kudina LP and Alexeeva NL (1992a). After-potentials and control of repetitive firing in human motoneurones. *Electroencephalography and Clinical Neurophysiology*, **85**, 345–53.

Kudina LP and Alexeeva NL (1992b). Repetitive doublets of human motoneurones: analysis of interspike intervals and recruitment pattern. *Electroencephalography and Clinical Neurophysiology*, **85**, 243–7.

Kudina LP and Churikova LI (1990). Testing excitability of human motoneurones capable of firing double discharges. *Electroencephalography and Clinical Neurophysiology*, **75**, 334–41.

Kuei JH, Shadmehr R, and Sieck GC (1990). Relative contribution of neurotransmission failure to diaphragm fatigue. *Journal of Applied Physiology*, **68**, 174–80.

Kugelberg E (1973). Properties of rat hind-limb motor units. In JE Desmedt (ed.), *New Developments In Electromyography and Clinical Neurophysiology*, pp. 2–13. Karger, Basel.

Kugelberg E (1976). Adaptive transformation of rat soleus motor units during growth. *Journal of the Neurological Sciences*, **27**, 269–89.

Kugelberg E and Lindegren B (1979). Transmission and contraction fatigue of rat motor units in relation to succinate dehydrogenase activity of motor unit fibres. *Journal of Physiology*, **288**, 285–300.

Kugelberg E and Thornell LE (1983). Contraction time, histochemical type, and terminal cisternae volume of rat motor units. *Muscle & Nerve*, **6**, 149–53.

Kugelberg E, Edstrom L, and Abbruzzese M (1970). Mapping of motor units in experimentally reinnervated rat muscle. Interpretation of histochemical and atrophic fibre patterns in neurogenic lesions. *Journal of Neurology, Neurosurgery and Psychiatry*, **33**, 319–29.

Kukulka CG and Clamann HP (1981). Comparison of the recruitment and discharge properties of motor units in human brachial biceps and adductor pollicis during isometric contractions. *Brain Research*, **219**, 45–55.

Kullberg S, Ramirez-Leon V, Johnson H, and Ulfhake B (1998). Decreased axosomatic input to motoneurons and astrogliosis in the spinal cord of aged rats. *Journal of Gerontology A*, **53**, B369–79.

Kuno M and Llinas R (1970a). Alterations of synaptic action in chromatolysed motoneurones of the cat. *Journal of Physiology*, **210**, 823–38.

Kuno M and Llinas R (1970b). Enhancement of synaptic transmission by dendritic potentials in chromatolysed motoneurones of the cat. *Journal of Physiology*, **210**, 807–21.

Kuno M, Miyata Y, and Munoz-Martinez EJ (1974). Differential reaction of fast and slow alpha-motoneurones to axotomy. *Journal of Physiology*, **240**, 725–39.

Kuo JJ, Siddique T, Fu R, and Heckman CJ (2005). Increased persistent Na$^+$ current and its effect on excitability in motoneurones cultured from mutant SOD1 mice. *Journal of Physiology*, **563**, 843–54.

Kust BM, Copray JC, Brouwer N, Troost D, and Boddeke HW (2002). Elevated levels of neurotrophins in human biceps brachii tissue of amyotrophic lateral sclerosis. *Experimental Neurology*, **177**, 419–27.

Kwong WH and Vrbova G (1981). Effects of low-frequency electrical stimulation on fast and slow muscles of the rat. *Pflügers Archiv*, **391**, 200–7.

Ladewig T, Kloppenburg P, Lalley PM, Zipfel WR, Webb WW, and Keller BU (2003). Spatial profiles of store-dependent calcium release in motoneurones of the nucleus hypoglossus from newborn mouse. *Journal of Physiology*, **547**, 775–87.

Lagerback PA and Kellerth JO (1985). Light microscopic observations on cat Renshaw cells after intracellular staining with horseradish peroxidase. I: The axonal systems. *Journal of Comparative Neurology*, **240**, 359–67.

Lagerback PA, Ronnevi LO, Cullheim S, and Kellerth JO (1981a). An ultrastructural study of the synaptic contacts of alpha 1-motoneuron axon collaterals. II: Contacts in lamina VII. *Brain Research*, **222**, 29–41.

Lagerback PA, Ronnevi LO, Cullheim S, and Kellerth JO (1981b). An ultrastructural study of the synaptic contacts of alpha-motoneurone axon collaterals. I: Contacts in lamina IX and with identified alpha-motoneurone dendrites in lamina VII. *Brain Research*, **207**, 247–66.

Laidlaw DH, Callister RJ, and Stuart DG (1995). Fiber-type composition of hindlimb muscles in the turtle, *Pseudemys (Trachemys) scripta elegans*. *Journal of Morphology*, **225**, 193–211.

Laidlaw DH, Bilodeau M, and Enoka RM (2000). Steadiness is reduced and motor unit discharge is more variable in old adults. *Muscle & Nerve*, **23**, 600–12.

Lance-Jones C and Landmesser L (1980). Motoneurone projection patterns in the chick hind limb following early partial reversals of the spinal cord. *Journal of Physiology*, **302**, 581–602.

Landmesser L (1978). The distribution of motoneurones supplying chick hind limb muscles. *Journal of Physiology*, **284**, 371–89.

Landmesser LT (2001). The acquisition of motoneuron subtype identity and motor circuit formation. *International Journal of Developmental Neuroscience*, **19**, 175–82.

Lännergren J (1975). Structure and function of twitch and slow fibres in amphibian skeletal muscle. In G Lennerstrand and P Bach-y-Rita (eds), *Basic Mechanisms of Ocular Motility and their Clinical Implications*, pp. 63–84. Pergamon Press, Oxford.

Lannergren J and Westerblad H (1986). Force and membrane potential during and after fatiguing, continuous high-frequency stimulation of single *Xenopus* muscle fibres. *Acta Physiologica Scandinavica*, **128**, 359–68.

Lannergren J and Westerblad H (1987). Action potential fatigue in single skeletal muscle fibres of *Xenopus*. *Acta Physiologica Scandinavica*, **129**, 311–18.

Lannergren J, Larsson L, and Westerblad H (1989). A novel type of delayed tension reduction observed in rat motor units after intense activity. *Journal of Physiology*, **412**, 267–76.

Larkum ME, Rioult MG, and Luscher HR (1996). Propagation of action potentials in the dendrites of neurons from rat spinal cord slice cultures. *Journal of Neurophysiology*, **75**, 154–70.

Larsson L (1992). Is the motor unit uniform? *Acta Physiologica Scandinavica*, **144**, 143–54.

Larsson L and Ansved T (1995). Effects of ageing on the motor unit. *Progress in Neurobiology*, **45**, 397–458.

Larsson L and Salviati G (1992). A technique for studies of the contractile apparatus in single human muscle fibre segments obtained by percutaneous biopsy. *Acta Physiologica Scandinavica*, **146**, 485–95.

Laskowski MB and Sanes JR (1987). Topographic mapping of motor pools onto skeletal muscles. *Journal of Neuroscience*, **7**, 252–60.

Laskowski MB and Sanes JR (1988). Topographically selective reinnervation of adult mammalian skeletal muscles. *Journal of Neuroscience*, **8**, 3094–9.

LaVelle A and LaVelle FW (1987). Chromatolysis. In G Adelman (ed.), *Encyclopedia of Neuroscience*, pp. 242–4. Birkhäuser, Boston, MA.

Lavoie PA (1982). Block of fast axonal transport *in vivo* by the local anesthetics dibucaine and etidocaine. *Journal of Pharmacology and Experimental Therapy*, **223**, 251–6.

Leberer E and Pette D (1986). Neural regulation of parvalbumin expression in mammalian skeletal muscle. *Biochemical Journal*, **235**, 67–73.

LeBlanc AD, Schneider VS, Evans HJ, Pientok C, Rowe R, and Spector E (1992). Regional changes in muscle mass following 17 weeks of bed rest. *Journal of Applied Physiology*, **73**, 2172–8.

Lee RH and Heckman CJ (1998a). Bistability in spinal motoneurons *in vivo*: systematic variations in persistent inward currents. *Journal of Neurophysiology*, **80**, 583–93.

Lee RH and Heckman CJ (1998b). Bistability in spinal motoneurons *in vivo*: systematic variations in rhythmic firing patterns. *Journal of Neurophysiology*, **80**, 572–82.

Lee RH and Heckman CJ (2001). Essential role of a fast persistent inward current in action potential initiation and control of rhythmic firing. *Journal of Neurophysiology*, **85**, 472–5.

Lee RH, Kuo JJ, Jiang MC, and Heckman CJ (2003). Influence of active dendritic currents on input-output processing in spinal motoneurons *in vivo*. *Journal of Neurophysiology*, **89**, 27–39.

Leksell L (1945). The action potential and excitatory effects of the small ventral root fibres to skeletal muscle. *Acta Physiologica Scandinavica*, **10** (Suppl 31), 1–84.

Lemon RN and Griffiths J (2005). Comparing the function of the corticospinal system in different species: Organizational differences for motor specialization? *Muscle & Nerve*, **32**, 261–79.

Lenman JAR and Ritchie AE (1977). *Clinical Electromyography*. Pitman Medical, London.

Levine ES, Litto WJ, and Jacobs BL (1990). Activity of cat locus coeruleus noradrenergic neurons during the defense reaction. *Brain Research*, **531**, 189–95.

Lev-Tov A and Fishman R (1986). The modulation of transmitter release in motor nerve endings varies with the type of muscle fiber innervated. *Brain Research*, **363**, 379–82.

Lev-Tov A, Pinter MJ, and Burke RE (1983). Posttetanic potentiation of group Ia EPSPs: possible mechanisms for differential distribution among medial gastrocnemius motoneurons. *Journal of Neurophysiology*, **50**, 379–98.

Lewin GR and Barde YA (1996). Physiology of the neurotrophins. *Annual Review of Neuroscience*, **19**, 289–317.

Lewis DM, Luck JC, and Knott S (1972). A comparison of isometric contractions of the whole muscle with those of motor units in a fast-twitch muscle of the cat. *Experimental Neurology*, **37**, 68–85.

Lewis DM, Rowlerson A, and Webb SN (1982). Motor units and immunohistochemistry of cat soleus muscle after long periods of cross-reinnervation. *Journal of Physiology*, **325**, 403–18.

Lexell J, Henriksson-Larsen K, and Sjostrom M (1983). Distribution of different fibre types in human skeletal muscles. 2. A study of cross-sections of whole m. vastus lateralis. *Acta Physiologica Scandinavica*, **117**, 115–22.

Lexell J, Jarvis J, Downham D, and Salmons S (1992). Quantitative morphology of stimulation-induced damage in rabbit fast-twitch skeletal muscles. *Cell and Tissue Research*, **269**, 195–204.

Li Y and Bennett DJ (2003). Persistent sodium and calcium currents cause plateau potentials in motoneurons of chronic spinal rats. *Journal of Neurophysiology*, **90**, 857–69.

Li Y, Gorassini MA, and Bennett DJ (2004a). Role of persistent sodium and calcium currents in motoneuron firing and spasticity in chronic spinal rats. *Journal of Neurophysiology*, **91**, 767–83.

Li Y, Harvey PJ, Li X, and Bennett DJ (2004b). Spastic long-lasting reflexes of the chronic spinal rat studied *in vivo*. *Journal of Neurophysiology*, **91**, 2236–46.

Lieber RL (2002). *Skeletal Muscle Structure, Function and Plasticity: The Physiological Basis of Rehabilitation*. Lippincott–Williams & Wilkins, Philadelphia, PA.

Lieber RL, Friden JO, Hargens AR, and Feringa ER (1986a). Long-term effects of spinal cord transection on fast and slow rat skeletal muscle. II: Morphometric properties. *Experimental Neurology*, **91**, 435–48.

Lieber RL, Johansson CB, Vahlsing HL, Hargens AR, and Feringa ER (1986b). Long-term effects of spinal cord transection on fast and slow rat skeletal muscle. I. Contractile properties. *Experimental Neurology*, **91**, 423–34.

Lieber RL, Loren GJ, and Friden J (1994). *In vivo* measurement of human wrist extensor muscle sarcomere length changes. *Journal of Neurophysiology*, **71**, 874–81.

Lind A and Kernell D (1991). Myofibrillar ATPase histochemistry of rat skeletal muscles: a 'two-dimensional' quantitative approach. *Journal of Histochemistry and Cytochemistry*, **39**, 589–97.

Linda H, Shupliakov O, Ornung G, *et al.* (2000). Ultrastructural evidence for a preferential elimination of glutamate-immunoreactive synaptic terminals from spinal motoneurons after intramedullary axotomy. *Journal of Comparative Neurology*, **425**, 10–23.

Lindsay AD and Binder MD (1991). Distribution of effective synaptic currents underlying recurrent inhibition in cat triceps surae motoneurons. *Journal of Neurophysiology*, **65**, 168–77.

Lindstrom P and Brismar T (1991). Mechanism of anoxic conduction block in mammalian nerve. *Acta Physiologica Scandinavica*, **141**, 429–33.

Lionikas A, Li M and Larsson L (2006). Human skeletal muscle, myosin function at physiological and non-physiological temperatures. *Acta Physiologica*, **186**, 151–8.

Lips MB and Keller BU (1998). Endogenous calcium buffering in motoneurones of the nucleus hypoglossus from mouse. *Journal of Physiology*, **511**, 105–17.

Lips MB and Keller BU (1999). Activity-related calcium dynamics in motoneurons of the nucleus hypoglossus from mouse. *Journal of Neurophysiology*, **82**, 2936–46.

Loeb GE (1987). Hard lessons in motor control from the mammalian spinal cord. *Trends in Neurosciences*, **10**, 108–13.

Loeb GE (1993). The distal hindlimb musculature of the cat: interanimal variability of locomotor activity and cutaneous reflexes. *Experimental Brain Research*, **96**, 125–40.

Lomo T (2003). What controls the position, number, size, and distribution of neuromuscular junctions on rat muscle fibers? *Journal of Neurocytology*, **32**, 835–48.

Lomo T and Rosenthal J (1972). Control of ACh sensitivity by muscle activity in the rat. *Journal of Physiology*, **221**, 493–513.

Lomo T, Westgaard RH, and Dahl HA (1974). Contractile properties of muscle: control by pattern of muscle activity in the rat. *Proceedings of the Royal Society of London, Series B*, **187**, 99–103.

Lomo T, Massoulie J and Vigny M (1985). Stimulation of denervated rat soleus muscle with fast and slow activity patterns induces different expression of acetylcholinesterase molecular forms. *Journal of Neuroscience*, **5**, 1180–7.

Lopez-Guajardo A, Sutherland H, Jarvis JC, and Salmons S (2000). Dynamics of stimulation-induced muscle adaptation: insights from varying the duty cycle. *Journal of Muscle Research and Cell Motility*, **21**, 725–35.

Lorist MM, Kernell D, Meijman TF, and Zijdewind I (2002). Motor fatigue and cognitive task performance in humans. *Journal of Physiology*, **545**, 313–19.

Lu B, Fu WM, Greengard P, and Poo MM (1993). Calcitonin gene-related peptide potentiates synaptic responses at developing neuromuscular junction. *Nature*, **363**, 76–9.

Lu QR, Sun T, Zhu Z, *et al.* (2002). Common developmental requirement for Olig function indicates a motor neuron/oligodendrocyte connection. *Cell*, **109**, 75–86.

Lucas SM, Ruff RL and Binder MD (1987). Specific tension measurements in single soleus and medial gastrocnemius muscle fibers of the cat. *Experimental Neurology*, **95**, 142–54.

Luff AR (1975). Dynamic properties of fast and slow skeletal muscles in the cat and rat following cross-reinnervation. *Journal of Physiology*, **248**, 83–96.

Luff AR (1981). Dynamic properties of the inferior rectus, extensor digitorum longus, diaphragm and soleus muscles of the mouse. *Journal of Physiology*, **313**, 161–71.

Luscher C, Streit J, Quadroni R, and Luscher HR (1994). Action potential propagation through embryonic dorsal root ganglion cells in culture. I. Influence of the cell morphology on propagation properties. *Journal of Neurophysiology*, **72**, 622–33.

Luscher HR and Shiner JS (1990). Computation of action potential propagation and presynaptic bouton activation in terminal arborizations of different geometries. *Biophysical Journal*, **58**, 1377–88.

Luscher HR, Ruenzel P, and Henneman E (1979). How the size of motoneurones determines their susceptibility to discharge. *Nature*, **282**, 859–61.

Luscher HR, Ruenzel P, and Henneman E (1983). Composite EPSPs in motoneurons of different sizes before and during PTP: implications for transmission failure and its relief in Ia projections. *Journal of Neurophysiology*, **49**, 269–89.

Luscher HR, Stricker C, Henneman E, and Vardar U (1989). Influences of morphology and topography of motoneurons and muscle spindle afferents on amplitude of single fiber excitatory postsynaptic potentials in cat. *Experimental Brain Research*, **74**, 493–500.

Lux HD, Schubert P, and Kreutzberg GW (1970). Direct matching of morphological and electrophysiological data in cat spinal motoneurones. In P Andersen and JKS Jansen (eds), *Excitatory Synaptic Mechanisms*, pp. 189–98. Universitetsforlaget, Oslo.

Lüttgau HC (1965). The effect of metabolic inhibitors on the fatigue of the action potential in single muscle fibres. *Journal of Physiology*, **178**, 45–67.

McCloskey DI (1981). Corollary discharges: motor commands and perception. In VB Brooks (ed.), *Handbook of physiology*, Section 1, Volume II, pp. 1415–47. American Physiological Society, Bethesda, MD.

McClung JR and Goldberg SJ (1999). Organization of motoneurons in the dorsal hypoglossal nucleus that innervate the retrusor muscles of the tongue in the rat. *Anatomical Record*, **254**, 222–30.

McComas AJ (1991). Invited review: motor unit estimation: methods, results, and present status. *Muscle & Nerve*, **14**, 585–97.

McComas AJ (1996). *Skeletal Muscle. Form and Function*. Human Kinetics, Champaign, IL.

McComas AJ, Galea V, and de Bruin H (1993). Motor unit populations in healthy and diseased muscles. *Physical Therapy*, **73**, 868–77.

McCurdy ML and Hamm TM (1992). Recurrent collaterals of motoneurons projecting to distal muscles in the cat hindlimb. *Journal of Neurophysiology*, **67**, 1359–66.

McCurdy ML and Hamm TM (1994). Topography of recurrent inhibitory postsynaptic potentials between individual motoneurons in the cat. *Journal of Neurophysiology*, **72**, 214–26.

MacDermid VE, Neuber-Hess MS, and Rose PK (2004). The temporal sequence of morphological and molecular changes in axotomized feline motoneurons leading to the formation of axons from the ends of dendrites. *Journal of Comparative Neurology*, **468**, 233–50.

McDonagh JC, Binder MD, Reinking RM, and Stuart DG (1980a). A commentary on muscle unit properties in cat hindlimb muscles. *Journal of Morphology*, **166**, 217–30.

McDonagh JC, Binder MD, Reinking RM, and Stuart DG (1980b). Tetrapartite classification of motor units of cat tibialis posterior. *Journal of Neurophysiology*, **44**, 696–712.

MacDonald SC, Fleetwood IG, Hochman S, *et al.* (2003). Functional motor neurons differentiating from mouse multipotent spinal cord precursor cells in culture and after transplantation into transected sciatic nerve. *Journal of Neurosurgery*, **98**, 1094–1103.

MacDougall JD, Elder GC, Sale DG, Moroz JR, and Sutton JR (1980). Effects of strength training and immobilization on human muscle fibres. *European Journal of Applied Physiology*, **43**, 25–34.

McHanwell S and Biscoe TJ (1981). The localization of motoneurons supplying the hindlimb muscles of the mouse. *Philosophhical Transactions of the Royal Society of London, Series B*, **293**, 477–508.

McLarnon JG (1995). Potassium currents in motoneurones. *Progress in Neurobiology*, **47**, 513–31.

McLennan IS (1994). Neurogenic and myogenic regulation of skeletal muscle formation: a critical re-evaluation. *Progress in Neurobiology*, **44**, 119–40.

McMahan UJ and Slater CR (1984). The influence of basal lamina on the accumulation of acetylcholine receptors at synaptic sites in regenerating muscle. *Journal of Cell Biology*, **98**, 1453–73.

McMahan UJ, Edgington DR, and Kuffler DP (1980). Factors that influence regeneration of the neuromuscular junction. *Journal of Experimental Biology*, **89**, 31–42.

McManaman JL, Oppenheim RW, Prevette D, and Marchetti D (1990). Rescue of motoneurons from cell death by a purified skeletal muscle polypeptide: effects of the ChAT development factor, CDF. *Neuron*, **4**, 891–8.

McMinn RM and Vrbova G (1967). Motoneurone activity as a cause of degeneration in the soleus muscle of the rabbit. *Quarterly Journal of Experimental Physiology*, **52**, 411–15.

McNulty PA, Falland KJ, and Macefield VG (2000). Comparison of contractile properties of single motor units in human intrinsic and extrinsic finger muscles. *Journal of Physiology*, **526**, 445–56.

McPhedran AM, Wuerker RB, and Henneman E (1965a). Properties of motor units in a heterogeneous pale muscle (m. gastrocnemius) of the cat. *Journal of Neurophysiology*, **28**, 85–99.

McPhedran AM, Wuerker RB, and Henneman E (1965b). Properties of motor units in a homogeneous red muscle (soleus) of the cat. *Journal of Neurophysiology*, **28**, 71–84.

McQuarrie IG (1978). The effect of a conditioning lesion on the regeneration of motor axons. *Brain Research*, **152**, 597–602.

McQuarrie IG and Jacob JM (1991). Conditioning nerve crush accelerates cytoskeletal protein transport in sprouts that form after a subsequent crush. *Journal of Comparative Neurology*, **305**, 139–47.

Ma J, Novikov LN, Wiberg M, and Kellerth JO (2001). Delayed loss of spinal motoneurons after peripheral nerve injury in adult rats: a quantitative morphological study. *Experimental Brain Research*, **139**, 216–23.

Macefield G, Hagbarth KE, Gorman R, Gandevia SC, and Burke D (1991). Decline in spindle support to alpha-motoneurones during sustained voluntary contractions. *Journal of Physiology*, **440**, 497–512.

Macefield VG, Gandevia SC, Bigland-Ritchie B, Gorman RB, and Burke D (1993). The firing rates of human motoneurones voluntarily activated in the absence of muscle afferent feedback. *Journal of Physiology*, **471**, 429–43.

Macefield VG, Fuglevand AJ, Howell JN, and Bigland-Ritchie B (2000). Discharge behaviour of single motor units during maximal voluntary contractions of a human toe extensor. *Journal of Physiology*, **528**, 227–34.

Maier A, Gambke B, and Pette D (1986). Degeneration-regeneration as a mechanism contributing to the fast to slow conversion of chronically stimulated fast-twitch rabbit muscle. *Cell and Tissue Research*, **244**, 635–43.

Maltenfort MG, Heckman CJ, and Rymer WZ (1998). Decorrelating actions of Renshaw interneurons on the firing of spinal motoneurons within a motor nucleus: a simulation study. *Journal of Neurophysiology*, **80**, 309–23.

Maltenfort MG, McCurdy ML, Phillips CA, Turkin VV, and Hamm TM (2004). Location and magnitude of conductance changes produced by Renshaw recurrent inhibition in spinal motoneurons. *Journal of Neurophysiology*, **92**, 1417–32.

Marsden CD, Meadows JC, and Merton PA (1971). Isolated single motor units in human muscle and their rate of discharge during maximal voluntary effort. *Journal of Physiology*, **217**, 12–13P.

Marsden CD, Meadows JC, and Merton PA (1983). 'Muscular wisdom' that minimizes fatigue during prolonged effort in man: peak rates of motoneuron discharge and slowing of discharge during fatigue. *Advances in Neurology*, **39**, 169–211.

Martin A, Carpentier A, Guissard N, van Hoecke J, and Duchateau J (1999). Effect of time of day on force variation in a human muscle. *Muscle & Nerve*, **22**, 1380–7.

Martin MR, Caddy KW, and Biscoe TJ (1977). Numbers and diameters of motoneurons and myelinated axons in the facial nucleus and nerve of the albino rat. *Journal of Anatomy*, **123**, 579–87.

Martin TP, Vailas AC, Durivage JB, Edgerton VR, and Castleman KR (1985). Quantitative histo-chemical determination of muscle enzymes: biochemical verification. *Journal of Histochemistry and Cytochemistry*, **33**, 1053–9.

Martin TP, Stein RB, Hoeppner PH, and Reid DC (1992). Influence of electrical stimulation on the morphological and metabolic properties of paralyzed muscle. *Journal of Applied Physiology*, **72**, 1401–6.

Martin-Caraballo M and Greer JJ (1999). Electrophysiological properties of rat phrenic motoneurons during perinatal development. *Journal of Neurophysiology*, **81**, 1365–78.

Matsuda Y, Oki S, Kitaoka K, Nagano Y, Nojima M, and Desaki J (1988). Scanning electron microscopic study of denervated and reinnervated neuromuscular junction. *Muscle & Nerve*, **11**, 1266–71.

Matteoli M, Haimann C, Torri-Tarelli F, Polak JM, Ceccarelli B, and De Camilli P (1988). Differential effect of alpha-latrotoxin on exocytosis from small synaptic vesicles and from large dense-core vesicles containing calcitonin gene-related peptide at the frog neuromuscular junction. *Proceedings of the National Academy of Sciences of the United States of America*, **85**, 7366–70.

Matthews PB (1981). Evolving views on the internal operation and functional role of the muscle spindle. *Journal of Physiology*, **320**, 1–30.

Matthews PB (1996). Relationship of firing intervals of human motor units to the trajectory of post-spike after-hyperpolarization and synaptic noise. *Journal of Physiology*, **492**, 597–628.

Matthews PB (1999). Properties of human motoneurones and their synaptic noise deduced from motor unit recordings with the aid of computer modelling. *Journal de Physiologie*, **93**, 135–45.

Mayer U (2003). Integrins: redundant or important players in skeletal muscle? *The Journal of Biological Chemistry*, **278**, 14587–90.

Mazza E, Nunez-Abades PA, Spielmann JM, and Cameron WE (1992). Anatomical and electrotonic coupling in developing genioglossal motoneurons of the rat. *Brain Research*, **598**, 127–37.

Meek MF, Van Der Werff JF, Nicolai JP, and Gramsbergen A (2001). Biodegradable p(DLLA-epsilon-CL) nerve guides versus autologous nerve grafts: electromyographic and video analysis. *Muscle & Nerve*, **24**, 753–9.

Meissner JD, Kubis HP, Scheibe RJ, and Gros G (2000). Reversible Ca^{2+}-induced fast-to-slow transition in primary skeletal muscle culture cells at the mRNA level. *Journal of Physiology*, **523**, 19–28.

Mendell LM and Arvanian VL (2002). Diversity of neurotrophin action in the postnatal spinal cord. *Brain Research Reviews*, **40**, 230–9.

Mendell LM and Henneman E (1971). Terminals of single Ia fibers: location, density, and distribution within a pool of 300 homonymous motoneurons. *Journal of Neurophysiology*, **34**, 171–87.

Mendell LM and Munson JB (1999). Retrograde effects on synaptic transmission at the Ia/motoneuron connection. *Journal de Physiologie*, **93**, 297–304.

Mendell LM, Munson JB and Scott JG (1976). Alterations of synapses on axotomized motoneurones. *Journal of Physiology*, **255**, 67–79.

Mendell LM, Collins WF 3rd, and Munson JB (1994). Retrograde determination of motoneuron properties and their synaptic input. *Journal of Neurobiology*, **25**, 707–21.

Merton PA (1954a). Interaction between muscle fibres in a twitch. *Journal of Physiology*, **124**, 311–24.

Merton PA (1954b). Voluntary strength and fatigue. *Journal of Physiology*, **123**, 553–64.

Metzger F, Wiese S, and Sendtner M (1998). Effect of glutamate on dendritic growth in embryonic rat motoneurons. *Journal of Neuroscience*, **18**, 1735–42.

Meunier FA, Schiavo G and Molgo J (2002). Botulinum neurotoxins: from paralysis to recovery of functional neuromuscular transmission. *Journal de Physiologie*, **96**, 105–13.

Michel RN, Cowper G, Chi MM, Manchester JK, Falter H, and Lowry OH (1994). Effects of tetrodotoxin-induced neural inactivation on single muscle fiber metabolic enzymes. *American Journal of Physiology*, **267**, C55–66.

Miledi R and Slater CR (1969). Electron-microscopic structure of denervated skeletal muscle. *Proceedings of the Royal Society of London, Series B*, **174**, 253–69.

Miledi R and Slater CR (1970). On the degeneration of rat neuromuscular junctions after nerve section. *Journal of Physiology*, **207**, 507–28.

Miles GB, Yohn DC, Wichterle H, Jessell TM, Rafuse VF, and Brownstone RM (2004). Functional properties of motoneurons derived from mouse embryonic stem cells. *Journal of Neuroscience*, **24**, 7848–58.

Miles GB, Dai Y, and Brownstone RM (2005). Mechanisms underlying the early phase of spike frequency adaptation in mouse spinal motoneurones. *Journal of Physiology*, **566**, 519–32.

Miller JB and Stockdale FE (1987). What muscle cells know that nerves don't tell them. *Trends in Neurosciences*, **10**, 325–9.

Miller TM and Heuser JE (1984). Endocytosis of synaptic vesicle membrane at the frog neuromuscular junction. *Journal of Cell Biology*, **98**, 685–98.

Mills KR (1991). Magnetic brain stimulation: a tool to explore the action of the motor cortex on single human spinal motoneurones. *Trends in Neurosciences*, **14**, 401–5.

Mills KR, Newham DJ, and Edwards RH (1982). Force, contraction frequency and energy metabolism as determinants of ischaemic muscle pain. *Pain*, **14**, 149–54.

Milner-Brown HS, Stein RB, and Yemm R (1973a). Changes in firing rate of human motor units during linearly changing voluntary contractions. *Journal of Physiology*, **230**, 371–90.

Milner-Brown HS, Stein RB, and Yemm R (1973b). The orderly recruitment of human motor units during voluntary isometric contractions. *Journal of Physiology*, **230**, 359–70.

Mishelevich DJ (1969). Repetitive firing to current in cat motoneurons as a function of muscle unit twitch type. *Experimental Neurology*, **25**, 401–9.

Mitchell JH and Schmidt RF (1983). Cardiovascular reflex control by afferent fibres from skeletal muscle receptors. In JT Shephard (ed.), *Handbook of Physiology*, Section 2, Volume III, pp. 623–58. American Physiological Society, Bethesda, MD.

Monster AW (1979). Firing rate behavior of human motor units during isometric voluntary contraction: relation to unit size. *Brain Research*, **171**, 349–54.

Monster AW and Chan H (1977). Isometric force production by motor units of extensor digitorum communis muscle in man. *Journal of Neurophysiology*, **40**, 1432–43.

Monster AW, Chan HC, and O'Connor D (1978). Activity patterns of human skeletal muscles: relation to muscle fiber type composition. *Science*, **200**, 314–7.

Moore JW, Stockbridge N, and Westerfield M (1983). On the site of impulse initiation in a neurone. *Journal of Physiology*, **336**, 301–11.

Morales FR, Boxer PA, Fung SJ, and Chase MH (1987). Basic electrophysiological properties of spinal cord motoneurons during old age in the cat. *Journal of Neurophysiology*, **58**, 180–94.

Moritani M, Kida H, Nagase Y, *et al*. (2003). Quantitative analysis of the dendritic architectures of single jaw-closing and jaw-opening motoneurons in cats. *Experimental Brain Research*, **150**, 265–75.

Mortimer JT (1981). Motor prostheses. In VB Brooks (ed.), *Handbook of Physiology*, Section 1, Volume II, pp. 155–87. American Physiological Society, Bethesda, MD.

Mosso A (1904). *Fatigue*. Swan Sonnenschein, London.

Mottram CJ, Jakobi JM, Semmler JG, and Enoka RM (2005). Motor-unit activity differs with load type during a fatiguing contraction. *Journal of Neurophysiology*, **93**, 1381–92.

Muir RB and Porter R (1973). The effect of a preceding stimulus on temporal facilitation at corticomotoneuronal synapses. *Journal of Physiology*, **228**, 749–63.

Mujika I and Padilla S (2001). Muscular characteristics of detraining in humans. *Medicine and Science in Sports and Exercise*, **33**, 1297–1303.

Mulle C, Benoit P, Pinset C, Roa M, and Changeux JP (1988). Calcitonin gene-related peptide enhances the rate of desensitization of the nicotinic acetylcholine receptor in cultured mouse muscle cells. *Proceedings of the National Academy of Sciences of the United States of America*, **85**, 5728–32.

Munson JB and McMahon SB (1997). Effects of GDNF on axotomized sensory and motor neurons in adult rats. *European Journal of Neuroscience*, **9**, 1126–9.

Munson JB, Sypert GW, Zengel JE, Lofton SA, and Fleshman JW (1982). Monosynaptic projections of individual spindle group II afferents to type-identified medial gastrocnemius motoneurons in the cat. *Journal of Neurophysiology*, **48**, 1164–74.

Munson JB, Foehring RC, Lofton SA, Zengel JE, and Sypert GW (1986). Plasticity of medial gastrocnemius motor units following cordotomy in the cat. *Journal of Neurophysiology*, **55**, 619–34.

Munson JB, Foehring RC, Mendell LM, and Gordon T (1997a). Fast-to-slow conversion following chronic low-frequency activation of medial gastrocnemius muscle in cats. II. Motoneuron properties. *Journal of Neurophysiology*, **77**, 2605–15.

Munson JB, Johnson RD, and Mendell LM (1997b). NT-3 increases amplitude of EPSPs produced by axotomized group Ia afferents. *Journal of Neurophysiology*, **77**, 2209–12.

Munson JB, Shelton DL, and McMahon SB (1997c). Adult mammalian sensory and motor neurons: roles of endogenous neurotrophins and rescue by exogenous neurotrophins after axotomy. *Journal of Neuroscience*, **17**, 470–6.

Murphy EH, Garone M, Tashayyod D, and Baker RB (1986). Innervation of extraocular muscles in the rabbit. *Journal of Comparative Neurology*, **254**, 78–90.

Nagy JI, Yamamoto T, and Jordan LM (1993). Evidence for the cholinergic nature of C-terminals associated with subsurface cisterns in alpha-motoneurons of rat. *Synapse*, **15**, 17–32.

Nakano H, Masuda K, Sasaki S, and Katsuta S (1997). Oxidative enzyme activity and soma size in motoneurons innervating the rat slow-twitch and fast-twitch muscles after chronic activity. *Brain Research Bulletin*, **43**, 149–54.

Nardone A, Romanò C, and Schieppati M (1989). Selective recruitment of high-threshold human motor units during voluntary isotonic lengthening of active muscles. *Journal of Physiology*, **409**, 451–71.

Narusawa M, Fitzsimons RB, Izumo S, Nadal-Ginard B, Rubinstein NA, and Kelly AM (1987). Slow myosin in developing rat skeletal muscle. *Journal of Cell Biology*, **104**, 447–59.

Needham DM (1926). Red and white muscle. *Physiological Reviews*, **6**, 1–27.

Neher E and Sakmann B (1976a). Noise analysis of drug induced voltage clamp currents in denervated frog muscle fibres. *Journal of Physiology*, **258**, 705–29.

Neher E and Sakmann B (1976b). Single-channel currents recorded from membrane of denervated frog muscle fibres. *Nature*, **260**, 799–802.

Nelson PG (1966). Interaction between spinal motoneurons of the cat. *Journal of Neurophysiology*, **29**, 275–87.

Nelson PG and Burke RE (1967). Delayed depolarization in cat spinal motoneurons. *Experimental Neurology*, **17**, 16–26.

Nemeth PM, Pette D, and Vrbova G (1981). Comparison of enzyme activities among single muscle fibres within defined motor units. *Journal of Physiology*, **311**, 489–95.

Nemeth PM, Solanki L, Gordon DA, Hamm TM, Reinking RM, and Stuart DG (1986). Uniformity of metabolic enzymes within individual motor units. *Journal of Neuroscience*, **6**, 892–8.

Nguyen QT and Lichtman JW (1996). Mechanism of synapse disassembly at the developing neuromuscular junction. *Current Opinion in Neurobiology*, **6**, 104–12.

Nicol CJ and Bruce DS (1981). Effect of hyperthyroidism on the contractile and histochemical properties of fast and slow twitch skeletal muscle in the rat. *Pflügers Archiv*, **390**, 73–9.

Nicolopoulos-Stournaras S and Iles JF (1983). Motor neuron columns in the lumbar spinal cord of the rat. *Journal of Comparative Neurology*, **217**, 75–85.

Nielsen J and Kagamihara Y (1993). Differential projection of the sural nerve to early and late recruited human tibialis anterior motor units: change of recruitment gain. *Acta Physiologica Scandinavica*, **147**, 385–401.

Nishimura H, Johnson RD, and Munson JB (1991). Rescue of motoneurons from the axotomized state by regeneration into a sensory nerve in cats. *Journal of Neurophysiology*, **66**, 1462–70.

Nissl F (1892). Über die veränderungen der Ganglienzellen am Facialiskern des Kaninchens nach ausreissung der Nerven. *Algemeine Zeitschrift für Psychiatrie*, **48**, 197–8.

Novitch BG, Wichterle H, Jessell TM, and Sockanathan S (2003). A requirement for retinoic acid-mediated transcriptional activation in ventral neural patterning and motor neuron specification. *Neuron*, **40**, 81–95.

Nunez-Abades PA, Spielmann JM, Barrionuevo G, and Cameron WE (1993). *In vivo* electrophysiology of developing genioglossal motoneurons in the rat. *Journal of Neurophysiology*, **70**, 1401–11.

Nussbaum MA, Clark LL, Lanza MA, and Rice KM (2001). Fatigue and endurance limits during intermittent overhead work. *AIHA Journal*, **62**, 446–56.

Oakley CR and Gollnick PD (1985). Conversion of rat muscle fiber types. A time course study. *Histochemistry*, **83**, 555–60.

O'Brien RA (1978). Axonal transport of acetylcholine, choline acetyltransferase and cholinesterase in regenerating peripheral nerve. *Journal of Physiology*, **282**, 91–103.

O'Donovan MJ, Pinter MJ, Dum RP, and Burke RE (1985). Kinesiological studies of self- and cross-reinnervated FDL and soleus muscles in freely moving cats. *Journal of Neurophysiology*, **54**, 852–66.

Odutola AB (1972). The organization of cholinesterase-containing systems of the monkey spinal cord. *Brain Research*, **39**, 353–68.

Ohira Y, Jiang B, Roy RR, *et al.* (1992). Rat soleus muscle fiber responses to 14 days of spaceflight and hindlimb suspension. *Journal of Applied Physiology*, **73**, 51S–7S.

Oppenheim RW (1991). Cell death during development of the nervous system. *Annual Review of Neuroscience*, **14**, 453–501.

Oppenheim RW and Nunez R (1982). Electrical stimulation of hindlimb increases neuronal cell death in chick embryo. *Nature*, **295**, 57–9.

Oppenheim RW, Prevette D, Yin QW, Collins F, and MacDonald J (1991). Control of embryonic motoneuron survival *in vivo* by ciliary neurotrophic factor. *Science*, **251**, 1616–18.

Oppenheim RW, Houenou LJ, Johnson JE, *et al.* (1995). Developing motor neurons rescued from programmed and axotomy-induced cell death by GDNF. *Nature*, **373**, 344–6.

Ornung G, Shupliakov O, Ottersen OP, Storm-Mathisen J, and Cullheim S (1994). Immunohistochemical evidence for coexistence of glycine and GABA in nerve terminals on cat spinal motoneurones: an ultrastructural study. *Neuroreport*, **5**, 889–92.

Ornung G, Shupliakov O, Linda H, *et al.* (1996). Qualitative and quantitative analysis of glycine- and GABA-immunoreactive nerve terminals on motoneuron cell bodies in the cat spinal cord: a postembedding electron microscopic study. *Journal of Comparative Neurology*, **365**, 413–26.

Ornung G, Ottersen OP, Cullheim S, and Ulfhake B (1998). Distribution of glutamate-, glycine- and GABA-immunoreactive nerve terminals on dendrites in the cat spinal motor nucleus. *Experimental Brain Research*, **118**, 517–32.

Palecek J, Lips MB, and Keller BU (1999). Calcium dynamics and buffering in motoneurones of the mouse spinal cord. *Journal of Physiology*, **520**, 485–502.

Parry DJ and Wilkinson RS (1990). The effect of reinnervation on the distribution of muscle fibre types in the tibialis anterior muscle of the mouse. *Canadian Journal of Physiology and Pharmacology*, **68**, 596–602.

Pattullo MC, Cotter MA, Cameron NE, and Barry JA (1992). Effects of lengthened immobilization on functional and histochemical properties of rabbit tibialis anterior muscle. *Experimental Physiology*, **77**, 433–42.

Pedersen BK, Steensberg A, Fischer C, *et al.* (2003). Searching for the exercise factor. Is IL-6 a candidate? *Journal of Muscle Research and Cell Motility*, **24**, 113–19.

Pellerin L (2003). Lactate as a pivotal element in neuron-glia metabolic cooperation. *Neurochemistry International*, **43**, 331–8.

Pernus F and Erzen I (1991). Arrangement of fiber types within fascicles of human vastus lateralis muscle. *Muscle & Nerve*, **14**, 304–9.

Perreault EJ, Day SJ, Hulliger M, Heckman CJ, and Sandercock TG (2003). Summation of forces from multiple motor units in the cat soleus muscle. *Journal of Neurophysiology*, **89**, 738–44.

Person RS and Kudina LP (1972). Discharge frequency and discharge pattern of human motor units during voluntary contraction of muscle. *Electroencephalography and Clinical Neurophysiology*, **32**, 471–83.

Personius KE and Balice-Gordon RJ (2000). Activity-dependent editing of neuromuscular synaptic connections. *Brain Research Bulletin*, **53**, 513–22.

Pestronk A, Drachman DB and Griffin JW (1980). Effects of aging on nerve sprouting and regeneration. *Experimental Neurology*, **70**, 65–82.

Peter JB, Barnard RJ, Edgerton VR, Gillespie CA, and Stempel KE (1972). Metabolic profiles of three fiber types of skeletal muscle in guinea pigs and rabbits. *Biochemistry*, **11**, 2627–33.

Peters EJ and Fuglevand AJ (1999). Cessation of human motor unit discharge during sustained maximal voluntary contraction. *Neuroscience Letters*, **274**, 66–70.

Petersen NT, Taylor JL, Butler JE, and Gandevia SC (2003). Depression of activity in the corticospinal pathway during human motor behavior after strong voluntary contractions. *Journal of Neuroscience*, **23**, 7974–80.

Petit J, Chua M, and Hunt CC (1993). Maximum shortening speed of motor units of various types in cat lumbrical muscles. *Journal of Neurophysiology*, **69**, 442–8.

Pette D (2002). The adaptive potential of skeletal muscle fibers. *Canadian Journal of Applied Physiology*, **27**, 423–48.

Pette D and Staron RS (1997). Mammalian skeletal muscle fiber type transitions. *International Review of Cytology*, **170**, 143–223.

Pette D and Staron RS (2000). Myosin isoforms, muscle fiber types, and transitions. *Microscopy Research and Technique*, **50**, 500–9.

Pette D and Vrbova G (1999). What does chronic electrical stimulation teach us about muscle plasticity? *Muscle & Nerve*, **22**, 666–77.

Pette D, Ramirez BU, Muller W, Simon R, Exner GU, and Hildebrand R (1975). Influence of intermittent long-term stimulation on contractile, histochemical and metabolic properties of fibre populations in fast and slow rabbit muscles. *Pflügers Archiv*, **361**, 1–7.

Pfaff S and Kintner C (1998). Neuronal diversification: development of motor neuron subtypes. *Current Opinion in Neurobiology*, **8**, 27–36.

Phillips CA, Repperger DW, Neidhard-Doll AT, and Reynolds DB (2004). Biomimetic model of skeletal muscle isometric contraction: I. an energetic-viscoelastic model for the skeletal muscle isometric force twitch. *Computers in Biology and Medicine*, **34**, 307–22.

Piehl F, Arvidsson U, Hokfelt T, and Cullheim S (1993). Calcitonin gene-related peptide-like immunoreactivity in motoneuron pools innervating different hind limb muscles in the rat. *Experimental Brain Research*, **96**, 291–303.

Pierotti DJ, Roy RR, Bodine-Fowler SC, Hodgson JA, and Edgerton VR (1991). Mechanical and morphological properties of chronically inactive cat tibialis anterior motor units. *Journal of Physiology*, **444**, 175–92.

Pinter MJ, Curtis RL, and Hosko MJ (1983). Voltage threshold and excitability among variously sized cat hindlimb motoneurons. *Journal of Neurophysiology*, **50**, 644–57.

Piotrkiewicz M, Hausmanowa-Petrusewicz I, and Mierzejewska J (1999). Motoneurons are altered in muscular dystrophy. *Journal de Physiologie*, **93**, 167–73.

Polgar J, Johnson MA, Weightman D, and Appleton D (1973). Data on fibre size in thirty-six human muscles. An autopsy study. *Journal of the Neurological Sciences*, **19**, 307–18.

Powers RK and Binder MD (1991a). Effects of low-frequency stimulation on the tension-frequency relations of fast-twitch motor units in the cat. *Journal of Neurophysiology*, **66**, 905–18.

Powers RK and Binder MD (1991b). Summation of motor unit tensions in the tibialis posterior muscle of the cat under isometric and nonisometric conditions. *Journal of Neurophysiology*, **66**, 1838–46.

Powers RK and Binder MD (1995). Effective synaptic current and motoneuron firing rate modulation. *Journal of Neurophysiology*, **74**, 793–801.

Powers RK and Binder MD (2000a). Relationship between the time course of the afterhyperpolarization and discharge variability in cat spinal motoneurones. *Journal of Physiology*, **528**, 131–50.

Powers RK and Binder MD (2000b). Summation of effective synaptic currents and firing rate modulation in cat spinal motoneurons. *Journal of Neurophysiology*, **83**, 483–500.

Powers RK and Binder MD (2001). Input-output functions of mammalian motoneurons. *Reviews of Physiology, Biochemistry and Pharmacology*, **143**, 137–263.

Powers RK and Binder MD (2003). Persistent sodium and calcium currents in rat hypoglossal motoneurons. *Journal of Neurophysiology*, **89**, 615–24.

Powers RK, Robinson FR, Konodi MA, and Binder MD (1992). Effective synaptic current can be estimated from measurements of neuronal discharge. *Journal of Neurophysiology*, **68**, 964–8.

Powers RK, Robinson FR, Konodi MA, and Binder MD (1993). Distribution of rubrospinal synaptic input to cat triceps surae motoneurons. *Journal of Neurophysiology*, **70**, 1460–8.

Powers RK, Sawczuk A, Musick JR, and Binder MD (1999). Multiple mechanisms of spike-frequency adaptation in motoneurones. *Journal de Physiologie*, **93**, 101–14.

Prakash YS, Zhan WZ, Miyata H, and Sieck GC (1995). Adaptations of diaphragm neuromuscular junction following inactivity. *Acta Anatomica (Basel)*, **154**, 147–61.

Prather JF, Powers RK, and Cope TC (2001). Amplification and linear summation of synaptic effects on motoneuron firing rate. *Journal of Neurophysiology*, **85**, 43–53.

Pratt CA and Jordan LM (1987). Ia inhibitory interneurons and Renshaw cells as contributors to the spinal mechanisms of fictive locomotion. *Journal of Neurophysiology*, **57**, 56–71.

Purves D and Sakmann B (1974a). The effect of contractile activity on fibrillation and extrajunctional acetylcholine-sensitivity in rat muscle maintained in organ culture. *Journal of Physiology*, **237**, 157–82.

Purves D and Sakmann B (1974b). Membrane properties underlying spontaneous activity of denervated muscle fibres. *Journal of Physiology*, **239**, 125–53.

Rack PMH and Westbury DR (1969). The effects of length and stimulus rate on tension in the isometric cat soleus muscle. *Journal of Physiology*, **204**, 443–60.

Rafuse VF and Gordon T (1996a). Self-reinnervated cat medial gastrocnemius muscles. I: comparisons of the capacity for regenerating nerves to form enlarged motor units after extensive peripheral nerve injuries. *Journal of Neurophysiology*, **75**, 268–81.

Rafuse VF and Gordon T (1996b). Self-reinnervated cat medial gastrocnemius muscles. II: analysis of the mechanisms and significance of fiber type grouping in reinnervated muscles. *Journal of Neurophysiology*, **75**, 282–97.

Rafuse VF and Gordon T (1998). Incomplete rematching of nerve and muscle properties in motor units after extensive nerve injuries in cat hindlimb muscle. *Journal of Physiology*, **509**, 909–26.

Rafuse VF, Pattullo MC, and Gordon T (1997). Innervation ratio and motor unit force in large muscles: a study of chronically stimulated cat medial gastrocnemius. *Journal of Physiology*, **499**, 809–23.

Rall W (1960). Membrane potential transients and membrane time constant of motoneurons. *Experimental Neurology*, **2**, 503–32.

Rall W (1969). Time constants and electrotonic length of membrane cylinders and neurons. *Biophysical Journal*, **9**, 1483–508.

Rall W (1977). Core conductor theory and cable properties of neurons. In ER Kandel (ed.), *Handbook of Physiology*, Section 1, Volume I, pp. 39–97. American Physiological Society, Bethesda, MD.

Rall W, Burke RE, Smith TG, Nelson PG, and Frank K (1967). Dendritic location of synapses and possible mechanisms for the monosynaptic EPSP in motoneurons. *Journal of Neurophysiology*, **30**, 1169–93.

Rall W, Burke RE, Holmes WR, Jack JJ, Redman SJ, and Segev I (1992). Matching dendritic neuron models to experimental data. *Physiological Reviews*, **72**, S159–86.

Ranatunga KW (1982). Temperature-dependence of shortening velocity and rate of isometric tension development in rat skeletal muscle. *Journal of Physiology*, **329**, 465–83.

Rankin LL, Enoka RM, Volz KA, and Stuart DG (1988). Coexistence of twitch potentiation and tetanic force decline in rat hindlimb muscle. *Journal of Applied Physiology*, **65**, 2687–95.

Ranvier L (1874). De quelques faits relatifs à l'histologie et à la physiologie des muscles striés. *Archives de Physiologie Normale et Pathologique*, **6**, 1–15.

Rasband MN and Shrager P (2000). Ion channel sequestration in central nervous system axons. *Journal of Physiology*, **525**, 63–73.

Redman S and Walmsley B (1983a). Amplitude fluctuations in synaptic potentials evoked in cat spinal motoneurones at identified group Ia synapses. *Journal of Physiology*, **343**, 135–45.

Redman S and Walmsley B (1983b). The time course of synaptic potentials evoked in cat spinal motoneurones at identified group Ia synapses. *Journal of Physiology*, **343**, 117–33.

Reed JZ, Butler PJ, and Fedak MA (1994). The metabolic characteristics of the locomotory muscles of grey seals (*Halichoerus grypus*), harbour seals (*Phoca vitulina*) and Antarctic fur seals (*Arctocephalus gazella*). *Journal of Experimental Biology*, **194**, 33–46.

Reggiani C, Bottinelli R, and Stienen GJ (2000). Sarcomeric myosin isoforms: fine tuning of a molecular motor. *News in Physiological Sciences*, **15**, 26–33.

Reichmann H and Pette D (1982). A comparative microphotometric study of succinate dehydrogenase activity levels in type I, IIA and IIB fibres of mammalian and human muscles. *Histochemistry*, **74**, 27–41.

Reichmann H, Srihari T, and Pette D (1983). Ipsi- and contralateral fibre transformations by cross-reinnervation. A principle of symmetry. *Pflügers Archiv*, **397**, 202–8.

Reid B, Slater CR, and Bewick GS (1999). Synaptic vesicle dynamics in rat fast and slow motor nerve terminals. *Journal of Neuroscience*, **19**, 2511–21.

Reid B, Martinov VN, Nja A, Lomo T, and Bewick GS (2003). Activity-dependent plasticity of transmitter release from nerve terminals in rat fast and slow muscles. *Journal of Neuroscience*, **23**, 9340–8.

Reinking RM, Stephens JA, and Stuart DG (1975). The motor units of cat medial gastrocnemius: problem of their categorisation on the basis of mechanical properties. *Experimental Brain Research*, **23**, 301–13.

Reis DJ and Wooten GF (1976). Blood flow in red and white muscle: relationship to metabolism development and behavior. *Progress in Brain Research*, **44**, 385–402.

Rekling JC, Funk GD, Bayliss DA, Dong XW, and Feldman JL (2000). Synaptic control of motoneuronal excitability. *Physiological Reviews*, **80**, 767–852.

Rennie MJ, Wackerhage H, Spangenburg EE, and Booth FW (2004). Control of the size of the human muscle mass. *Annual Review of Physiology*, **66**, 799–828.

Rexed B (1952). The cytoarchitectonic organization of the spinal cord in the cat. *Journal of Comparative Neurology*, **96**, 415–96.

Rexed B (1954). A cytoarchtectonic atlas of the spinal cord in the cat. *Journal of Comparative Neurology*, **100**, 297–379.

Rich MM and Lichtman JW (1989). *In vivo* visualization of pre- and postsynaptic changes during synapse elimination in reinnervated mouse muscle. *Journal of Neuroscience*, **9**, 1781–1805.

Richardson PM (1991). Neurotrophic factors in regeneration. *Current Opinion in Neurobiology*, **1**, 401–6.

Ridge RM and Betz WJ (1984). The effect of selective, chronic stimulation on motor unit size in developing rat muscle. *Journal of Neuroscience*, **4**, 2614–20.

Rivero JL, Talmadge RJ, and Edgerton VR (1998). Fibre size and metabolic properties of myosin heavy chain-based fibre types in rat skeletal muscle. *Journal of Muscle Research and Cell Motility*, **19**, 733–42.

Roberts AD, Billeter R, and Howald H (1982). Anaerobic muscle enzyme changes after interval training. *International Journal of Sports Medicine*, **3**, 18–21.

Robinson A, Tufft N, and Lewis DM (1991). A comparison of fibrillation in denervated skeletal muscle of the anaesthetized rat and guinea-pig. *Journal of Muscle Research and Cell Motility*, **12**, 271–80.

Rohmert W (1960). Ermittlung von Erholungpausen für statische Arbeit des Menschen. *Internationale Zeitschrift für Angewandte Physiologie, einschliesslich Arbeitsphysiologie*, **18**, 123–64.

Romanes GJ (1951). The motor cell columns of the lumbo-sacral spinal cord of the cat. *Journal of Comparative Neurology*, **94** 313–63.

Romanes GJ (1964). The motor pools of the spinal cord. *Progress in Brain Research*, **11**, 93–119.

Romanul FC (1964). Enzymes in muscle. I. Histochemical studies of enzymes in individual muscle fibers. *Archives of Neurology*, **11**, 355–8.

Romanul FC and Hogan EL (1965). Enzymatic changes in denervated muscle. I: Histochemical studies. *Archives of Neurology*, **13**, 263–73.

Romanul FC and Van der Meulen JP (1966). Reversal of the enzyme profiles of muscle fibres in fast and slow muscles by cross-innervation. *Nature*, **212**, 1369–70.

Rome LC, Funke RP, Alexander RM, *et al.* (1988). Why animals have different muscle fibre types. *Nature*, **335**, 824–7.

Romi F, Gilhus NE, and Aarli JA (2005). Myasthenia gravis: clinical, immunological, and therapeutic advances. *Acta Neurologica Scandinavica*, **111**, 134–41.

Ronnevi LO and Conradi S (1974). Ultrastructural evidence for spontaneous elimination of synaptic terminals on spinal motoneurons in the kitten. *Brain Research*, **80**, 335–9.

Roper J and Schwarz JR (1989). Heterogeneous distribution of fast and slow potassium channels in myelinated rat nerve fibres. *Journal of Physiology*, **416**, 93–110.

Rose PK and Cushing S (1999). Non-linear summation of synaptic currents on spinal motoneurons: lessons from simulations of the behaviour of anatomically realistic models. *Progress in Brain Research*, **123**, 99–107.

Rose PK and Odlozinski M (1998). Expansion of the dendritic tree of motoneurons innervating neck muscles of the adult cat after permanent axotomy. *Journal of Comparative Neurology*, **390**, 392–411.

Rose PK and Richmond FJ (1981). White-matter dendrites in the upper cervical spinal cord of the adult cat: a light and electron microscopic study. *Journal of Comparative Neurology*, **199**, 191–203.

Rose PK, MacDermid V, Joshi M, and Neuber-Hess M (2001). Emergence of axons from distal dendrites of adult mammalian neurons following a permanent axotomy. *European Journal of Neuroscience*, **13**, 1166–76.

Rotshenker S (1979). Synapse formation in intact innervated cutaneous-pectoris muscles of the frog following denervation of the opposite muscle. *Journal of Physiology*, **292**, 535–47.

Rotshenker S and Tal M (1985). The transneuronal induction of sprouting and synapse formation in intact mouse muscles. *Journal of Physiology*, **360**, 387–96.

Rotundo RL (2003). Expression and localization of acetylcholinesterase at the neuromuscular junction. *Journal of Neurocytology*, **32**, 743–66.

Roy RR, Meadows ID, Baldwin KM, and Edgerton VR (1982). Functional significance of compensatory overloaded rat fast muscle. *Journal of Applied Physiology*, **52**, 473–8.

Roy RR, Pierotti DJ, Flores V, Rudolph W, and Edgerton VR (1992). Fibre size and type adaptations to spinal isolation and cyclical passive stretch in cat hindlimb. *Journal of Anatomy*, **180**, 491–9.

Roy RR, Eldridge L, Baldwin KM, and Edgerton VR (1996). Neural influence on slow muscle properties: inactivity with and without cross-reinnervation. *Muscle & Nerve*, **19**, 707–14.

Roy RR, Ishihara A, Kim JA, Lee M, Fox K, and Edgerton VR (1999a). Metabolic and morphological stability of motoneurons in response to chronically elevated neuromuscular activity. *Neuroscience*, **92**, 361–6.

Roy RR, Talmadge RJ, Hodgson JA, Oishi Y, Baldwin KM, and Edgerton VR (1999b). Differential response of fast hindlimb extensor and flexor muscles to exercise in adult spinalized cats. *Muscle & Nerve*, **22**, 230–41.

Roy RR, Ishihara A, Moran MM, Wade CE, and Edgerton VR (2001). No effect of hypergravity on adult rat ventral horn neuron size or SDH activity. *Aviation, Space, and Environmental Medicine*, **72**, 1107–12.

Roy RR, Zhong H, Monti RJ, Vallance KA, and Edgerton VR (2002). Mechanical properties of the electrically silent adult rat soleus muscle. *Muscle & Nerve*, **26**, 404–12.

Royle SJ and Lagnado L (2003). Endocytosis at the synaptic terminal. *Journal of Physiology*, **553**, 345–55.

Rubinstein N, Mabuchi K, Pepe F, Salmons S, Gergely J, and Sreter F (1978). Use of type-specific antimyosins to demonstrate the transformation of individual fibers in chronically stimulated rabbit fast muscles. *Journal of Cell Biology*, **79**, 252–61.

Rushton WAH (1951). A theory on the effects of fibre size in medullated nerves. *Journal of Physiology*, **115**, 101–22.

Russo RE and Hounsgaard J (1999). Dynamics of intrinsic electrophysiological properties in spinal cord neurones. *Progress in Biophysics and Molecular Biology*, **72**, 329–65.

Rutherford OM and Jones DA (1988). Contractile properties and fatiguability of the human adductor pollicis and first dorsal interosseus: a comparison of the effect of two chronic stimulation patterns. *Journal of the Neurological Sciences*, **85**, 319–31.

Ryall RW (1981). Patterns of recurrent excitation and mutual inhibition of cat Renshaw cells. *Journal of Physiology*, **316**, 439–52.

Safronov BV and Vogel W (1995). Single voltage-activated Na^+ and K^+ channels in the somata of rat motoneurones. *Journal of Physiology*, **487**, 91–106.

Safronov BV and Vogel W (1996). Properties and functions of Na^+-activated K^+ channels in the soma of rat motoneurones. *Journal of Physiology*, **497**, 727–34.

Safronov BV, Wolff M, and **Vogel W** (2000). Excitability of the soma in central nervous system neurons. *Biophysical Journal*, **78**, 2998–3010.

Sah P (1996). Ca^{2+}-activated K^+ currents in neurones: types, physiological roles and modulation. *Trends in Neurosciences*, **19**, 150–4.

Sah P and **Faber ES** (2002). Channels underlying neuronal calcium-activated potassium currents. *Progress in Neurobiology*, **66**, 345–53.

Sakmann B and **Brenner HR** (1978). Change in synaptic channel gating during neuromuscular development. *Nature*, **276**, 401–2.

Sala C, Andreose JS, Fumagalli G, and **Lomo T** (1995). Calcitonin gene-related peptide: possible role in formation and maintenance of neuromuscular junctions. *Journal of Neuroscience*, **15**, 520–8.

Salmons S and **Henriksson J** (1981). The adaptive response of skeletal muscle to increased use. *Muscle & Nerve*, **4**, 94–105.

Salmons S and **Vrbova G** (1969). The influence of activity on some contractile characteristics of mammalian fast and slow muscles. *Journal of Physiology*, **201**, 535–49.

Sanders FK and **Whitteridge D** (1948). Conduction velocity and myelin thickness in regenerating nerve fibres. *Journal of Physiology*, **105**, 152–74.

Sanes JR (1983). Roles of extracellular matrix in neural development. *Annual Review of Physiology*, **45**, 581–600.

Sanes JR and **Jessell TM** (2000). The guidance of axons to their targets. In ER Kandel, JH Schwartz, and TM Jessell (eds), *Principles of Neural Science*, pp. 1063–86. McGraw-Hill, New York.

Sanes JR and **Lichtman JW** (1999). Development of the vertebrate neuromuscular junction. *Annual Review of Neuroscience*, **22**, 389–442.

Santana Pereira JA, de Haan A, Wessels A, Moorman AF, and **Sargeant AJ** (1995). The mATPase histochemical profile of rat type IIX fibres: correlation with myosin heavy chain immunolabelling. *Histochemical Journal*, **27**, 715–22.

Sargeant AJ (1987). Effect of muscle temperature on leg extension force and short-term power output in humans. *European Journal of Applied Physiology*, **56**, 693–8.

Sasaki K and **Otani T** (1961). Accommodation in spinal motoneurons of the cat. *Japanese Journal of Physiology*, **11**, 443–56.

Sawczuk A, Powers RK, and **Binder MD** (1995). Spike frequency adaptation studied in hypoglossal motoneurons of the rat. *Journal of Neurophysiology*, **73**, 1799–1810.

Sawczuk A, Powers RK, and **Binder MD** (1997). Contribution of outward currents to spike-frequency adaptation in hypoglossal motoneurons of the rat. *Journal of Neurophysiology*, **78**, 2246–53.

Scheibel ME and **Scheibel AB** (1970). Organization of spinal motoneuron dendrites in bundles. *Experimental Neurology*, **28**, 106–12.

Schiaffino S and **Reggiani C** (1996). Molecular diversity of myofibrillar proteins: gene regulation and functional significance. *Physiological Reviews*, **76**, 371–423.

Schiaffino S, Saggin L, Viel A, Ausoni S, Sartore S, and **Gorza L** (1986). Muscle fiber types identified by monoclonal antibodies to myosin heavy chains. In G Benzi, L Packer, and N Siliprandi (eds), *Biochemical Aspects of Physical Exercise*, pp. 27–34. Elsevier, Amsterdam.

Schiaffino S, Gorza L, Sartore S, *et al.* (1989). Three myosin heavy chain isoforms in type 2 skeletal muscle fibres. *Journal of Muscle Research and Cell Motility*, **10**, 197–205.

Schlue WR, Richter DW, Mauritz KH, and **Nacimiento AC** (1974). Responses of cat spinal motoneuron somata and axons to linearly rising currents. *Journal of Neurophysiology*, **37**, 303–9.

Schmalbruch H (1988). The effect of peripheral nerve injury on immature motor and sensory neurons and on muscle fibres. Possible relation to the histogenesis of Werdnig–Hoffmann disease. *Revue Neurologique*, **144**, 721–9.

Schmalbruch H, and Hellhammer U (1977). The number of nuclei in adult rat muscles with special reference to satellite cells. *Anatomical Record*, **189**, 169–75.

Schmalbruch H, al-Amood WS, and Lewis DM (1991). Morphology of long-term denervated rat soleus muscle and the effect of chronic electrical stimulation. *Journal of Physiology*, **441**, 233–41.

Schmitt TL and Pette D (1991). Fiber type-specific distribution of parvalbumin in rabbit skeletal muscle. A quantitative microbiochemical and immunohistochemical study. *Histochemistry*, **96**, 459–65.

Schomburg ED and Steffens H (2002). Only minor spinal motor reflex effects from feline group IV muscle nociceptors. *Neuroscience Research*, **44**, 213–23.

Schuler M and Pette D (1996). Fiber transformation and replacement in low-frequency stimulated rabbit fast-twitch muscles. *Cell and Tissue Research*, **285**, 297–303.

Schwaller B, Dick J, Dhoot G, *et al.* (1999). Prolonged contraction-relaxation cycle of fast-twitch muscles in parvalbumin knockout mice. *American Journal of Physiology*, **276**, C395–403.

Schwartz JH and De Camilli P (2000). Synthesis and trafficking of neuronal protein. In ER Kandel, JH Schwartz, and TM Jessell (eds), *Principles of Neural Science*, pp. 88–104. McGraw-Hill, New York.

Schwindt PC (1973). Membrane-potential trajectories underlying motoneuron rhythmic firing at high rates. *Journal of Neurophysiology*, **36**, 434–9.

Schwindt PC and Calvin WH (1973). Equivalence of synaptic and injected current in determining the membrane potential trajectory during motoneuron rhythmic firing. *Brain Research*, **59**, 389–94.

Schwindt P and Crill WE (1977). A persistent negative resistance in cat lumbar motoneurons. *Brain Research*, **120**, 173–8.

Schwindt P and Crill W (1980a). Role of a persistent inward current in motoneuron bursting during spinal seizures. *Journal of Neurophysiology*, **43**, 1296–318.

Schwindt PC and Crill WE (1980b). Properties of a persistent inward current in normal and TEA-injected motoneurons. *Journal of Neurophysiology*, **43**, 1700–24.

Schwindt PC and Crill WE (1982). Factors influencing motoneuron rhythmic firing: results from a voltage-clamp study. *Journal of Neurophysiology*, **48**, 875–90.

Scott WB, Lee SC, Johnston TE, and Binder-Macleod SA (2005). Switching stimulation patterns improves performance of paralyzed human quadriceps muscle. *Muscle & Nerve*, **31**, 581–8.

Seburn K, Coicou C, and Gardiner P (1994). Effects of altered muscle activation on oxidative enzyme activity in rat alpha-motoneurons. *Journal of Applied Physiology*, **77**, 2269–74.

Sejersted OM and Hargens AR (1995). Intramuscular pressures for monitoring different tasks and muscle conditions. *Advances in Experimental Medicine and Biology*, **384**, 339–50.

Sejersted OM and Sjogaard G (2000). Dynamics and consequences of potassium shifts in skeletal muscle and heart during exercise. *Physiological Reviews*, **80**, 1411–81.

Sekiya H, Kojima Y, Hiramoto D, Mukuno K, and Ishikawa S (1992). Bilateral innervation of the musculus levator palpebrae superioris by single motoneurons in the monkey. *Neuroscience Letters*, **146**, 10–12.

Sellin LC and Thesleff S (1980). Alterations in membrane electrical properties during long-term denervation of rat skeletal muscles. *Acta Physiologica Scandinavica*, **108**, 243–6.

Seneviratne U and de Silva R (1999). Lambert–Eaton myasthenic syndrome. *Postgraduate Medical Journal*, **75**, 516–20.

Serrano AL, Quiroz-Rothe E, and Rivero JL (2000). Early and long-term changes of equine skeletal muscle in response to endurance training and detraining. *Pflügers Archiv*, **441**, 263–74.

Serrano AL, Murgia M, Pallafacchina G, *et al.* (2001). Calcineurin controls nerve activity-dependent specification of slow skeletal muscle fibers but not muscle growth. *Proceedings of the National Academy of Sciences of the United States of America*, **98**, 13108–13.

Shall MS and Goldberg SJ (1992). Extraocular motor units: type classification and motoneuron stimulation frequency-muscle unit force relationships. *Brain Research*, **587**, 291–300.

Shapovalov AI and Grantyn AA (1968). [Suprasegmental synaptic effect on chromatolyzed motor neurons.] *Biofizika*, **13**, 260–9.

Sheffield-Moore M and Urban RJ (2004). An overview of the endocrinology of skeletal muscle. *Trends in Endocrinology and Metabolism*, **15**, 110–15.

Sherrington CS (1906). *The Integrative Action of the Nervous System.* Yale University Press, New Haven, CT.

Sickles DW and McLendon RE (1983). Metabolic variation among rat lumbosacral alpha-motoneurons. *Histochemistry*, **79**, 205–17.

Sickles DW and Oblak TG (1984). Metabolic variation among alpha-motoneurons innervating different muscle-fiber types. I. Oxidative enzyme activity. *Journal of Neurophysiology*, **51**, 529–37.

Sickles DW, Oblak TG and Scholer J (1987). Hyperthyroidism selectively increases oxidative metabolism of slow-oxidative motor units. *Experimental Neurology*, **97**, 90–105.

Sieck GC and Prakash YS (1995). Fatigue at the neuromuscular junction. Branch point vs. presynaptic vs. postsynaptic mechanisms. *Advances in Experimental Medicine and Biology*, **384**, 83–100.

Siegelbaum SA, Schwartz JH, and Kandel ER (2000). Modulation of synaptic transmission: second messengers. In ER Kandel, JH Schwartz, and TM Jessell (eds), *Principles of Neural Science*, pp. 229–52. McGraw-Hill, New York.

Simon M, Mann D, Coulton G, and Terenghi G (2002). Differential tyrosine kinase C mRNA distribution in extensor digitorum longus and soleus motoneurons in adult rats: effect of axotomy and neurotrophin-3 treatment. *Neuroscience Letters*, **320**, 9–12.

Simoneau JA and Pette D (1988). Species-specific effects of chronic nerve stimulation upon tibialis anterior muscle in mouse, rat, guinea pig, and rabbit. *Pflügers Archiv*, **412**, 86–92.

Simoneau JA, Lortie G, Boulay MR, Marcotte M, Thibault MC, and Bouchard C (1985). Human skeletal muscle fiber type alteration with high-intensity intermittent training. *European Journal of Applied Physiology*, **54**, 250–3.

Simoneau JA, Kaufmann M, and Pette D (1993). Asynchronous increases in oxidative capacity and resistance to fatigue of electrostimulated muscles of rat and rabbit. *Journal of Physiology*, **460**, 573–80.

Sjoberg J and Kanje M (1990). The initial period of peripheral nerve regeneration and the importance of the local environment for the conditioning lesion effect. *Brain Research*, **529**, 79–84.

Sjogaard G, Kiens B, Jorgensen K, and Saltin B (1986). Intramuscular pressure, EMG and blood flow during low-level prolonged static contraction in man. *Acta Physiologica Scandinavica*, **128**, 475–84.

Sjöström M, Downham DY, and Lexell J (1986). Distribution of different fibre types in human skeletal muscles: why is there a difference within a fascicle? *Muscle & Nerve*, **9**, 30–6.

Sjöström M, Lexell J, and Downham DY (1992). Differences in fiber number and fiber type proportion within fascicles. A quantitative morphological study of whole vastus lateralis muscle from childhood to old age. *Anatomical Record*, **234**, 183–9.

Sketelj J, Crne-Finderle N, and Brzin M (1992). Influence of denervation on the molecular forms of junctional and extrajunctional acetylcholinesterase in fast and slow muscles of the rat. *Neurochemistry International*, **21**, 415–21.

Smith JL, Betts B, Edgerton VR, and Zernicke RF (1980). Rapid ankle extension during paw shakes: selective recruitment of fast ankle extensors. *Journal of Neurophysiology*, **43**, 612–20.

Smith RS and Lannergren J (1968). Types of motor units in the skeletal muscle of *Xenopus laevis*. *Nature*, **217**, 281–3.

Sobue G, Sahashi K, Takahashi A, Matsuoka Y, Muroga T, and Sobue I (1983). Degenerating compartment and functioning compartment of motor neurons in ALS: possible process of motor neuron loss. *Neurology*, **33**, 654–7.

Sokoloff AJ, Siegel SG, and Cope TC (1999). Recruitment order among motoneurons from different motor nuclei. *Journal of Neurophysiology*, **81**, 2485–92.

Sokolove PG and Cooke IM (1971). Inhibition of impulse activity in a sensory neuron by an electrogenic pump. *Journal of General Physiology*, **57**, 125–63.

Solomon NP, Drager KD, and Luschei ES (2002). Sustaining a constant effort by the tongue and hand: effects of acute fatigue. *Journal of Speech, Language, and Hearing Research*, **45**, 613–24.

Son YJ and Thompson WJ (1995). Schwann cell processes guide regeneration of peripheral axons. *Neuron*, **14**, 125–32.

Son YJ, Trachtenberg JT, and Thompson WJ (1996). Schwann cells induce and guide sprouting and reinnervation of neuromuscular junctions. *Trends in Neurosciences*, **19**, 280–5.

Spector SA (1985). Effects of elimination of activity on contractile and histochemical properties of rat soleus muscle. *Journal of Neuroscience*, **5**, 2177–88.

Spector SA, Simard CP, Fournier M, Sternlicht E, and Edgerton VR (1982). Architectural alterations of rat hind-limb skeletal muscles immobilized at different lengths. *Experimental Neurology*, **76**, 94–110.

Spielmann JM, Laouris Y, Nordstrom MA, Robinson GA, Reinking RM, and Stuart DG (1993). Adaptation of cat motoneurons to sustained and intermittent extracellular activation. *Journal of Physiology*, **464**, 75–120.

Sréter FA, Pinter K, Jolesz F, and Mabuchi K (1982). Fast to slow transformation of fast muscles in response to long-term phasic stimulation. *Experimental Neurology*, **75**, 95–102.

Sréter FA, Lopez JR, Alamo L, Mabuchi K, and Gergely J (1987). Changes in intracellular ionized Ca concentration associated with muscle fiber type transformation. *American Journal of Physiology*, **253**, C296–300.

Stafstrom CE, Schwindt PC, Flatman JA, and Crill WE (1984). Properties of subthreshold response and action potential recorded in layer V neurons from cat sensorimotor cortex *in vivo*. *Journal of Neurophysiology*, **52**, 244–63.

Staron RS and Pette D (1990). The multiplicity of myosin light and heavy chain combinations in muscle fibers. In D Pette (ed.), *The Dynamic State of Muscle Fibers*, pp. 315–28. Walter de Gruyter, Berlin.

Starr KA and Wolpaw JR (1994). Synaptic terminal coverage of primate triceps surae motoneurons. *Journal of Comparative Neurology*, **345**, 345–58.

Stein JM and Padykula HA (1962). Histochemical classification of individual skeletal muscle fibers of the rat. *American Journal of Anatomy*, **110**, 103–23.

Stein RB, Bobet J, Oguztoreli MN, and Fryer M (1988). The kinetics relating calcium and force in skeletal muscle. *Biophysical Journal*, **54**, 705–17.

Stein RB, Gordon T, Jefferson J, *et al.* (1992). Optimal stimulation of paralyzed muscle after human spinal cord injury. *Journal of Applied Physiology*, **72**, 1393–1400.

Steinbach JH, Schubert D, and Eldridge L (1980). Changes in cat muscle contractile proteins after prolonged muscle inactivity. *Experimental Neurology*, **67**, 655–69.

Stephenson DG and Williams DA (1982). Effects of sarcomere length on the force-pCa relation in fast- and slow-twitch skinned muscle fibres from the rat. *Journal of Physiology*, **333**, 637–53.

Sterling P and Kuypers HG (1967). Anatomical organization of the brachial spinal cord of the cat. II: The motoneuron plexus. Brain Research, 4, 16–32.

Stotz PJ and Bawa P (2001). Motor unit recruitment during lengthening contractions of human wrist flexors. *Muscle & Nerve*, **24**, 1535–41.

St-Pierre D and Gardiner PF (1985). Effect of 'disuse' on mammalian fast-twitch muscle: joint fixation compared with neurally applied tetrodotoxin. *Experimental Neurology*, **90**, 635–51.

St-Pierre DM, Leonard D, Houle R and Gardiner PF (1988). Recovery of muscle from tetrodotoxin-induced disuse and the influence of daily exercise. 2: Muscle enzymes and fatigue characteristics. *Experimental Neurology*, **101**, 327–46.

Stuart DG and Enoka R (1983). Motoneurons, motor units, and the size principle. In RN Rosenberg and WD Willis (eds), *The Clinical Neurosciences: Neurobiology*, Section 5, pp. 471–517. Churchill Livingstone, New York.

Sulaiman OA and Gordon T (2000). Effects of short- and long-term Schwann cell denervation on peripheral nerve regeneration, myelination, and size. *Glia*, **32**, 234–46.

Sumner BE and Watson WE (1971). Retraction and expansion of the dendritic tree of motor neurones of adult rats induced *in vivo*. *Nature*, **233**, 273–5.

Sunderland S and Ray LJ (1950). Denervation changes in mammalian striated muscle. *Journal of Neurochemistry*, **13**, 159–77.

Sunnerhagen KS and Grimby G (2001). Muscular effects in late polio. *Acta Physiologica Scandinavica*, **171**, 335–40.

Sutherland H, Jarvis JC, Kwende MM, Gilroy SJ, and Salmons S (1998). The dose-related response of rabbit fast muscle to long-term low-frequency stimulation. *Muscle & Nerve*, **21**, 1632–46.

Sutherland H, Jarvis JC, and Salmons S (2003). Pattern dependence in the stimulation-induced type transformation of rabbit fast skeletal muscle. *Neuromodulation*, **6**, 176–89.

Suzuki H, Tsuzimoto H, Ishiko T, Kasuga N, Taguchi S, and Ishihara A (1991). Effect of endurance training on the oxidative enzyme activity of soleus motoneurons in rats. *Acta Physiologica Scandinavica*, **143**, 127–8.

Sweeney HL, Bowman BF, and Stull JT (1993). Myosin light chain phosphorylation in vertebrate striated muscle: regulation and function. *American Journal of Physiology*, **264**, C1085–95.

Swett JE, Eldred E, and Buchwald JS (1970). Somatotopic cord-to-muscle relations in efferent innervation of cat gastrocnemius. *American Journal of Physiology*, **219**, 762–6.

Swett JE, Wikholm RP, Blanks RHI, Swett AL, and Conley LC (1986). Motoneurons of the rat sciatic nerve. *Experimental Neurology*, **93**, 227–52.

Svirskis G and Hounsgaard J (1997). Depolarization-induced facilitation of a plateau-generating current in ventral horn neurons in the turtle spinal cord. *Journal of Neurophysiology*, **78**, 1740–2.

Szabo M, Salpeter EE, Randall W, and Salpeter MM (2003). Transients in acetylcholine receptor site density and degradation during reinnervation of mouse sternomastoid muscle. *Journal of Neurochemistry*, **84**, 180–8.

Tabary JC, Tabary C, Tardieu C, Tardieu G, and Goldspink G (1972). Physiological and structural changes in the cat's soleus muscle due to immobilization at different lengths by plaster casts. *Journal of Physiology*, **224**, 231–44.

Takahashi T (1990). Membrane currents in visually identified motoneurones of neonatal rat spinal cord. *Journal of Physiology*, **423**, 27–46.

Talmadge RJ, Roy RR, and Edgerton VR (1999). Persistence of hybrid fibers in rat soleus after spinal cord transection. *Anatomical Record*, **255**, 188–201.

Tam SL and Gordon T (2003). Mechanisms controlling axonal sprouting at the neuromuscular junction. *Journal of Neurocytology*, **32**, 961–74.

Tansey KE and Botterman BR (1996). Activation of type-identified motor units during centrally evoked contractions in the cat medial gastrocnemius muscle. II: Motoneuron firing-rate modulation. *Journal of Neurophysiology*, **75**, 38–50.

Tarabal O, Caldero J, Ribera J, *et al.* (1996). Regulation of motoneuronal calcitonin gene-related peptide (CGRP) during axonal growth and neuromuscular synaptic plasticity induced by botulinum toxin in rats. *European Journal of Neuroscience*, **8**, 829–36.

Tauc L (1982). Non vesicular release of neurotransmitter. *Physiological Reviews*, **62**, 857–93.

Tax AAM, Van der Gon JJD, Gielen CCAM, and Van den Tempel CMM (1989). Differences in the activation of M biceps brachii in the control of slow isotonic movements and isometric contractions. *Experimental Brain Research*, **76**, 55–63.

Taylor AM and Enoka RM (2004). Quantification of the factors that influence discharge correlation in model motor neurons. *Journal of Neurophysiology*, **91**, 796–814.

ter Haar Romeny BM, Denier van der Gon JJ, and Gielen CCAM (1984). Relation between location of a motor unit in the human biceps brachii and its critical firing levels for different tasks. *Experimental Neurology*, **85**, 631–50.

Termin A, Staron RS, and Pette D (1989). Myosin heavy chain isoforms in histochemically defined fiber types of rat muscle. *Histochemistry*, **92**, 453–7.

Tesch PA, Ekberg A, Lindquist DM, and Trieschmann JT (2004). Muscle hypertrophy following 5-week resistance training using a non-gravity-dependent exercise system. *Acta Physiologica Scandinavica*, **180**, 89–98.

Tetzlaff W, Bisby MA, and Kreutzberg GW (1988). Changes in cytoskeletal proteins in the rat facial nucleus following axotomy. *Journal of Neuroscience*, **8**, 3181–9.

Tetzlaff W, Zwiers H, Lederis K, Cassar L, and Bisby MA (1989). Axonal transport and localization of B-50/GAP-43-like immunoreactivity in regenerating sciatic and facial nerves of the rat. *Journal of Neuroscience*, **9**, 1303–13.

Tetzlaff W, Alexander SW, Miller FD, and Bisby MA (1991). Response of facial and rubrospinal neurons to axotomy: changes in mRNA expression for cytoskeletal proteins and GAP-43. *Journal of Neuroscience*, **11**, 2528–44.

Thaler J, Harrison K, Sharma K, Lettieri K, Kehrl J, and Pfaff SL (1999). Active suppression of interneuron programs within developing motor neurons revealed by analysis of homeodomain factor HB9. *Neuron*, **23**, 675–87.

Thaler JP, Koo SJ, Kania A, *et al.* (2004). A postmitotic role for Isl-class LIM homeodomain proteins in the assignment of visceral spinal motor neuron identity. *Neuron*, **41**, 337–50.

Thesleff S (1963). Spontaneous electrical activity in denervated rat skeletal muscle. In E Gutmann and P Hník (eds), *The Effect of Use and Disuse on Neuromuscular Function*, pp. 41–51. Czechoslovak Academy of Sciences, Prague.

Thomas CK and Grumbles RM (2005). Muscle atrophy after human spinal cord injury. *Biocybernetics and Biomedical Engineering*, **25**, 39–45.

Thomas CK and Ross BH (1997). Distinct patterns of motor unit behavior during muscle spasms in spinal cord injured subjects. *Journal of Neurophysiology*, **77**, 2847–50.

Thomas CK and Zijdewind I (2006). Fatigue of muscles weakened by death of motoneurons. *Muscle & Nerve*, **33**, 21–41.

Thomas CK, Stein RB, Gordon T, Lee RG, and Elleker MG (1987). Patterns of reinnervation and motor unit recruitment in human hand muscles after complete ulnar and median nerve section and resuture. *Journal of Neurology, Neurosurgery and Psychiatry*, **50**, 259–68.

Thomas CK, Bigland-Richie B, and Johansson RS (1991a). Force-frequency relationships of human thenar motor units. *Journal of Neurophysiology*, **65**, 1509–16.

Thomas CK, Johansson RS, and Bigland-Ritchie B (1991b). Attempts to physiologically classify human thenar motor units. *Journal of Neurophysiology*, **65**, 1501–8.

Thomas CK, Erb DE, Grumbles RM, and Bunge RP (2000). Embryonic cord transplants in peripheral nerve restore skeletal muscle function. *Journal of Neurophysiology*, **84**, 591–5.

Thomas CK, Sesodia S, Erb DE, and Grumbles RM (2003). Properties of medial gastrocnemius motor units and muscle fibers reinnervated by embryonic ventral spinal cord cells. *Experimental Neurology*, **180**, 25–31.

Thomas JS, Schmidt EM, and Hambrecht FT (1978). Facility of motor unit control during tasks defined directly in terms of motor unit behaviors. *Experimental Neurology*, **59**, 384–95.

Thomas PE and Ranatunga KW (1993). Factors affecting muscle fiber transformation in cross-reinnervated muscle. *Muscle & Nerve*, **16**, 193–9.

Thompson WJ, Sutton LA, and Riley DA (1984). Fibre type composition of single motor units during synapse elimination in neonatal rat soleus muscle. *Nature*, **309**, 709–11.

Thurbon D, Luscher HR, Hofstetter T, and Redman SJ (1998). Passive electrical properties of ventral horn neurons in rat spinal cord slices. *Journal of Neurophysiology*, **79**, 2485–502.

Tiret L, Le Mouellic H, Maury M, and Brulet P (1998). Increased apoptosis of motoneurons and altered somatotopic maps in the brachial spinal cord of Hoxc-8-deficient mice. *Development*, **125**, 279–91.

Titmus MJ and Faber DS (1990). Axotomy-induced alterations in the electrophysiological characteristics of neurons. *Progress in Neurobiology*, **35**, 1–51.

Todd G, Gorman RB, and Gandevia SC (2004). Measurement and reproducibility of strength and voluntary activation of lower-limb muscles. *Muscle & Nerve*, **29**, 834–42.

Tokizane T and Shimazu H (1964). *Functional Differentiation of Human Skeletal Muscle. Corticalization and Spinalization of Movement*. Charles C. Thomas, Springfield, IL.

Tomlinson BE and Irving D (1977). The numbers of limb motor neurons in the human lumbosacral cord throughout life. *Journal of the Neurological Sciences*, **34**, 213–19.

Totland GK and Kryvi H (1991). Distribution patterns of muscle fibre types in major muscles of the bull (Bos taurus). *Anatomy and Embryology*, **184**, 441–50.

Totosy de Zepetnek JE, Zung HV, Erdebil S, and Gordon T (1992). Innervation ratio is an important determinant of force in normal and reinnervated rat tibialis anterior muscles. *Journal of Neurophysiology*, **67**, 1385–403.

Tower SS (1937). Trophic control of non-nervous tissues by the nervous system: A study of muscle and bone Innervated from an isolated and quiescent regron of spinal cord. *Journal of. Comparative Neurology*, **67**, 241–61.

Troiani D, Filippi GM, and Bassi FA (1999). Nonlinear tension summation of different combinations of motor units in the anesthetized cat peroneus longus muscle. *Journal of Neurophysiology*, **81**, 771–80.

Tseng BS, Kasper CE, and Edgerton VR (1994). Cytoplasm-to-myonucleus ratios and succinate dehydrogenase activities in adult rat slow and fast muscle fibers. *Cell and Tissue Research*, **275**, 39–49.

Tweedle CD, Pitman RM, and Cohen MJ (1973). Dendritic stability of insect central neurons subjected to axotomy and de-afferentation. *Brain Research*, **60**, 471–6.

Tyler CM, Golland LC, Evans DL, Hodgson DR, and Rose RJ (1998). Skeletal muscle adaptations to prolonged training, overtraining and detraining in horses. *Pflügers Archiv*, **436**, 391–7.

Uemura M, Matsuda K, Kume M, Takeuchi Y, Matsushima R, and Mizuno N (1979). Topographical arrangement of hypoglossal motoneurons: an HRP study in the cat. *Neuroscience Letters*, **13**, 99–104.

Ulfhake B and Cullheim S (1981). A quantitative light microscopic study of the dendrites of cat spinal gamma -motoneurons after intracellular staining with horseradish peroxidase. *Journal of Comparative Neurology*, **202**, 585–96.

Ulfhake B and Cullheim S (1988). Postnatal development of cat hind limb motoneurons. III: Changes in size of motoneurons supplying the triceps surae muscle. *Journal of Comparative Neurology*, **278**, 103–20.

Ulfhake B and Kellerth JO (1981). A quantitative light microscopic study of the dendrites of cat spinal alpha-motoneurons after intracellular staining with horseradish peroxidase. *Journal of Comparative Neurology*, **202**, 571–83.

Ulfhake B and Kellerth JO (1982). Does alpha-motoneurone size correlate with motor unit type in cat triceps surae? *Brain Research*, **251**, 201–9.

Ulfhake B and Kellerth JO (1984). Electrophysiological and morphological measurements in cat gastrocnemius and soleus alpha-motoneurones. *Brain Research*, **307**, 167–79.

Ulmer HV, Knieriemen W, Warlo T, and Zech B (1989). Interindividual variability of isometric endurance with regard to the endurance performance limit for static work. *Biomedica Biochimica Acta*, **48**, S504–8.

Umemiya M and Berger AJ (1994). Properties and function of low- and high-voltage-activated Ca^{2+} channels in hypoglossal motoneurons. *Journal of Neuroscience*, **14**, 5652–60.

Unguez GA, Bodine-Fowler S, Roy RR, Pierotti DJ, and Edgerton VR (1993). Evidence of incomplete neural control of motor unit properties in cat tibialis anterior after self-reinnervation. *Journal of Physiology*, **472**, 103–25.

Unguez GA, Roy RR, Pierotti DJ, Bodine-Fowler S, and Edgerton VR (1995). Further evidence of incomplete neural control of muscle properties in cat tibialis anterior motor units. *American Journal of Physiology*, **268**, C527–34.

Unguez GA, Roy RR, Bodine-Fowler S, and Edgerton VR (1996). Limited fiber type grouping in self-reinnervation cat tibialis anterior muscles. *Muscle & Nerve*, **19**, 1320–7.

Vallbo AB and Wessberg J (1993). Organization of motor output in slow finger movements in man. *Journal of Physiology*, **469**, 673–91.

Van Cutsem M, Duchateau J, and Hainaut K (1998). Changes in single motor unit behaviour contribute to the increase in contraction speed after dynamic training in humans. *Journal of Physiology*, **513**, 295–305.

van der Laarse WJ, Diegenbach PC, and Maslam S (1984). Quantitative histochemistry of three mouse hind-limb muscles: the relationship between calcium-stimulated myofibrillar ATPase and succinate dehydrogenase activities. *Histochemical Journal*, **16**, 529–41.

van der Want JJ, Gramsbergen A, Ijkema-Paassen J, de Weerd H, and Liem RS (1998). Dendro-dendritic connections between motoneurons in the rat spinal cord: an electron microscopic investigation. *Brain Research*, **779**, 342–5.

van Dieen JH, Oude Vrielink HH, and Toussaint HM (1993). An investigation into the relevance of the pattern of temporal activation with respect to erector spinae muscle endurance. *European Journal of Applied Physiology*, **66**, 70–5.

van Duinen H, Lorist MM, and Zijdewind I (2005). The effect of caffeine on cognitive task performance and motor fatigue. *Psychopharmacology (Berlin)*, **180**, 539–47.

van Keulen LC (1979). Axon trajectories of Renshaw cells in the lumbar spinal cord of the cat, as reconstructed after intracellular staining with horseradish peroxidase. *Brain Research*, **167**, 157–62.

van Keulen L (1981). Autogenetic recurrent inhibition of individual spinal motoneurones of the cat. *Neuroscience Letters*, **21**, 297–300.

van Raamsdonk W, Smit-Onel M, Donselaar Y, and Diegenbach P (1987). Quantitative cytochemical analysis of cytochrome oxidase and succinate dehydrogenase activity in spinal neurons. *Acta Histochemica*, **81**, 129–41.

Vandenborne K, Elliott MA, Walter GA, et al. (1998). Longitudinal study of skeletal muscle adaptations during immobilization and rehabilitation. *Muscle & Nerve*, **21**, 1006–12.

Vanden Noven S, Wallace N, Muccio D, Turtz A, and Pinter MJ (1993). Adult spinal motoneurons remain viable despite prolonged absence of functional synaptic contact with muscle. *Experimental Neurology*, **123**, 147–56.

Vander Linden DW, Kukulka CG and Soderberg GL (1991). The effect of muscle length on motor unit discharge characteristics in human tibialis anterior muscle. *Experimental Brain Research*, **84**, 210–18.

Vanderhorst VG and Holstege G (1997a). Estrogen induces axonal outgrowth in the nucleus retroambiguus-lumbosacral motoneuronal pathway in the adult female cat. *Journal of Neuroscience*, **17**, 1122–36.

Vanderhorst VG and Holstege G (1997b). Organization of lumbosacral motoneuronal cell groups innervating hindlimb, pelvic floor, and axial muscles in the cat. *Journal of Comparative Neurology*, **382**, 46–76.

Vanderhorst VG, Terasawa E, and Ralston HJ 3rd (2002). Axonal sprouting of a brainstem-spinal pathway after estrogen administration in the adult female rhesus monkey. *Journal of Comparative Neurology*, **454**, 82–103.

Vandervoort AA (2002). Aging of the human neuromuscular system. *Muscle & Nerve*, **25**, 17–25.

Vanner SJ and **Rose PK** (1984). Dendritic distribution of motoneurons innervating the three heads of the trapezius muscle in the cat. *Journal of Comparative Neurology*, **226**, 96–110.

Veltink PH and **Alsté JA** (1992). Artificial electrical stimulation of myelinated nerve fibers. In A Pedotti and M Ferrarin (eds), *Restoration of walking for Paraplegics. Recent Advancements and Trends*, pp. 167–79. IOS Press, Amsterdam.

Venema HW (1988). Spatial distribution of fiber types in skeletal muscle: test for a random distribution. *Muscle & Nerve*, **11**, 301–11.

Viana F, Bayliss DA, and **Berger AJ** (1993). Multiple potassium conductances and their role in action potential repolarization and repetitive firing behavior of neonatal rat hypoglossal motoneurons. *Journal of Neurophysiology*, **69**, 2150–63.

Viana F, Bayliss DA, and **Berger AJ** (1994). Postnatal changes in rat hypoglossal motoneuron membrane properties. *Neuroscience*, **59**, 131–48.

Viana F, Bayliss DA, and **Berger AJ** (1995). Repetitive firing properties of developing rat brainstem motoneurones. *Journal of Physiology*, **486**, 745–61.

Vieira ER and **Kumar S** (2004). Working postures: a literature review. *Journal of Occupational Rehabilitation*, **14**, 143–59.

Vizoso AD and **Young JZ** (1948). Internode length and fibre diameter in developing and regenerating nerves. *Journal of Anatomy*, **82**, 110–35.

Vollestad NK, Sejersted OM, Bahr R, Woods JJ, and **Bigland-Ritchie B** (1988). Motor drive and metabolic responses during repeated submaximal contractions in humans. *Journal of Applied Physiology*, **64**, 1421–7.

Vult von Steyern F, Martinov V, Rabben I, Nja A, de Lapeyriere O, and **Lomo T** (1999). The homeodomain transcription factors Islet 1 and HB9 are expressed in adult alpha and gamma motoneurons identified by selective retrograde tracing. *European Journal of Neuroscience*, **11**, 2093–102.

Vyskocil F, Hnik P, Rehfeldt H, Vejsada R, and **Ujec E** (1983). The measurement of $[K^+]_e$ concentration changes in human muscles during volitional contractions. *Pflügers Archiv*, **399**, 235–7.

Wada M, Okumoto T, Toro K, *et al.* (1996). Expression of hybrid isomyosins in human skeletal muscle. *American Journal of Physiology*, **271**, C1250–5.

Walker DW and **Luff AR** (1995). Functional development of fetal limb muscles: a review of the roles of activity, nerves and hormones. *Reproduction, Fertility, and Development*, **7**, 391–8.

Walker SM and **Schrodt GR** (1974). I segment lengths and thin filament periods in skeletal muscle fibers of the Rhesus monkey and the human. *Anatomical Record*, **178**, 63–81.

Wallen P, Buchanan JT, Grillner S, Hill RH, Christenson J, and **Hokfelt T** (1989). Effects of 5-hydroxytryptamine on the afterhyperpolarization, spike frequency regulation, and oscillatory membrane properties in lamprey spinal cord neurons. *Journal of Neurophysiology*, **61**, 759–68.

Waller A (1850). Experiments on the section of the glossopharyngeal and hypoglossal nerves of the frog, and observation on the alteration produced thereby in the structure of their primitive fibres. *Philosophical Transactions of the Royal Society of London*, **140**, 423.

Walsh JV Jr, Burke RE, Rymer WZ, and **Tsairis P** (1978). Effect of compensatory hypertrophy studied in individual motor units in medial gastrocnemius muscle of the cat. *Journal of Neurophysiology*, **41**, 496–508.

Wang LC and **Kernell D** (2000). Proximo-distal organization and fibre type regionalization in rat hindlimb muscles. *Journal of Muscle Research and Cell Motility*, **21**, 587–98.

Wang LC and **Kernell D** (2001a). Fibre type regionalisation in lower hindlimb muscles of rabbit, rat and mouse: a comparative study. *Journal of Anatomy*, **199**, 631–43.

Wang LC and **Kernell D** (2001b). Quantification of fibre type regionalisation: an analysis of lower hindlimb muscles in the rat. *Journal of Anatomy*, **198**, 295–308.

Wang LC and **Kernell D** (2002). Recovery of type I fiber regionalization in gastrocnemius medialis of the rat after reinnervation along original and foreign paths, with and without muscle rotation. *Neuroscience*, **114**, 629–40.

Wang L, Copray S, Brouwer N, Meek MF, and **Kernell D** (2002). Regional distribution of slow-twitch muscle fibers after reinnervation in adult rat hindlimb muscles. *Muscle & Nerve*, **25**, 805–15.

Watson WE (1969). The response of motor neurones to intramuscular injection of botulinum toxin. *Journal of Physiology*, **202**, 611–30.

Waxman SG (1972). Regional differentiation of the axon: a review with special reference to the concept of the multiplex neuron. *Brain Research*, **47**, 269–88.

Webb P (1992). Temperatures of skin, subcutaneous tissue, muscle and core in resting men in cold, comfortable and hot conditions. *European Journal of Applied Physiology*, **64**, 471–6.

Weeks OI and **English AW** (1985). Compartmentalization of the cat lateral gastrocnemius motor nucleus. *Journal of Comparative Neurology*, **235**, 255–67.

Weiss P and **Hoag A** (1946). Competitive reinnervation of rat muscles by their own and foreign nerves. *Journal of Neurophysiology*, **9**, 413–8.

Wessberg J and **Vallbo AB** (1995). Coding of pulsatile motor output by human muscle afferents during slow finger movements. *Journal of Physiology*, **485**, 271–82.

Wessberg J and **Vallbo AB** (1996). Pulsatile motor output in human finger movements is not dependent on the stretch reflex. *Journal of Physiology*, **493**, 895–908.

Westbury DR (1982). A comparison of the structures of alpha and gamma-spinal motoneurones of the cat. *Journal of Physiology*, **325**, 79–91.

Westcott SL, Powers RK, Robinson FR, and **Binder MD** (1995). Distribution of vestibulospinal synaptic input to cat triceps surae motoneurons. *Experimental Brain Research*, **107**, 1–8.

Westerblad H, and **Allen DG** (1991). Changes of myoplasmic calcium concentration during fatigue in single mouse muscle fibers. *Journal of General Physiology*, **98**, 615–35.

Westerblad H, Bruton JD, Allen DG, and **Lannergren J** (2000). Functional significance of Ca^{2+} in long-lasting fatigue of skeletal muscle. *European Journal of Applied Physiology*, **83**, 166–74.

Westerblad H, Allen DG, and **Lannergren J** (2002). Muscle fatigue: lactic acid or inorganic phosphate the major cause? *News in Physiological Sciences*, **17**, 17–21.

Westerga J and **Gramsbergen A** (1992). Structural changes of the soleus and the tibialis anterior motoneuron pool during development in the rat. *Journal of Comparative Neurology*, **319**, 406–16.

Westerga J and **Gramsbergen A** (1993). Changes in the electromyogram of two major hindlimb muscles during locomotor development in the rat. *Experimental Brain Research*, **92**, 479–88.

Westgaard RH (1975). Influence of activity on the passive electrical properties of denervated soleus muscle fibres in the rat. *Journal of Physiology*, **251**, 683–97.

Westgaard RH and **de Luca CJ** (1999). Motor unit substitution in long-duration contractions of the human trapezius muscle. *Journal of Neurophysiology*, **82**, 501–4.

Westgaard RH and **Lomo T** (1988). Control of contractile properties within adaptive ranges by patterns of impulse activity in the rat. *Journal of Neuroscience*, **8**, 4415–26.

Wichterle H, Lieberam I, Porter JA, and **Jessell TM** (2002). Directed differentiation of embryonic stem cells into motor neurons. *Cell*, **110**, 385–97.

Wickham JB and **Brown JM** (1998). Muscles within muscles: the neuromotor control of intra-muscular segments. *European Journal of Applied Physiology*, **78**, 219–25.

Wickiewicz TL, Roy RR, Powell PL, and Edgerton VR (1983). Muscle architecture of the human lower limb. *Clinical Orthopaedics*, **179**, 275–83.

Wiedemann E, Eggert C, Illert M, Stock W, and Wilhelm K (1997). [Functional electromyography analysis of radial replacement operation.] *Orthopäde*, **26**, 673–83.

Wigston DJ and Sanes JR (1982). Selective reinnervation of adult mammalian muscle by axons from different segmental levels. *Nature*, **299**, 464–7.

Windhorst U (1996). On the role of recurrent inhibitory feedback in motor control. *Progress in Neurobiology*, **49**, 517–87.

Windisch A, Gundersen K, Szabolcs MJ, Gruber H, and Lomo T (1998). Fast to slow transformation of denervated and electrically stimulated rat muscle. *Journal of Physiology*, **510**, 623–32.

Wirth O, Gregory EW, Cutlip RG, and Miller GR (2003). Control and quantitation of voluntary weight-lifting performance of rats. *Journal of Applied Physiology*, **95**, 402–12.

Wise AK, Morgan DL, Gregory JE, and Proske U (2001). Fatigue in mammalian skeletal muscle stimulated under computer control. *Journal of Applied Physiology*, **90**, 189–97.

Witzmann FA, Kim DH, and Fitts RH (1982). Hindlimb immobilization: length-tension and contractile properties of skeletal muscle. *Journal of Applied Physiology*, **53**, 335–45.

Wolf SL, Ammerman J, and Jann B (1998). Organization of responses in human lateral gastrocnemius muscle to specified body perturbations. *Journal of Electromyography and Kinesiology*, **8**, 11–21.

Wolpaw JR and Tennissen AM (2001). Activity-dependent spinal cord plasticity in health and disease. *Annual Review of Neuroscience*, **24**, 807–43.

Wong-Riley MT (1989). Cytochrome oxidase: an endogenous metabolic marker for neuronal activity. *Trends in Neurosciences*, **12**, 94–101.

Wood SJ and Slater CR (1995). Action potential generation in rat slow- and fast-twitch muscles. *Journal of Physiology*, **486**, 401–10.

Wood SJ and Slater CR (1997). The contribution of postsynaptic folds to the safety factor for neuromuscular transmission in rat fast- and slow-twitch muscles. *Journal of Physiology*, **500**, 165–76.

Wood SJ and Slater CR (2001). Safety factor at the neuromuscular junction. *Progress in Neurobiology*, **64**, 393–429.

Woods JJ, Furbush F, and Bigland-Ritchie B (1987). Evidence for a fatigue-induced reflex inhibition of motoneuron firing rates. *Journal of Neurophysiology*, **58**, 125–37.

Yamuy J, Engelhardt JK, Morales FR, and Chase MH (1992a). Passive electrical properties of motoneurons in aged cats following axotomy. *Brain Research*, **570**, 300–6.

Yamuy J, Englehardt JK, Morales FR, and Chase MH (1992b). Active electrophysiological properties of spinal motoneurons in aged cats following axotomy. *Neurobiology of Aging*, **13**, 231–8.

Yang JS, Sladky JT, Kallen RG, and Barchi RL (1991). TTX-sensitive and TTX-insensitive sodium channel mRNA transcripts are independently regulated in adult skeletal muscle after denervation. *Neuron*, **7**, 421–7.

Yoshida S (1994). Tetrodotoxin-resistant sodium channels. *Cellular and Molecular Neurobiology*, **14**, 227–44.

Young SH and Poo MM (1983). Spontaneous release of transmitter from growth cones of embryonic neurones. *Nature*, **305**, 634–7.

Yue G and Cole KJ (1992). Strength increases from the motor program: comparison of training with maximal voluntary and imagined muscle contractions. *Journal of Neurophysiology*, **67**, 1114–23.

Zajac FE and Faden JS (1985). Relationship among recruitment order, axonal conduction velocity, and muscle-unit properties of type-identified motor units in cat plantaris muscle. *Journal of Neurophysiology*, **53**, 1303–22.

Zandwijk JPv, Bobbert MF, Baan GC, and Huijing PA (1996). From twitch to tetanus: performance of excitation dynamics optimized for a twitch in predicting tetanic muscle forces. *Biological Cybernetics*, **75**, 409–17.

Zeng J, Powers RK, Newkirk G, Yonkers M, and Binder MD (2005). Contribution of persistent sodium currents to spike-frequency adaptation in rat hypoglossal motoneurons. *Journal of Neurophysiology*, **93**, 1035–41.

Zengel JE, Reid SA, Sypert GW, and Munson JB (1985). Membrane electrical properties and prediction of motor-unit type of medial gastrocnemius motoneurons in the cat. *Journal of Neurophysiology*, **53**, 1323–44.

Zenker W and Hohberg E (1973). [Motor nerve fibres. The cross-sectional area of stem fibre and terminal branches.] *Zeitschrift für Anatomie und Entwicklungsgeschichte*, **139**, 163–72.

Zhang L and Krnjevic K (1987). Apamin depresses selectively the after-hyperpolarization of cat spinal motoneurons. *Neuroscience Letters*, **74**, 58–62.

Zijdewind I and Kernell D (1994a). Fatigue associated EMG behavior of the first dorsal interosseous and adductor pollicis muscles in different groups of subjects. *Muscle & Nerve*, **17**, 1044–54.

Zijdewind I and Kernell D (1994b). Index finger position and force of the human first dorsal interosseus and its ulnar nerve antagonist. *Journal of Applied Physiology*, **77**, 987–97.

Zijdewind I and Kernell D (2001). Bilateral interactions during contractions of intrinsic hand muscles. *Journal of Neurophysiology*, **85**, 1907–13.

Zijdewind I and Thomas CK (2001). Spontaneous motor unit behavior in human thenar muscles after spinal cord injury. *Muscle & Nerve*, **24**, 952–62.

Zijdewind I and Thomas CK (2003). Motor unit firing during and after voluntary contractions of human thenar muscles weakened by spinal cord injury. *Journal of Neurophysiology*, **89**, 2065–71.

Zijdewind I, Kernell D, and Kukulka CG (1995). Spatial differences in fatigue-associated electromyographic behaviour of the human first dorsal interosseus muscle. *Journal of Physiology*, **483**, 499–509.

Zijdewind I, Zwarts MJ, and Kernell D (1998). Influence of a voluntary fatigue test on the contralateral homologous muscle in humans? *Neuroscience Letters*, **253**, 41–4.

Zijdewind I, Toering ST, Bessem B, Van Der Laan O, and Diercks RL (2003). Effects of imagery motor training on torque production of ankle plantar flexor muscles. *Muscle & Nerve*, **28**, 168–73.

Ziskind-Conhaim L (1988). Electrical properties of motoneurons in the spinal cord of rat embryos. *Developmental Biology*, **128**, 21–9.

Zwaagstra B and Kernell D (1980). The duration of after-hyperpolarization in hindlimb alpha motoneurones of different sizes in the cat. *Neuroscience Letters*, **19**, 303–7.

Zwaagstra B and Kernell D (1981). Sizes of soma and stem dendrites in intracellularly labelled alpha-motoneurones of the cat. *Brain Research*, **204**, 295–309.

Index

(Page numbers followed by an F or T refer to information in a Figure or Table.)